Rethinking AIDS Prevention
Cultural Approaches

Edited by

Ralph Bolton
Pomona College
Claremont, California

and

Merrill Singer
Hispanic Health Council
Hartford, Connecticut

Gordon and Breach Science Publishers
USA • Switzerland • Australia • Belgium • France
Germany • Great Britain • India • Japan • Malaysia
Netherlands • Russia • Singapore

Copyright © 1992 by Gordon and Breach Science Publishers S.A., Y-Parc, Chemin de la Sallaz, 1400 Yverdon, Switzerland. All rights reserved.

First published 1992
Second printing 1993

Gordon and Breach Science Publishers

820 Town Center Drive
Langhorne, Pennsylvania 19047
United States of America

Post Office Box 90
Reading, Berkshire RG1 8JL
Great Britain

Private Bag 8
Camberwell, Victoria 3124
Australia

3-14-9, Okubo
Shinjuku-ku, Tokyo 169
Japan

58, rue Lhomond
75005 Paris
France

Emmaplein 5
1075 AW Amsterdam
Netherlands

Glinkastrasse 13-15
O-1086 Berlin
Germany

This material was originally published in Volume 14, Numbers 2–4 of the journal *Medical Anthropology*.

Library of Congress Cataloging-in-Publication Data

Rethinking AIDS prevention : cultural approaches / edited by Ralph Bolton and Merrill Singer.
 p. cm.
  "This material was originally published in volume 14, numbers 2–4 of the journal Medical anthropology"—T.p. verso
  Includes bibliographical references and index.
  ISBN 2-88124-552-8
  1. AIDS (Disease)—Prevention. 2. Medical anthropology. 3. AIDS (Disease)—Social aspects. I. Bolton, Ralph, 1939–
II. Singer, Merrill.
 RC607.A26R48 1992
 614.5'993—dc20

92-13820
CIP

Contents

Medical Anthropology, Vol. 14, pp. 139–143
Reprints available directly from the publisher
Photocopying permitted by license only

Introduction. Rethinking HIV Prevention: Critical Assessments of the Content and Delivery of AIDS Risk-Reduction Messages

Ralph Bolton and Merrill Singer

Key words: AIDS prevention, HIV, AIDS education, medical anthropology

In 1989, *Medical Anthropology* became the first journal in the field to devote an entire issue to anthropological research on the AIDS pandemic. As Lawrence S. Greene, the Editor-in-Chief, pointed out in a prefatory note at that time, "we anticipate further issues on this timely subject in the future." Indeed, even before that issue appeared, at the annual meeting of the Society for Applied Anthropology in Santa Fe, New Mexico in April of that year, the co-editors of the present issue met with Greene to begin to plan future special issues of the journal on the AIDS crisis. In our discussion we observed that despite growing involvement of anthropologists in AIDS research, too little attention was being focused directly on the critical task of improving the design of educational efforts aimed at stopping the transmission of HIV. As a result, we resolved to pull together an issue devoted to the topic of HIV prevention.

Anthropological research on AIDS encompasses a broad spectrum of inquiry (Bolton, Lewis, and Orozco 1991), and the results of these investigations have deepened our understanding of many dimensions of the epidemic. Such studies include: symbolic analyses of AIDS discourse; surveys of adolescent attitudes toward sexuality and AIDS, the response of health-care personnel toward AIDS patients, and general population knowledge, attitudes, and risk behaviors; ethnographies of drug using populations; discussions of ethical and methodological issues in AIDS research; experimental evaluation of the effectiveness of culturally specific AIDS prevention programs; and societal responses to the epidemic. All of these approaches have yielded important data and contributed valuable insights which should inform our efforts to cope more successfully with the AIDS crisis.

Nonetheless, we sense that much of our collected effort is too far removed from

RALPH BOLTON *is Professor of Anthropology at Pomona College, Claremont, CA 91711. He is Chair of the AIDS and Anthropology Research Group (an affiliate of the Society for Medical Anthropology) and a member of the AIDS and Anthropology Task Force of the American Anthropological Association. His current work focuses on cognitive mapping of the domain of sexuality and on the structure of sexual encounters.*

MERRILL SINGER *is Deputy Director of the Hispanic Health Council, 98 Cedar Street, Hartford, CT 06106. He is Chairperson of the American Anthropological Association Task Force on AIDS and is the Principal Investigator on Project COPE, A National AIDS Demonstration Research Project (NADR) funded by the National Institute on Drug Abuse.*

the needs and concerns of the men and women who are on the front lines of the battle to halt the transmission of HIV, those who design and implement on-the-ground programs of intervention intended to reduce high-risk behaviors. As anthropologists, we must raise the question of how we can help them to make their efforts more effective. We are all aware of the serious financial constraints faced by community organizations engaged in HIV prevention. These budgetary considerations make it all the more imperative for prevention activists to be as effective as possible.

Since 1989 biomedical research has produced therapeutic improvements which promise to extend the lives of those who are infected, and candidate vaccines that may eventually prevent infection from occurring are in various stages of development. Still, no biomedical fix is in sight and there are no guarantees that such a solution to AIDS will be forthcoming in the long run, let alone in the near future. Moreover, even if a vaccine or effective treatment were available, it is far from certain that they would be widely distributed and equally available to all populations, social classes, and subgroups across the globe. The prevention of new infections through education, therefore, must remain as one of our highest priorities. By training most anthropologists are not equipped to make serious contributions to potential biomedical solutions to the epidemic, but because of our expertise in social and cultural processes, we are singularly prepared to make major contributions to educational approaches to HIV prevention. After all, HIV prevention is first and foremost a problem in culture change. While the goal of prevention efforts is to reduce risk-taking by individuals, the processes whereby that goal is accomplished are necessarily social and they occur within specific cultural contexts. Although the papers in this volume deal with HIV prevention in enormously different target populations, all of them emphasize the importance of basing prevention programs on a thorough comprehension of the social and cultural systems of the people for whom the program is intended.

Bolton's paper offers a critical assessment of the role of promiscuity in the epidemic and of a prevention strategy which attempts to reduce HIV transmission by advising people to reduce the number of their sexual partners. This strategy, he argues, is derived from moralistic approaches to AIDS which ignore sexual values and behavioral realities and exemplifies the unwarranted application of epidemiologic concepts and findings to the design of prevention programs. The unintended consequence of the partner-reduction message has been to reduce the salience of safe-sex messages, thereby compromising their effectiveness. His analysis suggests that at least in sex-positive subcultures the outcome of this strategy has been to increase rather than decrease HIV transmission. Bolton recommends the elimination of references to multiple partners as a risk factor in AIDS prevention messages.

In her paper, Schoepf describes the action-research in which she has been involved in Zaire, one of the epicenters of the AIDS pandemic in Africa. She points to the need to de-medicalize AIDS prevention and to develop community-based interpersonal methods of AIDS education which empower people to make risk-reduction behavioral changes. The case study reported in this paper demonstrates the important point that while cultural knowledge is essential in designing prevention programs, cultural explanations for the failure of prevention programs must not be accepted at face value. Schoepf and her associates in Zaire found that although cultural impediments to the use of condoms do exist, traditional beliefs and values did not stand as insurmountable obstacles to promoting condom use. By enlisting traditional healers in AIDS prevention, Schoepf and her African colleagues were able to induce a process of cosmological reinterpretation which made condoms more culturally acceptable.

The safer-sex approach to risk-reduction has proven to be highly effective in promoting behavioral changes in the domain of sexuality, especially among gay men in Europe and the U.S. Instead of focussing on the dangers of sexuality, this approach emphasizes the positive values of sexual pleasure and the importance of empowering individuals and communities to make changes in their sexual practices which simultaneously reduce the risk of HIV transmission and enhance sexual fulfillment. In their paper, Taylor and Lourea describe a dynamic model which can be used by AIDS educators to generate safe-sex interventions that are sensitive to the individual, cultural, and social attributes of specific target audiences. Based on the authors' extensive experience in offering safe-sex workshops and other performances, this paper, which is unique in the prevention literature, offers valuable, detailed advice on how to design safer-sex interventions.

While the first three papers in this volume are concerned solely with the sexual transmission of HIV, the paper by Singer, Jia, Schensul, Weeks, and Page examines HIV prevention among injection drug users (IDUs) for whom multiple transmission routes exist, thereby complicating the prevention process. The authors of this paper convincingly challenge the homogenous portrayal of IDUs commonly found in the media. By comparing the participants in their studies in Hartford, Connecticut and Miami, Florida, they reveal major differences in the beliefs and behavioral patterns of these two populations. Given these differences, they argue that to be effective prevention strategies must be grounded in an ethnographically holistic awareness of the local context. Their analysis underscores, too, the importance of providing in each setting multiple types of interventions, such as street outreach education, bleach distribution, drug treatment programs, and sterile needle exchange projects, among others. These authors have been engaged for a number of years in implementing and testing the efficacy of many of these strategies in reducing risk behavior and seroconversion among IDUs, their sex partners, noninjection cocaine users, and professional sex workers.

Susser and González discuss their work on a prevention project carried out among homeless men living in a shelter in New York City. Given the enormous difficulties in survival confronted by the homeless, HIV prevention in this context presents special problems. The authors argue that in this setting to effect changes in risk behavior it is necessary first to initiate a process of re-evaluation and re-creation of a sense of identity. Their innovative approach to prevention involved engaging these homeless men in the making of a video addressing HIV infection among shelter residents. In collectively writing a script for the video, the participants not only became better informed about AIDS, but they also generated valuable information on the drawbacks and possibilities of various prevention strategies. This action research triggered a response of group self-help. Fostering such responses, the authors note, should be a primary goal of anthropologists working on HIV prevention.

In the final paper, Bolton, Vincke, Mak, and Dennehy explore the connections between alcohol consumption and risky sex. In the prevention literature the conclusion that drinking increases sexual risk-taking appears to be firmly entrenched, and most prevention programs convey the message that sex and alcohol are a dangerous combination. The authors conclude that this claim rests on a shaky empirical foundation. In their research among Belgian gay men they failed to find significant relationships between alcohol variables and sexual risk-taking; moreover, their review of the scientific literature suggests that most studies of this hypothesis have failed to replicate the findings of the early research on this subject. They advance several hypotheses to account for this "vanishing" co-factor of risky sex, including the possibility that such a relationship may exist in limited socio-cultural contexts. However, they argue that rethinking the alcohol message is essential and that it may be necessary to turn the former message upside down. By allowing alcohol to serve as an excuse for risky behavior, we may inadvertently encourage risk taking; by telling people that alcohol does not cause risky behavior, we may encourage them to take responsibility for their actions.

The papers in this volume challenge some of the most basic assumptions in HIV prevention. They question conventional wisdom on fundamental issues. We hope that they will stimulate debate and research on how to improve the content and delivery of HIV prevention messages. Despite the diversity of settings represented in these papers, a common theme emerges: *prevention works best when it promotes change through individual and community empowerment strategies informed by holistic understandings of the local context, when it acknowledges the positive contributions of local cultural values to the process of change, and when it incorporates an array of options that permit individuals to transform their lives in ways that enhance their physical, emotional, and material well-being.* Prevention efforts fail when they revictimize and stigmatize those who do not accept messages incompatible with their basic values and needs, when they blame those whose behavior suggests recalcitrance or relapse from risk standards established by health "experts," when they are based on top-down rather than community-designed and implemented approaches, and when they are shaped by the moralistic and authoritarian models advocated by political, religious, and medical leaders whose agendas may be inimical to the best interests of the clients of many prevention programs.

HIV prevention in the 1990s may be even more difficult than it was in the 1980s. We ignore at our peril the lessons of the first decade of the epidemic. As anthropologists we need to use our special vantage point to help rethink prevention. Fortunately, this process has begun. In October 1991, approximately 30 anthropologists who are actively involved in AIDS research, programming, and policy issues, gathered together in Atlanta, Georgia for a conference on AIDS and Anthropology in the United States. With the support and active participation of the Centers for Disease Control and many CDC staff, the conference served as a state-of-the-art review of anthropological contributions to AIDS prevention research and community AIDS education and empowerment efforts. It was evident at this conference, as well as at several smaller anthropological conferences on AIDS that took place at the University of Pennsylvania, Hunter College, the New School for Social Research, and at other sites during 1991, that anthropology demonstrates a number of notable strengths in responding to the AIDS crisis. Many of these strengths are displayed in the papers included in this collection. Moreover, the anthropological imprint can already be discerned in numerous AIDS prevention projects within the United States and across the globe. While the number of anthropologists directly involved in responding to the epidemic remains comparatively small, their impact has been felt to a far greater degree than in many areas of applied research and program/policy design.

However, it is also clear that there is much work to be done and many gaps remain in anthropological AIDS understanding and involvement. During the Atlanta conference, for example, it was evident that we lack critical knowledge about issues like the sexual behavior and attitudes of many (if not all) populations; the culture of service providers and the effect of this culture on AIDS service provision; the role of social relations structured around class, gender and ethnicity on participation in risky behaviors; the means of effectively involving so-called hard-to-reach populations like the homeless, sex partners of IVDUs, and gay men from ethnic minority communities; the configuration of life history factors (e.g. child abuse, domestic violence) that generate and shape risk behaviors; the contributions of anthropological insight to secondary prevention and treatment; and the operational understanding of cultural and gender appropriateness in prevention programs. A similar range of issues could be developed for AIDS efforts in the Third World. Items like these constitute the agenda for AIDS and anthropology as we move into the second decade of the epidemic.

REFERENCES CITED

Bolton, R., M. Lewis, and G. Orozco
   1991   AIDS Literature for Anthropologists: A Working Bibliography. The Journal of Sex Research 28(2):307–346.

Medical Anthropology, Vol. 14, pp. 145–223
Reprints available directly from the publisher
Photocopying permitted by license only

AIDS and Promiscuity: Muddles in the Models of HIV Prevention

Ralph Bolton

AIDS has been blamed on promiscuity and the promiscuous, and a major goal of many HIV-prevention programs has been to induce people to reduce the number of their sexual partners. Despite the salience of this concept in the AIDS discourse of scientists, policymakers, the media, religious leaders, and the gay community, critical analysis of the role of promiscuity in this epidemic has been lacking. Following a review of promiscuity in various genres of AIDS discourse, this article discusses promiscuity in American society and in HIV-prevention campaigns. The relative risks associated with monogamy, abstinence and promiscuity are examined, and the author concludes that the partner-reduction strategy, instead of contributing to a reduction in HIV transmission has been an impediment to AIDS prevention efforts, exacerbating the problem by undermining the sex-positive approaches to risk reduction that have proven effective. Responsibility for this misguided strategy is attributed to a moralistic approach to AIDS and to the misapplication of epidemiological concepts and inappropriate social science models to the task of promoting healthy forms of sexuality.

Key words: AIDS, sexual behavior, promiscuity, HIV prevention

INTRODUCTION

AIDS is about promiscuity. In the voluminous material on this epidemic, promiscuity stands out as the key concept, dominating and linking together diverse genres of thought and discourse about AIDS. Sometimes it is in the foreground, its presence explicit, even shrill, constituting the core of the discourse, the central symbol or variable around which the facts of AIDS are organized and interpreted. At other times it is in the background, its presence more subtle, *sotto voce*, quiet, implicit. But named or not, the concept of promiscuity is present, lurking or parading, exercising a powerful influence on how people respond to this modern-day scourge.[1]

Given the pervasiveness of this concept in AIDS discourse, then, it is surprising that so little critical attention has been focussed on it, that so little effort has gone into analyzing in depth the role played by promiscuous behavior and the concept of promiscuity in this epidemic.[2,3] What should not be surprising in light of the salience of promiscuity is that the role it plays is multifaceted and shifting. In this

RALPH BOLTON, *Professor of Anthropology at Pomona College, Claremont, CA 91711, is Chair of the AIDS and Anthropology Research Group (an affiliate of the Society for Medical Anthropology) and a member of the AIDS and Anthropology Task Force of the American Anthropological Association. His current work focusses on cognitive mapping of the domain of sexuality and on the structure of sexual encounters.*

paper I shall explore some of the complexities surrounding the issue of promiscuity in relation to AIDS.[4]

Some Essential Terms and Definitions

What is promiscuity? This is a messy concept, one whose boundaries are fuzzy and, indeed, elastic. As Holleran (1988:113) notes, "Everyone has his/her own definition of promiscuity." Often attributed to Alfred Kinsey is the humorous—and astute—observation that "the promiscuous person is anyone who is getting more than you are." Wanting something more precise, we can turn to the Oxford English Dictionary for a formal definition of the term, of course. There we discover that "promiscuous" refers to the grouping or massing of members or elements of different kinds together without order, making no distinctions, undiscriminating, that it is a term of contempt or deprecation. The OED discussion in the domain of sexuality cites McLennan, Lang, and Spencer and indicates that it is an attribute of "some races of low civilization." Obviously, our anthropological ancestors of the 19th Century were not alien to the concept of promiscuity.[5]

But this is not much help, of course, and we fall back on ordinary understandings of the term, which means simply having many sexual partners, at its broadest extension, or, more narrowly, having more than the culturally-approved number of such partners. Since in American culture, the traditionally dominant sexual ideology, which Davis (1983) refers to as "Jehovanist," restricts sex to the relationship between husband and wife in a monogamous marriage, someone who has one premarital, nonmarital, extramarital, or postmarital (post-divorce?) sexual encounter might be considered promiscuous. As Murdock (1949:263) pointed out: "Our own culture includes a blanket taboo against fornication, an over-all prohibition of all sexual intercourse outside of the marital relationship."

That the concept is closely tied to marriage is evident when we ask what the antonym for promiscuity is. Quite clearly in AIDS discourse, the term used most often to contrast with promiscuity is "monogamy," which every beginning anthropology student knows refers to a form of marriage in which one male and one female are united. In its technical usage, as Robin Fox (1967, 1983) has insisted, monogamy has nothing to do with sex, just with marriage. However, the term is also employed in discussions of nonhuman animal behavior to refer to mating patterns that involve a single male and a single female for life, or at least for the breeding season.

Thus, a person is either monogamous (i.e., married and faithful) or promiscuous (i.e., married but unfaithful or unmarried and unchaste); the English lexicon in this domain does not permit any other option. To be sure, there is one other possibility, namely abstinence from sex. Here again, a confusion of terminology exists, with celibacy (defined as the state of being unmarried) usually being used to designate abstinence, further demonstrating the conflation of sex and marriage. In view of the baggage of pejorative connotations that promiscuity carries, quite understandably there has been a casting about in recent years for suitable euphemisms, with all of the proposed alternatives being awkward and not very satisfactory. A simple, nonpejorative synonymous noun for promiscuity is difficult to find in English. Not yet widely disseminated or accepted is the neologism "polypartnering." A person "has multiple partners" or "is sexually active" (Does this imply that someone who is monogamous is "sexually inactive" or "sexually passive"? Shades of Calvin Coolidge?), or he/she "engages in casual sex" or "is nonmonogamous."

This raises the issue of definitions of sex, which is something we all recognize when we see or do it but when we try to define it we run into trouble. If we are looking for the application of the term to a type of behavior, the OED is not very helpful since the closest it comes to dealing with this subject refers to "the class of phenomena with which the difference between male and female is concerned." Ironically, even textbooks on human sexuality generally refrain from trying to define "sex" in relation to behavior. According to the glossary of one textbook, to give just one example, sex is "biological maleness and femaleness" (Luria, Friedman, and Rose 1987:G19). Roffman (1991:4) has pointed out that in American culture sex generally equals intercourse and that it "almost always implies penile/vaginal penetration."

By implication, then, if sex involves male and female and equals penile/vaginal penetration, sex between individuals of the same gender is impossible, and gays and lesbians could not be promiscuous, no matter how many partners they might have. But if a broader view of sex is taken to include any activity involving genital or erotic stimulation (i.e., both intercourse and outercourse), and if marriage between individuals of the same gender is not possible, then *all* gay and lesbian couplings must be, by definition, promiscuous.[6] And by now the conceptual morass (no pun intended) we confront when examining the connections between promiscuity and AIDS is apparent.

Additional Considerations: Sexologists on Promiscuity

Seeking to extricate ourselves from this terminological and conceptual tangle, we can turn to professional sexologists for guidance. What do they have to say on this subject? Taking an opportunistic sample of 19 human sexuality textbooks as my sources, I examined sexologists' usage of promiscuity. While the term is sufficiently significant to be referenced in the index of 17 of these books, in most cases its usage is confined to a few restricted contexts.

In these sources two different approaches are taken to define promiscuity. One approach simply designates the number of sexual partners as the determining criterion, e.g., "Promiscuous: A term used to refer to someone who engages in sexual activity with many different people" (Hyde 1982:587). "Many" is left indeterminate, of course. The other approach incorporates additional criteria into the definition. For example, Byer and Shainberg (1991:611) state that promiscuity is "indiscriminate, transient, sexual intercourse with many people for the relief of sexual tensions rather than for feelings of affection." By this definition one could have many partners and still not be promiscuous if one had "feelings of affection" for them, though I doubt that that is what the authors intended.

Many authors note that the term is not scientifically useful because of its vagueness and its pejorative, derogatory, and subjective usage (e.g., McCary 1979:247; Byer and Shainberg 1991:545–546; Katchadourian 1985:370–371), but this does not deter some textbook writers from using the term, especially in certain contexts. Notable among these contexts are discussions of diseases such as cervical cancer and VD (McCary and McCary 1982:542,560), incest (Geer, Heiman, and Leitenberg 1984:433), prostitution (Mahoney 1983:487, Katchadourian and Lunde 1972:439), the "swinging singles scene" (Masters, Johnson and Kolodny 1985:402–403), swinging (Mahoney 1983:286) and, of course, homosexuality. The term is more likely to be used in discussions of gay men than of heterosexuals. Heterosexual promiscuity is more generally discussed under the more neutral rubrics of "nonmarital sex," "premarital sex," and "extramarital sex". Some authors, however, do attempt to counter the stereotype of "gay promiscuity" (Hyde 1990:426) or to explain it (Masters, Johnson, and Kolodny (1988:434; Luria, Friedman, and Rose 1987:441). Allgeier and Allgeier (1984:339, 1988:322, 1991:335) index promiscuity only in relation to their discussion and rejection of the claim that access by adolescents to contraceptives leads to promiscuity, while Hyde (1979:248) indexes the term only to dismiss the idea of "rampant promiscuity" among the young.

Judgments grounded in sex negativity rather than scientific objectivity are rife in these texts, which almost never take into account cross-cultural evidence on polypartnering (see, for example, Ford and Beach 1980[1951]; Frayser 1985; Symons 1979).[7] Involvement with multiple partners often is interpreted as a result of personality defects such as feelings of inadequacy (Jones 1984:434), immaturity (Rice 1989:314), and neurotic conflicts (Katchadourian 1985:308). Numerous authors underscore the view that promiscuity is not caused by a heightened sex drive (Jones 1984:434; McCary and McCary 1982:542; Rice 1989:314).

Unbalanced as they are by the richness of understandings of promiscuity contained in the works of authors such as Symons (1979) and Holleran (1988), the impoverished nature of these discussions on promiscuity reflects the pervasive ideological fog on this issue which even sexologists are seemingly unable or unwilling to penetrate.[8] The stakes involved in understanding promiscuity took a quantum leap, however, when HIV entered the picture. Nathan Fain, already in 1982, captured the essence of the problem when he wrote, "One word is like a hand grenade in the whole affair: promiscuity" (p. 19).

PROMISCUITY IN GENRES OF AIDS DISCOURSE

As noted above, the concept of promiscuity surfaces in a variety of genres of AIDS discourse: the scientific, the political, and the religious and in presentations on AIDS by the media and in the literature of the gay community. Let us look at each of these in turn.

Scientific Discourse: Epidemiology and Etiology

In the very first scientific publication on what was to become AIDS, the report on five cases of pneumocystis pneumonia in Los Angeles, indeed in the first sentence, promiscuity is alluded to in identifying the men as "all active homosexuals" (Gottlieb et al. 1988:68 [1981]). [9] And in their final paragraph the authors state: "Two of the 5 reported having frequent homosexual contacts with various partners" (p. 70). Thus, the stage was set for the subsequent emphasis on promiscuity as an element in the epidemic. Even before there was solid epidemiological evidence implicating promiscuity as a factor in the chain of causation of AIDS, stereotypical understandings of the lives of gay men generated the hypothesis that AIDS was caused by promiscuity. Gay men were reputedly notoriously promiscuous, and as AIDS was recognized in individuals who were not homosexual, they were assigned to other "risk groups" which could also be linked to the notion of promiscuity. Although the pre-AIDS IV drug literature emphasized that drug use resulted in lack of sexual interest, drug usage in this country is generally associated in popular thought with sexual permissiveness, with indiscriminate coupling, and with prostitution, and so it was not difficult to assimilate intravenous drug users to what Murray and Payne (1988) call the "promiscuity paradigm." Haitians and Africans, all black, were surely promiscuous (Hrdy 1987); after all, American racial dogmas have usually attributed hypersexuality, nonmonogamy, and unstable family life to people of color regardless of domicile in the U.S. or abroad (Worth 1990:122). [10] Indeed, hypersexuality is often alleged for minorities and "others" of all kinds; for example, as Adam (1978:45) has noted, it is "a trait attributed to Jews by anti-Semites." To protect the promiscuity thesis, undetected homosexual activity, or failing evidence for that, heterosexual promiscuity, anal intercourse or unusual sexual practices were invoked, and blame was frequently fixed on prostitution (see Fumento 1989). Prostitutes are, of course, promiscuous by occupational definition.

Thus, what all of these categories (gay men, drug abusers, Africans, Haitians, people of color, and prostitutes) shared was promiscuity, real or imagined. The general promiscuity hypothesis began to be challenged only with the discovery of AIDS cases among infants, hemophiliacs, and the recipients of blood transfusions who did not fit into any of the promiscuous "risk groups." [11] These were truly "innocent victims." Of what were they "innocent"? This term in Western tradition when applied to children refers primarily to the absence of carnal knowledge. Their innocence is of sex and promiscuity.

Standing alone, promiscuity could no longer be the sole cause of AIDS since promiscuity is nowhere a new invention, whereas AIDS appeared to be a new disease. Nor could homosexuality stand as the cause. But it was agreed that promiscuity among gay men in San Francisco and New York was on a scale unprecedented in world history (Grmek 1990:169), and that the homosexual community was the "amplifier of the outbreak of AIDS" because while homosexuality was "probably as old as mankind . . . commercialized homosexual sex" (i.e., bathhouses) was a new phenomenon, which greatly increased easy access to sexual partners (Francis 1983: 139–140).

Several etiological theories of AIDS incorporated promiscuity as a crucial component even though they differed in their interpretation of how promiscuity produced disease. One early theory, the "immune overload" theory, suggested that due to being overworked the immune system eventually collapsed. An immune system that has been stressed, in this scenario, by repeated episodes of diseases, primarily

STDs, can no longer respond (Marx 1986b[1982]). The plausibility of this theory was enhanced by studies which indicated that gay men had higher incidences of many such diseases (e.g., syphilis, gonorrhea, hepatitis B, amebiasis) because of their "promiscuity" and because of "exotic" sexual practices such as rimming and fisting. Another version of this theory focused on the potential impact on the immune system from anal intercourse. It argued that the frequent desposition of semen in the rectum by multiple partners could be the cause because of the immune suppressing properties of semen (Richards, Bedford, and Witkin 1986[1984]); Leibowitch 1985; Fettner and Check 1984; Fromer 1983; Antonio 1986; Siegal and Siegal 1983). Such speculation was especially suitable for "explaining" AIDS among gay men, but the paradigm required stretching to cover other "risk groups." Not much stretching was required for Africans and Haitians and even drug users, all of whom were also presumed to be hypersexual and immunocompromised by high rates of disease, exotic tropical diseases in the case of the Africans and Haitians. The theory required considerably more stretching for transfusion cases and hemophiliacs and, to the breaking point, for infants (McCombie 1990:11).

The major alternative theory was that AIDS was a communicable disease spread by sexual practices and sharing contaminated needles.[12] In this model, which quickly gained hegemony following the isolation of the retrovirus we now know as HIV, promiscuity's role is to permit the transmission of the etiologic agent (Essex 1986[1985]). It should be noted that echoes of the former paradigm can still be heard in discussions of AIDS etiology, most notably in the work of Peter Duesberg and his defenders. Duesberg (1987) rejects HIV as the cause of AIDS without specifying an alternative, but his discussions emphasize lifestyle considerations, including promiscuity, as do those of other critics of the retroviral theory (Rappoport 1988; Gregory and Leonardo 1986).

Epidemiological evidence in support of the role of promiscuity in causing AIDS was not long in coming. Over the years since the start of the epidemic, study after study has reported a statistical association between number of sexual partners and AIDS, and later with HIV infection. The first study (Marmor et al. 1982) focused on men in New York City and compared AIDS patients who had Kaposi's sarcoma with healthy control subjects. In addition to inhaled nitrite use and frequency of sexually transmitted diseases, a key difference between AIDS patients and controls was the number of different sexual partners reported by each group. Subjects with AIDS were more likely than the controls to have had 10 or more different partners in a typical month prior to the onset of symptoms (Turner, Miller, and Moses 1989). A follow-up study by Jaffe and associates (1983:129) found that subjects with AIDS averaged 61 different sexual partners in the preceding year in contrast to the reported average of 25 for controls.[13] Thus, as Turner, Miller, and Moses point out, even before the viral cause of AIDS was known, research showed that AIDS was associated with a large number of sexual partners.

Studies continue to be published with data supportive of a correlation between number of sexual partners and HIV infection (Darrow et al. 1987, 1988; Piot et al. 1988; Curran et al. 1988; Turner, Miller and Barker 1988). Curran et al. (1985:1355) noted that "an increased number of sexual partners was the most consistent risk factor associated with acquisition of infection or AIDS in homosexual men." And they added that "large numbers of heterosexual partners are risk factors for AIDS in heterosexual men" in Central Africa.[14] While most studies report significant associations between AIDS/HIV and promiscuity, not all of them do. An early study done in Denmark, for example, found no relationship between these variables (Melbye et al. 1984). But many recent studies as well have failed to document a correlation between "number of partners" and HIV infection or AIDS (e.g., Merino et al. 1990; Collier, Barnes, and Handsfield 1986; Schechter et al. 1989; Rietmeijer et al. 1989; Simonsen et al. 1990; van Griensven et al. 1990; McCoy et al. 1990; Lifson et al. 1990 [Kaposi's sarcoma specifically]; Padian et al. 1987) or found mixed results, e.g., Burcham et al. (1989), who found no correlation with the number of lifetime sexual partners but did find one with the number of recent partners (Ss with 10 or more partners had a higher risk of seroconversion than those with 0–9). Nonetheless, because so many studies early in the epidemic did find an association, promiscuity became firmly entrenched in epidemiological discourse as a major risk factor. Counting sexual partners, especially of gay men, became a prime preoccupation of epidemiologists.

In light of the prominence of promiscuity in the epidemiological literature, its pervasive presence as a key variable in mathematical modelling of the course of the epidemic is understandable (e.g., Ahlgren, Gorny, and Stein 1990; Bongaarts 1988; Weyer and Eggers 1990; Lin 1991; Sattenspiel and Castillo-Chavez 1990; Sattenspiel et al. 1990; Koopman et al. 1988; Jacquez et al. 1988; May, Anderson, and Blower 1990). In this literature, "contact rate" is the term used to refer to a measure which includes data on the number of partners, rate of partnership formation, and partnership duration (Office of Science and Technology Policy 1988). Given the crucial importance of the impact of safe sex on HIV transmission, it is interesting to note that the modelers tend to ignore this variable (Hunt et al. 1990).[15] In most of the research, a "contact" seems to mean unprotected penetrative sex. Thus, promiscuity and risk become conflated. Leslie and Brunham (1990) discuss the limitations inherent in the assumptions of classic epidemiological modelling for providing projections that are meaningful for real-life populations in the HIV epidemic.

For the most part, the term "promiscuity" has been eschewed in scientific writings on AIDS epidemiology. It is largely absent from publications emanating from the CDC, despite the widespread usage of the term traditionally in medical texts to denote sex with multiple partners (Oppenheimer 1988). But not all AIDS scientists managed to abolish it from their vocabulary. Weyer and Eggers (1990) and Essex (1986:3[1985]), for example, mention "highly promiscuous" individuals or homosexuals. Sonnabend's use of the term "profound promiscuity" in his discussion of the etiology of AIDS published in the Journal of the American Medical Association prompted a rejoinder from two gay physicians who objected to use of the term because of its judgmental character and noted that it was "not suitable to the scientific medical literature" (Fain 1984:3). Oppenheimer (1988) hypothesizes that the research emphasis on "promiscuity" and "lifestyle" (which are largely synonymous in this context) would not have occurred if the first AIDS cases had not been discovered in gay men, about whom medical researchers had fewer qualms in making judgmental assessments; it also resulted in paying less theoretical attention from the outset to cases involving women (except prostitutes) and heterosexuals generally.

Gay Community Discourse

Most observers of the gay community are quick to point out that lifestyles within the community vary greatly and that the stereotype of hyper-promiscuity among gay men in America does not apply to all gay men, some of whom are monogamous, some even exclusively (both behaviorally and ideologically) monogamous (McWhirter and Mattison 1984; Bell and Weinberg 1978; Blumstein and Schwartz 1983; Franklin 1988; Tuller 1988; Kurdek and Schmitt 1988). With that said, however, there can be no doubt that promiscuity and an ethos of sexual freedom have been important features of gay life, and for outsiders, it was undoubtedly what was being labelled indirectly by the term "gay lifestyle." When applied by nongays to gays, "gay lifestyle" is largely a metaphor for promiscuity.

In the years following the onset of the contemporary gay liberation movement in 1969 with the riots in New York City at the Stonewall Inn, gay men, having fought to free themselves from the assumptions and constraints of heterosexism, joined the sexual revolution which was part of the American scene at that time (Marotta 1981; Altman 1982). The sexual ideology which dominated American gay culture during the 1970s is expressed in Wittman's "Gay Manifesto," in which he rejected the exclusiveness and possessiveness of heterosexual relationships (cited in Lee 1988:28). Sexuality in a myriad of forms became the core of the emergent gay culture of the 1970s, at least in most major cities of the Western world (Lang 1990:175).

To explain what some regard as the sexual excesses (sexual pluralism) of gay men is not difficult. Historical factors related to oppression with a subsequent release from major constraints in the late 1960s and the 1970s were certainly instrumental, as are some life cycle considerations in individuals' coming to terms with their variant sexual orientation. In addition, one can also draw on sociobiological understandings and suggest that gay men as men are doing what straight men would do if the opportunity structures were as readily available to them (Symons 1979). The 1970s saw a masculinization of gay men, and this rejection of a stereotyped femininity may have intensified gay identification with male sexual prowess as manifested in promiscuous conquests (Gough 1989).

Still, gay men in the U.S. are socialized into American culture in which there obviously exists considerable ambivalence about promiscuity—both an attraction to it and a disdain for its excesses and limitations. This ambivalence is a reflection of the discrepancy, to be discussed below, between the ideology of fidelity and the behavioral reality of promiscuity—guilt, perhaps, mingled with pride related to a counter ideology of infidelity which co-exists with the dominant ethos. This conflict is captured wonderfully in a PBS documentary on the development of the hepatitis B vaccine in the series called *Quest for the Killers*. A woman is shown interviewing a gay man in Greenwich Village in the late 1970s, asking him about the number of sexual partners he has had in the past six months. He first seems to be aghast that she is asking that question; then he waffles. So she prompts him to calculate it by figuring how many he has during an average week. He begins to look very sheepish as he replies that he has five partners per day three times per week, for a total of 60 per month and 360 for six months. The scene in this program is also an instance of the media playing up the stereotype; the incident is not balanced or nuanced by questions of how typical or atypical the man is.

Concern over promiscuity existed in the gay community prior to AIDS. Gay physicians, in particular, were worried about the health consequences of such behavior (Gorman 1986:162). For example, the National Coalition of Gay STD Services issued a brochure in 1981 which contained guidelines and recommendations for healthful sexual activity. That brochure discussed the risks of having multiple sexual partners and of anonymous sex.[16] But by the late 1970s calls for an end to promiscuity were being made outside the medical context by gay men who were dissatisfied with the endless round of one-night stands. Most notable in this regard is the work of Larry Kramer, author of the novel entitled *Faggots* (1978). Toward the end of the novel, which chronicles gay life in New York City in the 1970s, the protagonist states:

You've already fucked half of New York . . . I've fucked the other half. You told me you were in the bars since you were seventeen, you had your muscles at twenty-three. There isn't a scene you haven't seen or done. And you're only thirty. Why can't you imagine something better? I dare you to change! And try for something better!

The novel, which deplored the dominant sexual ethos of gay men, was controversial, but it expressed a concern that was shared by some segments of the community.

Shortly thereafter, AIDS struck, and the debate over promiscuity intensified. One of the reasons behind the hesitant and confused response of the gay community to the AIDS crisis in the beginning was a suspicion that AIDS (then known as GRID, Gay-Related Immunodeficiency) was being concocted by erotophobic enemies as an attack on gay society and its culture. Throughout the 1980s the pros and cons of promiscuity were widely discussed as gay men adjusted to the presence of AIDS. Kramer (1985, 1989) continued his frontal assaults. His play (1985), *The Normal Heart*, became the most celebrated dramatic response to AIDS. Its success was due in no small measure to the fact that it conformed to the dominant sexual ideology of the heterosexual world. Straights could watch this play without flinching. In this work, as Crimp (1988:247) notes, Kramer's view is:

that gay men should stop having so much sex, that promiscuity kills. But this common sense is, of course, conventional moral wisdom: it is not safe sex, but monogamy that is the solution. The play's message is therefore not only reactionary, it is lethal, since monogamy per se provides no protection whatsoever against a virus that might already have infected one partner in a relationship.

The conflict and contradictions between safe sex and promiscuity approaches to sex in the age of AIDS are laid bare in Crimp's statement (see also D'Eramo 1988). Other plays were more sex-positive, e.g., William Hoffman's *As Is* (1985) and Robert Chesley's *Night Sweat* (1984), and less commercially successful.

Seeking to understand the natural disaster which had struck their community and to deal with individual personal tragedies caused by AIDS, many gay men sought refuge in regrets about the zipless fucking of their past, while others rejected such self-blame ("*Je ne regrette rien*") as a manifestation of self-hate (Bérubé 1988). As Holleran (1988:6–7) says, "Promiscuity was the *lingua franca*, the Esperanto, of the male homosexual community . . . Men are now weeping in doctors' offices over the fact that they were once promiscuous. . . . (Now that it is denied to them, people realize how romantic promiscuity was.)."

The gay community is divided between separatists and integrationists, and promiscuity is one of the issues of contention. While separatists generally adhere to the sexual ethos generated in the early years of gay liberation, assimilationists argue that gay survival requires an accommodation to the dominant sexual ideology of monogamy. This position is advanced most systematically by Kirk and Madsen (1989) who argue that gay "misbehavior," which includes anonymous sex and promiscuity, is a major cause of "America's fear and hatred of gays." If this is true, it could be argued that it is because gay promiscuity is open and unapologetic, whereas every effort is made to keep straight promiscuity closeted or hidden behind a facade of ideological moralizing. But even nonassimilationists who are not sex-negative, have sometimes espoused an anti-promiscuity position. For example, early in the epidemic, Callen and Berkowitz (1988:166[1983]) wrote: "Sex and 'promiscuity' have become the dogma of gay male liberation. Have we modified the belief that we could dance our way to liberation into the belief that we could somehow fuck our way there? If sex is liberating, is more sex necessarily more liberating?. . . The party that was the '70s is over. Taking ignorance to the baths and backrooms is not sexual freedom—it's oppression."[17,18]

Another manifestation of erotophobic anti-promiscuity that emerged in the 1980s was the sexual addiction movement. The sexual revolution of the 1960s and 1970s resulted in the depathologization of many forms of nonprocreative sex, and indeed, to a pathologization of insufficient or inadequate sex. But in the early 1980s efforts began to re-pathologize sexual behavior, especially "too much sex" or "sexual compulsion" (Coleman 1991). Therapists, armed with this new label for an old behavior pattern, managed to convince many gay men, frightened by the spectre of AIDS, that they suffered from this disorder and were in need of therapeutic intervention (Quadland and Shattls 1987). In addition, groups modelled on Alcoholics Anonymous sprang up in most gay communities in the U.S. (Bardach 1991). Guides to staying well in the AIDS age include discussions of how to deal with sexual compulsivity (Froman 1990). In an article entitled "The Myth of Sexual Compulsivity," Levine and Troiden (1988) have examined the validity of this "pathology," brilliantly exposing its conceptual flaws and sociocultural underpinnings.

This overview of discourse on promiscuity in the gay community is necessarily highly abbreviated, but nonetheless it provides evidence of how pervasive and how divisive this topic had become within the community which had been hit hardest and earliest by AIDS.

Public Policy Discourse

Promiscuity has been deeply embedded in a number of AIDS public policy discussions, and sexual morality is often the basis for decisions about legislation and funding on AIDS topics. The dominant approach of the Reagan administration and its conservative supporters was to stop AIDS by eliminating the immorality of promiscuity.

The first major pronouncement on AIDS by the Reagan administration was the document prepared by Surgeon General C. Everett Koop. Though less moralistic in tone than statements by other high administration officals, Koop used the term "promiscuous" in his summary:

The most certain way to avoid getting the AIDS virus and to control the AIDS epidemic in the United States is for individuals to avoid promiscuous sexual practices, to maintain mutually faithful monogamous sexual relationships and to avoid injecting illicit drugs.[19] (p. 27)

In discussing "single teen-age girls", Koop states:

They have been taught to say NO to sex! They have been taught to say NO to drugs! By saying NO to sex and drugs, they can avoid AIDS which can kill them! The same is true for teenage boys who should also not have rectal intercourse with other males. It may result in AIDS. (p. 18)

As a pragmatist and as the authority responsible for the nation's health, Koop was aware, however, that preaching about abstinence and fidelity was not sufficient to stop the sexual transmission of HIV (Koop 1988[1987]). To the dismay of ideologues in the Reagan administration, he went on to emphasize the importance of using condoms:

. . . for those who are abstinent or those who have a mutually faithful monogamous sexual relationship, AIDS presents no problem. But for sexually active individuals who are neither abstinent nor have a mutually faithful monogamous relationship, we have little to offer except condoms. [Koop 1987:2111]

The debate over the content of AIDS prevention messages was nowhere more vitriolic than in the context of guidelines for education in schools. Education Secretary William Bennett and Domestic Policy Advisor Gary Bauer were the leading critics of Koop and the most vociferous proponents of a policy of chastity; their aim was to legislate morality.[20] Bennett is reported having stated in a television documentary in 1987 that "AIDS may give us an opportunity to discourage [teen sex], and that would be a good thing" (Haffner 1988:94). The CDC guidelines for AIDS education in schools listed as its first objective to encourage young people who have not engaged in sexual intercourse to "abstain from sexual intercourse until they are ready to establish a mutually monogamous relationship within the context of marriage" or if they have already had intercourse to stop doing so until ready for such a relationship (Quackenbush and Nelson 1988:436). Secondarily the guidelines recommended condoms for those who would not abstain.[21] Thus chastity became the official policy of the U.S. Government.

Federal funding of HIV prevention programs was seriously hampered by severe content restrictions imposed on granting agencies by Congress, led by homophobic legislators such as Jesse Helms and William Dannemeyer, who preferred controlling the epidemic by coercive measures, including quarantine, rather than by education (Bayer 1989:170). For them, advocating safe sex meant condoning and encouraging sodomy and promiscuity. The 1988 Helms Amendment explicitly prohibited expending any funds for education which "promotes homosexuality or promiscuity" (Patton 1990:56; Osborn 1989:408).[22]

At the local level, promiscuity was the issue involved in efforts to shut down bathhouses, since these were sites which facilitated anonymous, promiscuous sex. The Battle of the Baths, which was waged most intensely in San Francisco and New York, was a symbolic attack on promiscuity, not a public policy matter that would have a significant impact in reducing HIV transmission (Institute of Medicine 1986:128–129). As Bayer (1989:71) has pointed out, it served mainly as "a powerful statement about the dangers of promiscuity."[23] In 1986, the Public Health Service endorsed efforts by local and state authorities to close bathhouses and other commercial sex establishments which permitted anonymous sexual contacts or sex with multiple partners (Nichols 1989:183).

Promiscuity is also implicated in the policy issues surrounding prostitution, which once again came under attack as a source of disease (Brandt 1987; D'Emilio and Freedman 1988).[24] Promiscuous by profession and subject to control by the criminal justice system, sex workers were quickly singled out as targets for forced HIV antibody testing. The Public Health Service recommended in 1987 that prostitutes be counseled and tested (Bayer 1989:186), but it did not recommend testing of clients, despite the finding that a prostitute was more likely to become infected by a client than vice versa. Obviously, public officials and health authorities considered some forms of promiscuity more dangerous than others, notably the promiscuity of stigmatized groups.[25]

Finally, AIDS-related research on sexuality has been stymied by opposition based on the claim that such research would lead to promiscuous behavior. Thus, plans for a national sex survey were scuttled despite the urgent need to have better data on the sexual practices of the American population in order to improve the efficacy of prevention programs (Miller, Turner, and Moses 1990). Another study, of teenage sexuality, was cancelled by the Secretary of Health and Human Services, Louis W. Sullivan, because it might "encourage casual sex" (Marshall 1991; Rutten 1991). This decision was prompted by Dannemeyer's attacks which targeted the issues of both homosexuality and promiscuous sex. How, one might ask, would a survey of several thousand individuals result in greater promiscuity? The concern was not for the behavior of those interviewed but rather the impact on society generally which might occur with revelations about how widespread promiscuous behavior is. Getting funding for sex research not committed *a priori* to a sex-negative agenda has been virtually impossible during the first decade of AIDS (Bolton 1992; Carrier and Bolton 1991).

Religious Discourse

In recent years sexuality has become a flashpoint of controversy and factionalism in many religious communities in the United States. It is clearly an important subtext in the conflict between pro-choice and anti-choice antagonists in the struggle over abortion, but beyond that, re-interpreting the role of sexuality in human life has become a major concern of various Christian denominations as they attempt to deal with the social changes of the second half of the 20th century. Nonmarital sexuality in general and homosexuality in particular have posed especially serious difficulties for religious leaders as they face the transparent discrepancies between social realities and traditional theological doctrines on sexuality.

Liberal denominations have moved in the direction of accepting nonmarital sex, whether heterosexual or homosexual, as compatible with a Christian or Jewish morality. The ordination of gay and lesbian ministers and rabbis and the performance of the blessing of gay unions are no longer earthshaking events, even if they do continue to evoke considerable dissent. But the ideal in almost all cases continues to be one of fidelity and love within a monogamous relationship, and "recreational" sexuality continues to be condemned.

AIDS has provided leverage to both sides in the struggle over sexuality. It offered conservative moralists a weapon; this was especially true early in the epidemic when "God's Wrath" was asserted as the cause of AIDS (Kopelman 1988; Ross 1988). AIDS was seen as divine vengeance for humanity's rampant immorality (i.e., promiscuity and homosexuality). And it was used to promote the anti-sexual agenda of the Religious Right, with some proponents of this ideology actively lobbying against government funding for AIDS research because they argued that a cure for AIDS was undesirable since it would promote promiscuity (Altman 1986; Patton 1985b; Shilts 1987). In essence, the Religious Right saw in AIDS an opportunity to undo the "sexual revolution" which had taken place despite their opposition and which they abhorred. This interpretation, of course, can still be heard expounded by fundamentalist televangelists, but it has faded somewhat as more has been learned about the biological etiology of AIDS, as awareness of heterosexual transmission of AIDS has increased, and, perhaps not least, as the hypocrisy of some of the most vehement proponents of fundamentalist doctrines (e.g., Jim Bakker, Marvin Gorman, and Jimmy Swaggart) has been exposed by their own alleged or documented sexual infidelities.

The proponents of religious reassessment of sexuality have also used AIDS, but they argue that acceptance of homosexuality and of committed nonmarital sex will help to fight AIDS by promoting stable, faithful relationships.

Media Discourse

Media treatment of the promiscuity dimension of AIDS has varied considerably depending on the genre of coverage of AIDS issues. A thorough review of AIDS in the media is beyond the scope of this paper, but some observations on the media and promiscuity are in order.[26] Both understatement and overstatement were in evidence during the first decade of the epidemic.

On television, promiscuity was generally glossed over in dramatic presentations. Movies made for TV tended to portray individuals who were "innocent victims" of AIDS. Even when the main characters were gay men, as in *An Early Frost*, *Our Sons* and *Andre's Mother*, they were depicted as close approximations to mainstream values of monogamy. Often when promiscuity was mentioned in these works, it was to deny that the characters had been promiscuous. Given the intent of these productions to create sympathetic understanding of persons affected by AIDS, attributing promiscuity to the characters might have been considered counter-productive.

The history of AIDS documentaries is more mixed. Those which discussed AIDS and sexuality often included segments on casual sex scenes, both straight and gay, and on prostitution, of course. Here the message being delivered was that promiscuity is a cause of AIDS and dangerous. Without a thorough content analysis of AIDS programming it is impossible to be sure, but it appears that over the decade there has been a decline in emphasis on promiscuity as AIDS cases increase in heterosexuals and as the proportion of cases related to homosexuality declines.

News stories were more likely than these other formats to sensationalize promiscuity on television. The "big story" was the revelation of Rock Hudson's illness and death, in which promiscuity was not a prominent issue, perhaps because he was in a relationship and because his "outing" as homosexual was sensational enough. The promiscuity of other AIDS "victims" was played up, however, and their promiscuity made into a *cause célèbre*. For example, following the publication of Shilts' (1987) book, the story of Gaetan Dugas, Patient Zero, was given extensive coverage and the role of his sexual escapades in spreading AIDS around the continent was highlighted (Grmek 1990:18–20; Williamson 1989). The same was true of Fabian Bridges, an HIV-infected male prostitute, who was reported to be deliberately infecting clients. Indeed, in both of these cases the promiscuous individual was blamed for continuing to have sex knowingly and intentionally without concern for the consequences to his partners, thereby linking promiscuity with psychopathology (Bersani 1988) and sickness with crime (Quam 1990:34). This approach was taken also in some entertainment programs, e.g., an episode of *Midnight Caller*, in which an HIV-infected bisexual man continues to be promiscuous (Gross 1991).

Advertising, too, deserves to be mentioned here. Despite recommendations from health officials that commercials and PSAs for condoms be broadcast, major networks continue to refuse to accept ads for condoms, since promotion of condoms might be interpreted as an endorsement of promiscuity. Promiscuity itself, of course, is salient in television programming, and ads for promiscuity in the form of phone sex (heterosexual only) are to be found on many channels. Indeed, the Presidential Commission on the Human Immunodeficiency Virus Epidemic (1988) listed the entertainment industry's portrayal of promiscuous sex in a glamorous light as an obstacle to HIV prevention efforts.

At the onset of the epidemic, coverage in the print media was scant at best.[27] In part this was due to the reluctance of editors and publishers to deal with sexuality in "family-oriented" magazines and newspapers (Kinsella 1989:2). Homosexuality and promiscuity were considered inappropriate topics. Media attention picked up when there were "innocent victims" to report on. But in the beginning, AIDS coverage in at least one newspaper was considerable, i.e., The San Francisco Chronicle, and the reporter, Randy Shilts, a gay man who had been a bathhouse regular and even a bathhouse employee (Kinsella 1989:170). His coverage of the epidemic was intended to scare his readers into abandoning promiscuity, on the premise that promiscuity equals death.

Occasionally, news coverage indicated that AIDS was a problem only for those in the "fast-lane" (i.e., promiscuous), attempting to reassure readers, presumed to be monogamous heterosexuals (the "general public"), that it was not a danger to them. Publication of the Masters and Johnson book which declared that heterosexuals were not at serious risk, for instance, received extensive news coverage. At other times, the message was "now everyone is at risk." Stories which predicted that AIDS spelled the end of the sexual revolution (the same prediction made earlier during the period of herpes hysteria) obviously focused on promiscuity (Schneider 1988:98).

With these observations as background, I shall now turn to examine the realities of promiscuity in contemporary American culture.

PROMISCUITY IN AMERICAN SOCIETY: THE REALITY

Heterosexual Attitudes and Values

Numerous scholars have documented shifts in the American sexual ideology during the 20th century, from a restrictive to a more permissive model (Frayser 1985, 1991), from a Jehovanist to a Naturalist paradigm (Davis 1983), from an erotophobic to a pleasure esthetic (Bronski 1984), and from an emphasis on danger to an emphasis on desire (Vance 1984; Rubin 1984; DuBois and Gordon 1984; Echols 1984). But despite these changes, the romantic ideal of sex confined to a faithful, monogamous heterosexual relationship between a man and a woman in love remains firmly entrenched in American sexual ideology (Blumstein and Schwartz 1983:271).

Indeed, even the traditional double standard persists, though it may have lessened (Sprecher 1989; Rubin 1991; Blumstein and Schwartz 1983), despite the critiques of feminists and the changing role of women in society. Linguistic evidence for this is abundant when one examines terms for promiscuous behavior as applied to men and women. A woman who is promiscuous is referred to as a slut, whore, tramp, loose—she sleeps around. A promiscuous man is a stud, a "woman's man," a Don Juan or Casanova—he sows his wild oats. The evaluative connotations of these two sets of terms differ; it's the rare woman who would revel in being called a slut, and the rare man who would not take pride in being called a stud. Pejorative labels for the promiscuous are largely reserved for women and gay men; they do not apply to heterosexual males. Historically, they have been used as a weapon for controlling the sexuality of women and minorities. And they continue to be so used (Worth 1990).

When one turns from overarching abstractions to sexual particulars, however, it is clear that traditional attitudes and values have become greatly attenuated. Evidence is overwhelming that a majority of Americans find premarital sex acceptable, and those who disapprove tend to be older individuals. A 1985 poll by the Roper Organization indicated 36% disapprove of premarital sex while 61% approve. Among individuals between 18 and 29 years, the corresponding figures were 20% to 78% (Byer and Shainberg 1991:32). A recent study of college students found that 91% of the men and 84% of the women approved of premarital intercourse (Rubinson and De Rubertis 1991). While their elders may attempt to control the sexuality of the young, teenagers mostly accept the idea that they have a right to be sexual. According to Rubin (1991:60), "If there are two words that describe the sexual sensibility of today's youth, they are 'tolerance' and 'entitlement' . . . it's the language of love and romance, not commitment and marriage, that defines the boundaries of sexuality for most teenagers." Attitudes toward premarital sex do vary to some degree depending on the level of emotional commitment involved (Frayser 1985:410). Of considerable importance is how much this permissive stance cuts across all groups in society. For example, religiosity does not appear to have much impact on premarital sexual behavior and attitudes (Sack, Keller, and Hinkle 1984) nor on patterns of sexual promiscuity generally (Blumstein and Schwartz 1983).

Attitudes and values toward extramarital sex remain less permissive than those toward premarital sex. Rubinson and De Rubertis (1991), in their study of college students, found that acceptance of extramarital sex had declined between 1972 and 1987 from 12% to 3%. In data gathered from students in my own college course on human sexuality, the statistics are similar: only 3.7% approve somewhat of extramarital sex, while 19.0% disapprove somewhat and 66.4% disapprove strongly. Other studies over the years have reported that approximately 70–74% of adults consider extramarital sex to be always wrong and another 12–16% consider it almost always wrong (Luria, Friedman, and Rose 1987). Thus, it would appear that the sexual revolution had a profound impact on attitudes toward premarital sex but relatively little influence on norms for adultery (Glenn and Weaver 1979).

Attitudes toward promiscuity do not transmit HIV, of course, only behavior can. Confirming what we know about the lack of isomorphism between attitudes and behavior from research on other domains, one recent study found that sexual ideology accounts for only 10–15% of the variance in sexual experience levels (Troiden and Jendreck 1987). Let us look, then, at nonmonogamous behavior in American society.

Heterosexual Behavior Patterns

If the ideal in American society is "no sex before marriage, no sex outside marriage, and marriage until death do us part," the statistical evidence suggests that the number of individuals in the society who conform to this ideal is extremely low. Although all sex research is beset with measurement problems (Abramson 1990; Coyle, Boruch, and Turner 1991; Turner, Miller, and Moses 1989; Miller, Turner, and Moses 1990; Catania et al. 1990a, 1990b; McLaws et al. 1990; Reinisch, Sanders, and Ziemba-Davis 1988; Turner 1989), many studies document the extent to which sexual ideology and sexual behavior diverge.

Nonconsensual Sex: Child Abuse and Rape.   Beginning with the most serious violation of the traditional code, childhood sexual abuse, research provides incidence estimates that indicate widespread sexual activity. After reviewing the studies on this topic, Zierler et al. (1991) claim that between 28 and 36% of children under the age of 14 years experience sexual abuse. In their own investigation, they found that 50% of the women and 20% of the men acknowledged a history of rape or forced sex before the age of 18 years. National estimates, they note, are "that one in four girls and one in six boys are sexually assaulted before the age of 18" (p. 575). Reported rapes in the U.S. reached a level of 92,000 cases in 1988, and in view of the fact that most rapes are not reported to authorities, this number grossly understates the problem of nonconsensual sexual behavior (Allgeier and Allgeier 1991). *Premarital Sex.* Teenage sexuality has come under scrutiny in recent years, not so much because of the dangers posed by the AIDS epidemic but rather because of the "epidemic" of unwanted pregnancies among unmarried adolescents (Rubin 1991; Miller, Turner, and Moses 1990). Approximately one million teenagers become pregnant each year in the U.S. Half of them have abortions. Two and one half million teenagers contract a sexually transmitted disease each year. This evidence of teenage sexual behavior is not in dispute, but what is the subject of acrimonious debates is how to deal with this issue. Sex education, high school clinics, and condom distribution are favored by some (e.g., Willis 1988; Rodman, Lewis, and Griffith 1988; Krauthammer 1988; Dryfoos 1988; Edelman 1988; Trudell and Whatley 1991), while the opponents of such programs argue that these approaches will lead to greater promiscuity when the goal should be to insist on abstinence (e.g., Anchell 1988; Conservative Family Campaign 1988 [1986–1987]; LaHaye 1988; Macdonald 1988; Kuharski 1988; Sanderson and Wilson 1991).

Data show that, as of 1979, 40% of American women are sexually active before the age of 16 and that by 19 years of age over 70% have experienced intercourse. Indeed, by age 19, over 50% have had multiple partners. Of men 17 years of age, 20% indicate that they have had six or more partners (Turner, Miller, and Moses 1989:98–101; see also Biggar, Brinton, and Rosenthal 1989; Clement 1990; Turner 1989). In the 1980s the percentages have risen still higher (Brooks-Gunn and Furstenberg 1990). While the average age of first intercourse nationally is approximately 16 years, it may be as low as 12 in some urban areas. In addition, it should be noted that several studies have reported sexual activity to orgasm between males for approximately 17% to 37% of all adolescents (Kipke, Futterman, and Hein 1990:1154).

How many partners do sexually-active unmarried individuals have? Based on two national surveys done in 1987 and 1988, Turner, Miller, and Moses (1989:106) estimate the percentages by age clusters of men and women who abstain or who have three or more partners as follows:

TABLE I. Number of partners in last year of unmarried men and women in the United States.

Age Group	Men		Women	
	No Partner (%)	3+ Partners (%)	No Partner (%)	3+ Partners (%)
18–24	16.5	40.7	19.0	15.5
25–34	12.4	26.9	13.2	7.9
35–49	13.5	28.5	25.5	7.5
50–64	22.3	29.0	60.2	1.2
65+	74.0	4.2	93.7	0.0

Abstinence, then, is definitely not part of being unmarried in American society. *Extramarital Sex.*   Adultery is widespread in American society, despite the attitudes and values reported above. Studies of the incidence of such behavior have been reviewed by Thompson (1983). Kinsey's research first brought to public attention how extensively the norm of marital fidelity is violated; he and his associates estimated that 50% of married men and 26% of married women had engaged in extramarital sex (Kim 1969). More recent work suggests that those figures understate the current situation, especially for women. Getting accurate data on rates is difficult, of course, but it is quite likely that 50–65% of married men and 45–55% of married women have participated in extramarital sex prior to the age of 40 years (Thompson 1983:6–7).[28] It is difficult to know how many different partners married men and women who engage in extramarital sex have. One study, skewed toward white, college-educated respondents, found that during the relationship 11% of husbands had had 2–5 partners, 6% had had 6–20 partners, and 2% had had more than 20 partners, while 8% of the wives had had 2–5 partners, 3% had had 6–20 partners, and 1% had had more than 20 partners during the relationship (Turner, Miller, and Moses 1989:112). Another study indicated that 4–6% of married men and 1–2% of married women between the ages of 25 and 49 admitted to having more than one partner during the previous year (Turner, Miller, and Moses 1989:107–108).

A discussion of extramarital sexual behavior would be incomplete without reference to married men who have sex with men. Inasmuch as bisexual men have been found to be less likely to use protection during sex than gay men, the extramarital activities of these men is of concern (Gagnon 1990:189–194; Petrow 1990). In AIDS research, bisexual men are usually lumped with gay men. One of the few studies on the sexual behavior of bisexual men (Earl 1990) found that bisexual men averaged between 3.5 and 6.25 partners per month, and in almost all cases, wives were not aware of their mate's extramarital sex. It is virtually impossible to estimate the percentage of married men who are bisexual and promiscuous, but the number is undoubtedly considerable. Fay et al. (1989), on the basis of surveys done in 1970 and 1988, calculate that approximately 1.5% of men in the sample are currently married men and have engaged in sex with another man during the preceding year. They also calculate that 8% of the men in the study are currently married and have had during their lifetime occasional or fairly frequent homosexual contact, and 1.1% of the male population are currently married and have had 10 or more male partners since the age of 20.

Divorce and Postmarital Sex.   Even if premarital and extramarital sex were nonexistent, the ideal of having sex with only one partner in a lifetime would be vitiated by the realities of divorce in American society. Given the divorce rate in the U.S., the American marriage pattern has frequently been characterized as one of "serial monogamy." As Gagnon (1990:207) says: "The cycle of coupling, uncoupling, and recoupling is now accepted as the dominant sexual pattern in the United States." Martin and Bumpass (1989) calculated that two-thirds of all first marriages in the United States end in some manner other than the death of one of the partners. In essence, only one-third of first marriages survive. Their estimate is based on data that go beyond the official statistics to include separations as well as divorces. Their analysis, furthermore, suggests that while marital disruption rates plateaued in the

1980s, this phenomenon is not the result of either a change in values or AIDS but rather a consequence of having reached an upper limit related to structural constraints.

There is undoubtedly a link between sexuality and marital stability. Certainly, infidelity is a common component in decision making leading to divorce. Dissatisfaction with monogamous marital sex may result in sexual exploration which in turn may lead to divorce due to jealousies or to having found a more exciting sexual partner, although some research suggests that the quality of marital sex is not itself correlated with extramarital sex (Spanier and Margolis 1983).

Associated with the high divorce rate one finds the phenomenon of many heterosexual adults living for extended periods without a mate, even though 70% of them eventually do remarry. During such periods of matelessness, abstinence from sex is not especially notable. Allgeier and Allgeier (1991:463) cite research which shows that only 20% of separated and 26% of divorced individuals indicate that they abstained during the previous year; moreover, including the abstainers, those who were divorced averaged 2.41 partners during that period while those who were separated average 1.31. Indeed, divorced individuals had a higher number of lifetime partners (11.75) than had single, married, or widowed individuals. Promiscuity, then, not fidelity in marriage, is conspicuously present throughout all stages of the heterosexual life cycle, mythology and ideology notwithstanding.

Gay Male Behavior

Sexual values and attitudes within the gay community have been discussed above.[29] Here I shall merely report on behavioral data. Dramatic changes have occurred in gay male sexual behavior since the beginning of the epidemic, and much of what we know about the types and frequencies of specific sexual behaviors is the result of research done in response to AIDS. The number of partners gay men have may be somewhat exaggerated in studies because of the lack of representativeness of the samples which have examined such behavior (Harry 1986). Done mostly with nonrandom samples which necessarily recruit individuals who are more open about their sexual orientation and more likely to live in gay communities in major metropolitan areas, this research may underestimate the prevalence of coupled gay men and overestimate promiscuity. Individuals who live in suburban and rural areas may have different behavior patterns which reflect their personal predispositions as well as differences in the opportunity structures provided by their environment (Lynch 1987).

Prevalence of Homosexualty. Kinsey shocked the national consciousness by revealing that homosexuality was widespread in American society. His findings that approximately 37% of American males had had homosexual contact to orgasm at some point in their lives, that 10% had been almost exclusively homosexual for at least three years between the ages of 16 and 55, and that 4% had been exclusively homosexual throughout their entire lives provided the first serious estimates of the prevalence of such behavior. More recent studies have yielded lower estimates. Fay et al. (1989) analyzed two national samples, data collected in 1970 and 1988, and concluded that 20.3% of adult men have had at least one homosexual experience, 11.3% had their last such experience before the age of 16, and 6.7% had their last such experience after they were 19 years of age. They calculate that men who have sex with other men occasionally or fairly often constitute 3.3% of the adult male population, a figure which is only slightly lower than the estimate used by the Public Health Service in making projections about the number of Americans infected by HIV. Fay et al. caution that their estimate must be viewed as a lower bound for the real prevalence of homosexual behavior. Given the pressures of homophobia, intensified by AIDS (Nardi and Bolton 1991), the odds are high that their calculations seriously underestimate the prevalence of homosexual behavior. It is important to note that they based their estimate on a survey done in 1970, i.e., before the impact of gay liberation had been felt, and one done in 1988, i.e., after gay men were being blamed for AIDS and subject to increasing discrimination (William F. Buckley had published in respectable newspapers by this time his proposal to tattoo gay men on the buttocks). For both surveys, it is rather amazing that as many men as did so were willing to reveal to an unknown interviewer their homosexual conduct. If the surveys had been done in 1980, one might have more confidence that they represented the true prevalence of homosexual behavior (although in 1980 the gay community was recovering from the Anita Bryant "save the children" campaign).

Gay Relationships.   A minority of gay men are in monogamous relationships at any given time, but relationships are both sought and maintained by many gay men during their lives. Weinberg and Williams (1974:283) found that a majority of their gay respondents had had an exclusive relationship with another male during their lifetime. In another study, 41.4% of 1038 respondents said "Yes" in response to the question, "Do you have a lover?" Fully 87.7% of those without a current lover indicated that they would like to have one and 59.9% of these indicated that they would like to live with the lover. Of those with a lover, 59.3% were currently living together (Spada 1979).

Roles within gay relationships do not mimic those in heterosexual marriages (Peplau 1988). There is rarely conformity to one partner fulfilling a "masculine role" and the other a "feminine" role. Gay relationships tend to be more egalitarian, with decision making and activities shared (McWhirter and Mattison 1984). They may also involve more openness and honesty, especially with respect to sexuality, and gay men seem to place greater value on personal autonomy without sacrificing closeness and intimacy (Peplau and Cochran 1988). Statements of gay men about their relationships have been found to parallel those indicated by heterosexuals about their relationships with respect to how intimate and satisfying they assessed the relationships to be.

Gay Nonmonogamy.   This value on autonomy is nowhere more apparent than in the domain of sexuality. Sexual exclusivity is generally not a characteristic of gay relationships. Every study on this issue has found that sexually-exclusive relation-ships are a small minority of those found among gay men (e.g., Reece and Segrist 1988). Gay relationships may begin with a desire for fidelity on the part of one or both partners and may be monogamous during some portion of the duration of the relationship, but Blumstein and Schwartz (1983) found that within the first two years of a relationship 66% had not been completely monogamous; the corresponding figures were 89% for relationships of 2–10 years' duration and 94% for those that had lasted 10 years or longer. They conclude that gay men "have no trouble incorporating casual sex into their relationships" (p. 301). This finding is consistent with one of the major findings of McWhirter and Mattison (1984:285) who wrote:

The majority of couples in our study, and all of the couples together for longer than five years, were not continuously sexually exclusive with each other. Although many had long periods of sexual exclusivity, it was not the ongoing expectation for most. We found that gay men expect mutual emotional dependability with their partners and that relationship fidelity transcends concerns about sexuality and exclusivity.

In other words, emotional monogamy not sexual monogamy is characteristic of gay relationships (Marcus 1988:25).

This is not to say that promiscuity does not pose problems for gay relationships; in the how-to books published for gay couples in recent years, one finds extended discussions of how gay men handle extra-relationship sex. Although in some cases such encounters are considered "cheating" (as among most heterosexuals), in many cases clearcut rules are established concerning when, where, and with whom (e.g., mutual friends may be off-limits) such casual encounters are to be tolerated.

Gay "Divorce". The durability of gay relationships varies; certainly gay men participate in the cycle of coupling, uncoupling, and recoupling that Gagnon (1990) described as a characteristic of contemporary American heterosexuality. Only for gay men the cycling may be faster, on average, since in most cases for them there are neither offspring nor legal constraints and other societal pressures to decelerate the process (Bell and Weinberg 1978). Nonetheless, McWhirter and Mattison's (1984) research on gay couples found that nearly one third had lasted longer than 10 years, and they note that couples who have been together 40–50 years are not rare (see also Marcus 1988). Research by Reece and Segrist (1988) indicates importantly that the durability of gay relationships is not related, however, to promiscuity/sexual plurality.

It is clear from all extant research that gay men have by and large rejected the tight linkage between sex and marriage that is intrinsic to the Jehovanist sexual ideology and the hypocrisy that it appears to engender and that is so strikingly evident in the heterosexual data which show a wide gulf between ideals and behavior.

Number of Sexual Partners. Some definitions of promiscuity suggest that lack of discrimination in choice of partners is involved. Assertions about this supposed feature of promiscuity are of course intended to be pejorative. One could interpret the phenomenon, if it existed, from a different perspective by suggesting that it involves a more democratic approach to sexuality in which the individual refuses to discriminate against potential sex partners who do not possess an array of qualities desired in an ideal partner. Both homosexuals and heterosexuals vary in the breadth of the range of potential partners who meet the minimum criteria for sexual acceptability. In both gay and straight bars, at closing time people look more beautiful than earlier. But, in fact, gay men are often exceedingly demanding with respect to the set of standards that must be met by a potential sex partner or lover. This, of course, is what "attitude" is all about. When one examines gay personals, one discovers long lists of prerequisite attributes specified (e.g., height, body build, hair color, personal habits and hobbies, specific sexual preferences, genital configurations). Indeed, given such exhaustive specifications, from a probabilistic standpoint it is astonishing that any connections are made at all (Lumby 1988; Lee 1988; Laner and Kamel 1988; Sergios and Cody 1988).

But, of course, they are, and the AIDS epidemic has brought to public attention, in both the scientific literature and the general press, the "dirty" secret of gay men's "profound" promiscuity, with "shocking" statistics of men having had 500 to 1,000 or more sexual partners. Out of fear of societal recriminations and retribution, there have been some efforts to downplay these figures, but Bell and Weinberg (1978:82) writing before the epidemic, after reviewing the literature and in light of their own research, concluded that "little credence can be given to the supposition that homosexual men's 'promiscuity' has been overestimated."

Before reporting on the number of gay men's sexual partners, however, we need to pause to ask, What is a sexual partner? and What is a sexual contact? Herdt and Boxer (1991:175) point to problems with the construct itself, noting that it is fuzzy, and Patton (1985a:181) inquires: "What if you have anonymous sex six times a week and have sex with your long-term lover five times in the same week? Is that eleven contacts or seven? Some studies even sort out this problem by asking about number of partners, but then jerking off your buddy gets counted the same as fisting your lover." In fact, more attention to this concept is needed. What constitutes a partner? What actions must be engaged in before someone qualifies as a "sexual partner"? Unless greater specificity is provided, "number of sexual partners" is rather devoid of substance. Lack of attention to this issue is probably due to an assumption by scientists as well as the public that sex equals penetration, a heterosexist bias found in much AIDS research even among those studying gay men. At a minimum, in examining number of partners, a distinction must be made between penetrative and nonpenetrative sex partners since only the latter has meaningful implications with respect to HIV prevention and since there is no linear relationship between these two measures of number of partners (Davies et al. 1991; Hunt et al. 1990).

Martin and Vance (1984) note that all sex research, from Kinsey to the present, has been plagued with difficulties in obtaining reliable data on numbers of sexual contacts. Pre-epidemic data for gay men are reported by Doll et al. (1990a). Their data were gathered from 4910 gay and bisexual men in 1978 and 1979, but inasmuch as the respondents were recruited from clients at STD clinics in five metropolitan areas, they undoubtedly give inflated values. The number of non-steady partners varied considerably by city with the means ranging from a low of 18.1 for St. Louis to a high of 36.1 for San Francisco during a four-month period. The median figures ranged from 8 to 30. Bell and Weinberg (1978) reported data on number of lifetime partners: 28% of white men and 19% of Black men had had 1000 or more partners, 15% and 14% had had 500–999, and 17% and 11% had had 250–499; only 9% and 17% had had fewer than 25 sexual partners. The average ages of their respondents were 37 for whites and 27 for Blacks.

Overall, while gay men may have neither more nor less sex than their heterosexual counterparts, the evidence is abundant that it is distributed among a large number partners rather than concentrated.

Summing Up

Taking into consideration all of the versions of promiscuous behavior described above (premarital, nonmarital, extramarital, postmarital), it is apparent that a significant proportion of all sexual activity in the United States does not conform to the dominant sexual ideology held by Americans, and, indeed, that the model itself is not subscribed to in the case of some specific elements such as premarital sex.[30,31] It is impossible given the quantity and quality of available data to calculate the percentage of the totality of sexual behavior that is accounted for by promiscuity, of course, but the CDC has indicated that approximately 23 million Americans have more than one sexual partner during a given year (Moran et al. 1990). Approximately 120 million report a single partner during the year, but in any subsequent year an undetermined number of 120 million will have additional partners. Therefore, 23 million is a lower bound of the total number for whom promiscuity is a current risk factor for becoming infected with HIV—if safe sex guidelines are not being followed.

Promiscuity, then, is a fact of life, embarrassing because it conflicts with American ideals, yet undeniable. What is denied by almost everyone, regardless of the number of their sexual partners, is that he or she is promiscuous.[32] One reason so many people can have many sexual partners without considering themselves promiscuous is a simple matter of timing. As long as one is having sex with only one partner during a given timespan, one is not promiscuous. Serial "relationships", however ephemeral, negate application of the term "promiscuous" to self. Sex within a relationship is acceptable, apparently, but many of these relationships are fleeting, thereby offering promiscuity without guilt.

ANTI-PROMISCUITY IN PREVENTION CAMPAIGNS

It is this landscape of discourse on promiscuity and of sexual attitudes, values, and behavior, then, that provided the terrain for campaigns to prevent the transmission of HIV. By early 1983, scientists at a CDC-convened workshop were recommending that gay men and heterosexuals should "minimize the number of their sexual partners, and refrain from anonymous sexual contacts" (Marx 1986a:23[1983]; Curran et al. 1985). Subsequently the CDC would be forced by legislation to include only abstinence as the recommendation for gay men to reduce their risk of HIV infection (Citizens Commission on AIDS 1989).

The Message: "Love Faithfully"

From the outset of the epidemic, AIDS prevention materials showed an anti-promiscuity bent, and except for the voices of a few resisters in the gay community in the first years of the epidemic, almost no one questioned the wisdom of emphasizing promiscuity as a risk factor. "More than anything else," write Reiss and Leik (1989), "the American public has been bombarded with the message to keep the number of sexual partners to one or a very few." "The most aggressive leadership possible is necessary to promote mutually faithful sexual relationships and, where that fails, safer sex practices," wrote Potts (1988:9), and that is the direction HIV prevention has taken. In the words of two Mayo Clinic physicians: "Personal purity is the prophylaxis which we, as physicians, are especially bound to advocate. Continence may be a hard condition (to some harder than to others), but it can be borne, and it is our duty to urge this lesson upon young and old who seek our advice in matters sexual" (Vaughn and Li 1988:267 [1986]). However, reduction in number of partners was conspicuously absent from the recommendations regarding the content of educational programs proposed by the panels convened by the Institute of Medicine in 1986 to consider how to deal with the epidemic; their recommendations stressed changes in sexual practices, not number of partners (Institute of Medicine 1986).

Nonetheless, given the epidemiological findings of associations between numbers of partners and AIDS, the recommendation made by many to limit the number of partners seemed to make sense to those who designed prevention campaigns. The strategy was two-pronged, to get people to have fewer partners and to have them reduce their involvement in behaviors that were thought to be conducive to transmitting the disease; though at this point the virus had not been identified, the possibility of an infectious agent being responsible was seriously considered, and therefore what was known about the transmission of hepatitis B was transferred to the new disease. Reducing the number of partners was also good advice from the perspective of other etiological theories involving immune system overload from semen. Moreover, until condoms were proven to be impermeable to HIV, reliance on barrier protection alone seemed unwise (Goldsmith 1988[1987]), although doctors were recommending use of condoms to patients even before proof was in (Tovey 1988[1987]) because of their effectiveness in preventing the transmission of other viruses. It was not until 1986 that the first report on the effectiveness of condoms in relation to HIV was published (Conant et al. 1988[1986], a delay which was surely due in part to the preference for an anti-promiscuity prevention message.

Although there are a few exceptions, the overwhelming majority of pamphlets and posters dealing with AIDS recommend limiting the number of partners, even, it should be noted with some irony, some distributed by the association of bathhouse owners, Independent Gay Health Clubs of America (IGHC). The wording of the message has varied little over the years; examples follow:

1. "Reduce the number of sexual partners you have" (Independent Gay Health Clubs 1985);

2. "Reduce your number of sexual partners. Sex with multiple partners definitely increases your risk of disease" (AIDS Project Los Angeles 1983);

3. "Limit the number of sexual partners you have" (Gay & Lesbian Community Services Center, Los Angeles n.d.);

4. ". . . you should be careful in your selection of sexual partners. Sex with multiple partners, sex with people in high risk groups, and sex with highly promiscuous partners increases your chance of exposure" (United Way, Los Angeles n.d.);

5. "The risk of infection increases according to the number of sexual partners

one has, male or female. The more partners you have, the greater the risk of becoming infected with the AIDS virus" (Surgeon General's Report on Acquired Immune Deficiency Syndrome, U.S.P.H.S. n.d.);

6. "Don't have sex with multiple partners, or with persons who have multiple partners (including prostitutes). The more partners you have, the greater your risk" (American Red Cross 1986);

7. "Do not have sex with multiple partners, including prostitutes . . . The more partners you have, the greater your chances of catching AIDS" (U.S. Dept. of Health and Human Services 1986);

8. "Limit sex to ONE partner" (Minority AIDS Project, L.A. n.d.);

9. "Know your partner. Avoid having many sex partners and avoid sexual contact with others who do" (U.S. Public Health Service 1984).

It should be noted, moreover, that the advice to reduce the number of one's sexual partners usually is the first recommendation listed, thereby giving it primacy. It should be observed, in addition, that in most of these materials the recommendation is to "reduce the number of partners" rather than to become monogamous, a tacit recognition of the improbability that the latter message would be effective and presumably an attempt to avoid the appearance of moralizing. The same message appeared in other formats as well; for instance, public service announcements and posters often denounced causal sex (Watney 1989b).

The questions that need to be addressed are: Was this good advice then? Is this good advice now? During the early phase of the epidemic, this advice may have been correct, since by reducing the number of partners one lowered the odds of having sex with someone who was infected. (Presumably unsafe sex inasmuch as the safe sex concept was in its infancy.) Safe sex guidelines were new, not widely disseminated, and their implementation spotty. Moreover, it could be argued that it was not known how successful appeals to "play safely" would be, and therefore having fewer partners would be reasonable advice. Additionally, the evidence was not yet in with respect to the types of sexual behaviors which most efficiently transmitted the virus; we now know that most sexual behaviors other than unprotected vaginal or anal penetration rarely, if ever, are implicated in transmission. But in the early days even kissing was suspect behavior. Under those knowledge conditions, perhaps anything other than advocacy for abstinence was permissive.

In retrospect, however, it may have been unwise to complicate the message, to follow the two-pronged strategy; certainly this is true after the mid-1980s when enough was known about the behaviors most likely to transmit HIV. Having fewer partners provided no protection if one of those partners was infected. In fact, although there was uncertainty about the safe sex guidelines in some details, they have held up remarkably well over the years; indeed, most of them erred on the conservative side, except for those that said "use condoms whenever possible" instead of saying "use condoms *always* with penetrative sex." Thus, it might have been more effective from the start to say one could have sex with as many people as one wanted as long as it was safe sex. To attack both sexual practices and promiscuity may have resulted in less protection than attacking only unsafe practices alone would have. More on this below.

As the virus spread, as the number of infected increased, reduction in the

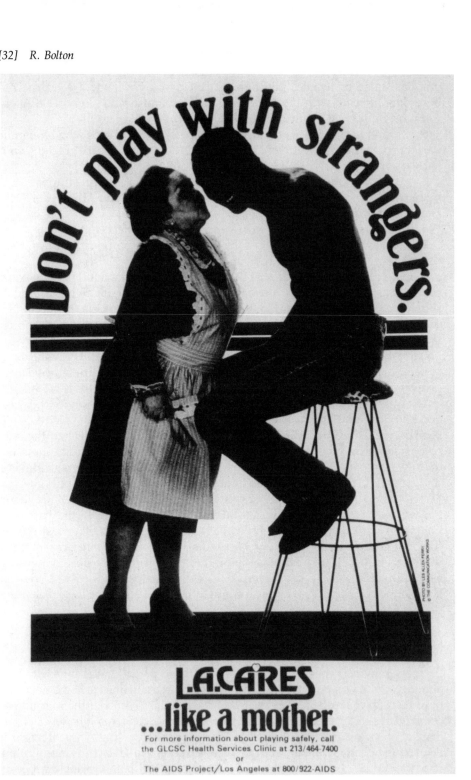

Figure 1.

AIDS

IS AN EQUAL OPPORTUNITY DISEASE!!!

TOO MANY BLACK MALES, FEMALES AND BABIES HAVE DIED FROM AIDS.

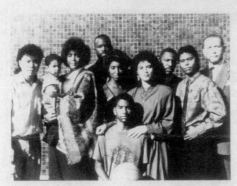

- Limit Sex to one partner
- Use Latex Condoms (rubbers) that have **Nonoxynol-9.**
- Don't exchange body fluids.
- Don't share needles
- Reduce alcohol intake and mind-altering drugs.
- Reduce stress or worry. Exercise and get plenty of rest.
- Eat well-balanced meals.

· People can be infected with the **AIDS virus and look healthy.**

AIDS can be spread sexually from men to men, from men to women, from women to men.

· Babies can be born with the virus if the mother is infected.

REMEMBER–THERE IS NO CURE FOR AIDS.
Prevention is the only way to stop this disease.

WANT TO KNOW MORE? ASK US:
Contact: MINORITY AIDS PROJECT

(213) 936-4949
IN YOUR AREA CALL:

Other Referrals
800/922-AIDS

Spanish Hotline
800/222-SIDA

Figure 2.

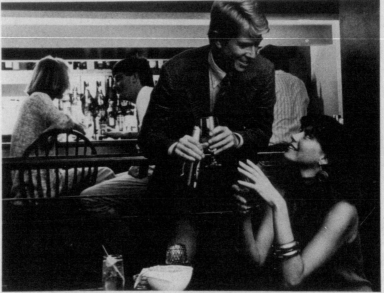

Figure 3.

The other night Charlie brought home a quart of milk, a loaf of bread and a case of AIDS.

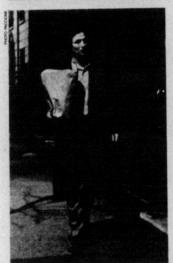

Charlie always felt his bisexual affairs were harmless enough.

But Charlie did catch the AIDS virus. That's why his family's at risk. His wife risks losing her husband, and when she has sex with him, her own life. If she becomes pregnant she can pass the AIDS virus to her baby.

Charlie could have protected himself. Saying "No" could have done it, or using a condom.

Right now there's no vaccine for AIDS, and no cure in sight. With what we know today, and with the precautions that can be taken, no

AIDS one has to come home with a story like Charlie's.

If you think you can't get it, you're dead wrong.

NEW YORK CITY DEPARTMENT OF HEALTH. FOR MORE INFORMATION CALL: 1 (718) 485-8111

Figure 4.

If You're Wondering Whether To Wait For Sex, Wait Till You Read This.

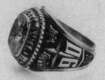

The only 100% sure protection against AIDS is no sex at all. So it's only smart to wait till you're older to have sex. And then it's safest to stay with one partner—who is also faithful to you—for a long time. And always, always use a condom.

   Don't ever share needles for drugs, ear-piercing or tattoos, either. Stay safe, and you have an excellent chance of loving longer. For more information, call the AIDS Hotline in Northern California at 1-800-367-2437, or in Southern California at 1-800-922-2437.

AIDS.
It's Up To You.
State of California AIDS Education Campaign

Figure 5.

The Faithful Have Nothing To Fear.

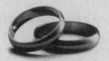

Not everyone has to worry about AIDS. You're safe if you're in a long-term sexual relationship with someone who is just as faithful to you. And if neither of you is using needles for drugs. For more facts and further reassurance, call the AIDS Hotline in Northern California at 1-800-367-2437, or in Southern California at 1-800-922-2437.

AIDS.
It's Up To You.

State of California AIDS Education Campaign

Figure 6.

number of partners made less and less sense. The odds grew that one would have sex with an infected person even as one reduced the number of one's partners. One observer in 1985 argued that the reduction concept was ill-advised *unless* the reduction was down to one exclusive partner (Handsfield 1988[1985]). He gave two examples. In Seattle, he said, approximately one-third of gay men are infected; if they reduce the number of their partners from 10 to 2 per annum, they still have a 55% risk of being infected. He does not mention what the odds were if they followed his advice that they become monogamous. In San Francisco, the same reduction, he noted, would still result in an 89% chance of exposure to the virus. Thus, reducing the number of partners did not eliminate risk unless it was accompanied by safe sex.

Resistance to limiting the number of partners was certain to arise because the sexual liberation for which gay men had fought so hard included the right to be promiscuous. Promiscuity was a key feature of gay culture as it evolved, and attempts to extirpate promiscuity could be interpreted as an attack on gay culture and gay liberation, much more so than an emphasis on eradicating risky practices could be. It is doubtful that AIDS prevention planners carefully examined the role of promiscuity in gay society. Promiscuity created community. *Communitas* was experienced in bars and baths, in the streets and in bed. The personal was political, as feminists would say. It was sex, after all, that gay men had in common; it was their sexuality that differentiated them from the larger society. Cruising was the favorite pasttime for many, and sexual adventures were conversational center-pieces. "Tricks" became friends. What made gay life exciting was the adventure, the open-ended nature of life, the possibilities that awaited each new day. "So many men, so little time" was an often heard lament. Calling for a reduction in the number of sexual partners implied a radical restructuring of all of gay social life; compared to that, advising people to put on a condom was a small detail of little overall consequence, except to save lives, of course.[33] It implied a withdrawal to hearth and home and conjured up images of heterosexual domesticity which to many gay men was anathema, the place from which they had escaped in order to create a less stiffling, more stimulating environment.

The phrase "number of partners" itself would call to mind the term "numbers" which in gay language referred to casual sex partners—and a famous gay novel, *Numbers*, by John Rechy (1967). Numbers had meaning in gay culture. As Patton (1990:47) notes: Promiscuity was always a loose concept among gay men—often as much a symbolic badge of belonging as it was a numerical concept." Sexuality provided the underpinnings of the status structure of gay society, and numbers were medals of honor; tricks were a means of counting coup. A reduction in sexual partners would certainly reduce connectedness among gay men and alter, if not destroy, the social structure of gay society. To make up for this loss, other mechanisms did arise in the 1980s. AIDS organizations, until they became bureau-cratic and heterosexualized, provided a new context for *communitas*, and there was a proliferation of other activities and organizations—sports clubs, men's choruses, and gay churches, among others, which provided opportunities for sublimation, as well as new venues for picking up a trick or lover for those who were "numerically" unreformed (Patton 1990:43). But could they replace promiscuity?

In sum, the advice to reduce the number of partners did not take into account the dominant culture of those whose behavior was being targeted for change; it catered to the ideology of the heterosexual majority and the segment of the gay community that was anti-promiscuous (e.g., the Larry Kramers), but if these people were already monogamous it made no sense to privilege their values—they would not be in need of the message, presumably. There are reasons to believe that the strategy was wrong and counterproductive, as we shall note below. Yet even today, risk-reduction materials continue to promote an anti-promiscuity line. In this discussion I have emphasized the anti-promiscuity campaign directed toward gay men, but I would like to stress that the same pattern is apparent in the campaigns directed toward other populations, heterosexual teenagers, for example, the majority of whom also adhere to an ethos which accepts the expression of their sexuality outside the institution of marriage.

Related to the anti-promiscuity, anti-casual sex advice, was the suggestion that a person "know" his partner. This, too, was and is misguided advice. It created the perception that it was safe to have sex with people one knew because they couldn't possibly be infected: only strangers posed a threat. What exactly was one to know about his partner? Given that a high percentage of individuals in major gay centers had had many partners, one was hardly to discover that they were virgins, that you were their first partner. Their health was an area one should get to know, but since the virus has a long latency period, perfectly healthy people are potentially dangerous. I am unaware of studies that show how recipients of the message "know your partner" actually interpreted this advice. Anecdotally it would seem that for many people it meant not having sex on a first date, a tactic which might slow down the spread of HIV by a week or two. What the advice also failed to consider was the fact that people do lie—about their sexual histories, about their drug habits, and about their HIV status. The results of a Roper Poll found that "91% of Americans believe that people are 'sometimes less than truthful' with their partners about their sexual histories" (Anonymous 1991:20). Another study offered even more poignant data on this point. In a large sample of college students, Cochran and Mays (1990) found that 20% of the men indicated that they would lie about HIV test results, telling a prospective partner that they had tested negative when they had not even been tested, and 47% of the men and 42% of the women would underreport to a partner the number of sexual partners they had had. In addition, 25% of the men and 10% of the women would not confess to being involved with another person, and by much larger margins they would never confess to having had a casual sex contact (Anonymous 1988). Huggins et al. (1991) report that men are most likely to tell lovers about a positive HIV test, less likely to tell a regular partner, and unlikely to tell a casual sex partner. This suggests that one must know one's partner very well before one can have confidence in one's knowledge of his or her serostatus. "Know your partner" is dangerous advice, not at all a valid substitute for safe sex precautions.

The point of this discussion is obvious. It never did matter whom one had sex with or how many people one had sex with; what mattered then and what matters now is what kind of sex one has. Ekstrand and Coates (1990) claim that unprotected anal intercourse and multiple sex partners are "the only firmly established major risk factors for seroconversion in the male-to-male relationships;" Volberding (1988:26) states that "high risk sexual practices include activity with numerous partners," and, inexplicably, some investigators still measure "risk reduction" using only number of partners as their outcome indicator. But, in fact, number of partners is *not* a major risk factor. It is a red herring. Any unprotected vaginal or anal intercourse is potentially dangerous. Clearly, the epidemiological and the moral discourse on AIDS that centered on promiscuity rendered prevention efforts less effective than they should have been, distracting attention from what should have been the message pure and simple, "play safely."

But if protection alone, safe sex, is sufficient, why was it necessary to include any mention of promiscuity? There must have operated some implicit assumptions that many of the people at risk would not adopt safe sex techniques, that the only way to reduce their risk would be to get them to lower the number of partners with whom they had unsafe sex. The fallacy of that position for gay men in places where HIV was already established is indisputable. It is a fallacy even in places where the prevalence is low (e.g., among heterosexuals in most places in the U.S.), because it is this emphasis on probabilitisic thinking rather than on safe sex that leads to the growing incidence of HIV. (For an especially egregious example of this approach in "safe sex advice" books, see Ulene 1987.) From a logical standpoint, reducing partner numbers may (it also may not, as we shall see) slow down the rate of growth, but only safe sex can stop it.

The Impact of the Anti-Promiscuity Message

Has the anti-promiscuity message had an impact on sexual behavior? Have people reduced the number of sexual partners? Have they become chaste, monogamous, faithful? Has it resulted in a sexual "counterrevolution" during the past decade? How effective has this approach been in reducing the transmission of HIV? These are crucial questions, and the answers should determine our assessment of the wisdom or folly of the moralistic, sex-negative orientation to HIV prevention that has prevailed in AIDS discourse during the 1980s.

Reduction in Number of Partners: Gay Men.   In the case of gay men, there is abundant evidence that the anti-promiscuity message coincided with a reduction in the number of sex partners. Study after study has shown that gay men became "less" promiscuous. Becker and Joseph (1988) reviewed the scientific literature (36 studies) on behavioral changes in response to AIDS. Invariably, the studies of gay men which reported on this subject noted declines in the average number of partners the subject had. Studies published since that review continue to document the decline in number of partners (e.g., Ekstrand and Coates 1990; Kuiken et al. 1990; McKirnan and Peterson 1989; Siegel et al. 1988, 1989; van Griensven et al. 1989; Bauman and Siegel 1987; Pollak and Moatti 1990).

Determining the extent of the reduction is difficult because of the differing methods used in these studies to measure the decline. In some studies, informants are merely asked whether they have reduced their number of partners, and in others, mainly longitudinal, prospective studies, they are asked to report how many partners they had during a period of one month or six months. A few examples must suffice here. Winkelstein et al. (1987b) reported a decline of 60% or more over two years (1984–1986) in San Francisco in the number of men who had had 10 or more partners during each six-month period. McKusick et al. (1985) reported a decline in the average number of partners per month from 6.3 (1982) to 4.9 (1983) to 3.9 (1984) for nonmonogamous men in their cohort (also San Francisco). During the same period there was a reduction in the number of new partners from 4.7 to 3.5 to 2.5. In New York City, Martin's (1987) respondents reported an average of 78% decline in the number of extra-domestic partners between 1980–1981 and 1984–1985, from a yearly median of 36 to a median of 8. Emmons et al. (1986) reported that 76.5% of their respondents in Chicago claimed that they had attempted to reduce the number of their sex partners since the epidemic began, and 24.4% avoided anonymous partners during the preceding month. Golubjat-nikov, Pfister, and Tillotson (1983) reported a decline in Madison, Wisconsin from 6.8 partners per month in 1982 to 3.2 in 1983. Carne et al. (1987) reported for Middlesex, England a decline in the median number of sex partners per month from 3 in 1984–1985 to 1 in 1986. Also for the UK, Burton et al. (1988[1986]) found that 48% of their respondents had decreased the number of partners from the year before, while 10% had more partners; they found 19% with no partner the previous month, 41% with 1 partner, 35% with 2–5 partners, 4% with 6–10 partners and 2% with 11–20 partners. Siegel et al. (1988) reported for New York City that 80% had reduced the number of their partners since learning about AIDS and 77% reduced the number of anonymous contacts, but they also found that the decline between 1984 and 1986–88 was modest (10%). In some studies the decline was not general but pertained only to the number of partners with whom the respondent had unprotected anal intercourse (e.g., Kuiken et al. 1990, for Amsterdam between 1984 and 1988).

Indeed, it would appear that much of the decline in metropolitan areas of the U.S. and Europe occurred before 1985–1986, i.e., before professional health educators took over prevention efforts from grass-roots groups (Patton 1990; Burton et al. 1988[1986]; Wiktor et al. 1990). Bochow (1990), for example, found no change in number of partners between 1987 and 1988 in West Germany and West Berlin (>20 partners per year: 15%, 1987; 14%, 1988; <6 partners: 52%, 1987, 53%, 1988). Doll et al. (1990b), for San Francisco, found no decline between 1983–84 and 1986–87 in the median number of partners in episodes involving unprotected sex during a 4-month period (at both times it was 1).

Further presumptive evidence of a decline in promiscuity is the fact that sex in traditional venues such as bathhouses decreased early in the epidemic, i.e., before such institutions were closed officially (Kolata 1986[1983]; McKusick et al. 1985).

One early partner reduction strategy that some gay men experimented with was especially disastrous. Many gay men before AIDS and since have sets of "fuck buddies," men with whom they are not romantically involved but with whom they have sex from time to time. They know each other fairly well sometimes and therefore may dispense with precautions. With AIDS, there was an attempt by some to turn these sets into closed circles, i.e., groups of men among whom sex would be allowed, but members would be prohibited from having sex outside the circle. Unfortunately, this meant that if one of the members was already infected, or if one of them secretly strayed and became infected, the virus spread throughout the entire group. Some of these groups were entirely wiped out by this strategy which emphasized reducing the numbers and knowing your partner rather than safe-sex techniques.

The reductions, while significant and in some investigations impressive, by no means involved the elimination of promiscuity. By most standards, one would have to say that the number of partners gay men continued to have was high enough to warrant extreme concern if safe sex were not being practiced in their encounters. One must certainly ask what the use is in reducing the number of partners from 100 to 50 per year, or from 25 to 5? (Nichols 1986).

It is interesting to note that the reductions in promiscuity indicated above were accompanied during the 1980s by an explosion of a new form of promiscuity: phone sex. If one can judge by the amount of space devoted to advertisements in gay publications, long-distance promiscuity more than compensated for proximate promiscuity—and with absolute safety. Indeed, the phone and the modem introduced limitless possibilities (constrained only by budget, time, and imagination) for interacting sexually with a multitude of partners, risk-free.

Abstinence as a Response: Gay Men.   While CDC guidelines prohibit federally funded HIV prevention programs from recommending anything other than abstinence for gay men, this option was never considered seriously by anyone close to the scene, and the evidence suggests that this alternative was not a significant response to AIDS among gay men. Most studies do not report significant increases in abstinence. Bochow (1990), for example found 4% in his sample who abstained in both 1987 and 1988. And this figure is probably close to the actual rate of abstinence in most gay communities.

Some studies have found higher rates, but in those abstinence is usually defined as no sex during the last month, and we know that for many reasons men may cycle in and out of an abstinent lifestyle of one month's duration and still not be abstinent, only temporarily inactive. That cycling has probably not been significantly impacted by the AIDS epidemic. In France, Pollak and Moatti (1990) found an increase between 1985 and 1986 from 5% to 8% in the number of men who had not had any sexual partner during the previous six months; the 8% level was then maintained through 1988. Siegel et al. (1988) found rates of 7–10% abstinence during the most recent typical month in their sample but no significant change in the rate between 1984 and 1986. Martin (1987) found no change in abstinence between recalled pre-AIDS data and 1985 data. Valdiserri et al. (1989) did find six-month abstinence rates of 7.4% to 9.1% in their samples in Pittsburgh in 1986–1987, and McKusick et al. (1985) found an increase in the percentage of men in their cohort who had not had sex the previous month (6%, 1982; 8%, 1983; 10%, 1984). There may have been a period early in the epidemic when some men became sexually incapacitated because of AIDS fear. But it is also likely that the increase in sexual inactivity reported by McKusick and associates was due to an increased frequency of AIDS-related illness episodes occurring among these men in San Francisco in that era; this interpretation is bolstered by the fact that the rate increase in abstinence occurred not only among nonmonogamous men but also among those who had a primary partner. After the HIV antibody test was available, it was found that some seropositive people go through a period of abstinence as they adjust to the knowledge of their status, but they then return again to sexual activity

(Turner 1989). Kuiken et al. (1990) report a drop of 40% in the sexual activity of seropositives during the first two years after seroconversion, an effect which disappears within two years. In other words, this was abstinence forced by circumstances not by choice; this rise in abstinence is likely to continue in communities with high seroprevalence rates as a larger proportion of the HIV-infected men become symptomatic.

Holleran (1988:119) was correct when he said, "all those who think abstinence will be practiced by the majority of people during the age of AIDS—all those who think promiscuity has ceased—are deluded." In fact, he understated the case; abstinence is practiced by a tiny minority.

Monogamy as a Response: Gay Men.   There were predictions that AIDS would force gay men to settle down into stable, sexually-exclusive monogamous relationships. To what extent has this happened? Most studies refute the prediction, showing essentially little or no change in the proportion of gay men who are in monogamous relationships. Siegel et al. (1988) found only 10% monogamous in both 1984 and 1986 in New York City, and they discovered that those who moved out of monogamy were more likely to move toward having multiple partners than in the direction of abstinence. McKusick et al. (1985) showed stability in the prevalence of monogamy from 1983 to 1984 in San Francisco (26% vs. 25%); a similar proportion is evident in Valdiserri et al.'s (1988) data for Pittsburgh where they found 25% had had sex with only a single partner during the previous six months. Bochow (1990) found no change from 1987 to 1988 in his data (24% to 22%). McKirnan and Peterson (1989) compare their 1986 data to pre-AIDS estimates of monogamy and conclude that there has been no change in monogamy (31% in 1970, 32% in 1986) nor in "stable close relationships" (presumably not sexually exclusive: 46% in 1970; 44% in 1986). Interestingly, they also reported that being in a relationship was only modestly correlated with number of sexual partners (r = −.29), suggesting that relationships themselves have little impact on promiscuity, which is consistent with the earlier discussion of the nature of gay relationships. McKirnan and Peterson (1989:166) conclude that their data "strongly indicate that, contrary to popular belief, there has been little or no change in relationship patterns among gay men due to the AIDS crisis." Emmons et al. (1986) found that 49.5% of their cohort were in a "primary relationship" in 1984–1985, but they do not indicate how many of those relationships involved sexual exclusivity. A few studies did find some increase in the number of such relationships (e.g., Joseph et al. [1987] report an increase from 17.6% at baseline in 1984–1985 to 24.6% six months later; van Griensven et al. [1989] found an increase from 5% to 15% between July 1985 and December 1986; Pollak and Moatti's [1990] data showed an increase from 10% to 25% between 1985 and 1987, but 50% at both times were not closed relationships).

Apparently gay men found it no easier or no more desirable to establish and maintain monogamous relationships after AIDS than they did before. They may also have been aware that fear of disease is neither a good nor a sufficient basis for entering into a relationship (Anonymous 1990). Love and a desire for emotional intimacy are prerequisites as much for gay relationships as for straight marriages.

Though the prevalence of monogamy among gay men did not change, something else did, namely the ideology. More lip service, at least, was given to the value of having a relationship. This was reflected in a spate of books published in the 1980s that were essentially manuals intended to promote coupledom among gay men (e.g., Marcus 1988; Isensee 1990; Berzon 1988) as well as in numerous academic works on the subject of gay relationships (e.g., De Cecco 1988; McWhirter and Mattison 1984). On this topic, behavior and ideology began to diverge and mirror the analogous inconsistency between straight behavior and ideology. Patton (1990:47) made the astute observation that "Men in long-term relationships who had always had multiple partners and who formerly projected an image of themselves as promiscuous, now talked more publicly of their long-term relationships, while often retaining the same number of partners."

In many ways, HIV had a negative impact on relationship stability and formation. Couples often experienced stresses on their relationships when antibody testing showed that one partner was negative and the other positive; and illness itself, of one or both partners, caused additional strains, sufficient to sever bonds that were not strong enough to bear additional pressure (Huggins et al. 1991). And when searching for a partner, the antibody test created a new acceptability criterion: HIV serostatus. Personal ads began to specify that the partner should be HIV− or HIV+ (presumably to match the antibody status of the advertiser). Instead of facilitating a rush to monogamy, AIDS merely created new impediments.

Changes in High-Risk Behavior.   Since the focus of this paper is on promiscuity and reductions in number of partners, I will only briefly discuss changes in prevalence of high-risk sexual behaviors. Several excellent reviews of the multitude of studies which document such changes among gay and bisexual men have been published (e.g., Turner, Miller, and Moses 1989; Stall, Coates, and Hoff 1988; Becker and Joseph 1988). Almost all studies reviewed showed significant increases in the use of condoms when engaging in anal intercourse; in some case the increases were dramatic over a short period. Burton et al. (1988[1986]) found 59% of the men in his UK sample already using condoms in 1986. Studies published after these reviews continue to find increases in safer-sex practices and declines, though sometimes less extensive, in risky practices. Doll et al. (1990b), for instance, report a decline between 1983–1984 and 1986–1987 from 17% to 2.2% of respondents who had engaged in unprotected receptive anal sex (the highest-risk behavior) during a 4-month period with nonsteady partners and from 42.2% to 12.3% with steady partners. Ekstrand and Coates (1990) document a similar decline, down from 37% to 2% for insertive anal intercourse and 34% to 4% for receptive anal intercourse (unprotected) between 1984 and 1988. Detels et al. (1989) report an increase over two years in those who always used condoms in anal intercourse from 3% to 28.5%. As important as increases in condom use, however, is the finding of many studies of an overall decrease in anal intercourse as well as a rise in the proportion of such sexual behavior which is protected (e.g., Kuiken et al. 1990; Fitzpatrick et al. 1989; Huggins et al. 1991; van Griensven et al. 1989; Valdiserri et al. 1989). The amount of change in specific practices varies by locale, and it tends to be greatest in the epicenters of the epidemic, which is hardly surprising since those locales had been "flooded with intervention programs" (Catania et al. 1989), including some sex-positive ones (see Taylor and Lourea 1992, this issue; also Gorman and Mallon 1989). Bochow (1990) points out that change is determined in part by how closely one is affected by AIDS in one's own environment.

What is quite clear in the data is that most gay men made changes in specific sexual practices more readily than they reduced the number of their partners. In other words, they maintained their sexual ethos and changed the less meaningful elements, which was the correct course to take from a prevention perspective. Bochow (1990:183) states: "An important finding of [our] first survey showed that the tendency to cling to notions of sexual freedom prevails over rigid renunciation and denial of erotic diversity—a finding that is further confirmed by the replication study."

Some Implications of the Changes in Gay Male Promiscuity. It is difficult to assess the impact that the reduction in partner numbers actually had on HIV transmission because we are rarely given the necessary information in the studies that have been done to make such an assessment. For example, we rarely are told who reduced their partners. Was it the most promiscuous or the least promiscuous (Peto 1988[1986])? In some studies the median for two time periods is provided rather than the mean since it is presumably a better measure of change, but we need to know the distributions. If the most promiscuous halved the number of their partners, the reduction might be significant, but it may be that the impact is minimal because few people have reduced their numbers while the most promiscuous still have many partners. Pollak and Moatti's (1990) data suggest that it was the most promiscuous and the least promiscuous who reduced the number of their partners: those with none or one partner went from 21% in 1985 to 35% in 1988, and those with more than 20 per six-months period went from 10% to 6%; between these extremes there was little change. How do we interpret this? It means that most people did not change much at all, that those with many partners still had many, except for some whose reduction may have been the result of having been infected early and who were now experiencing illness or dying; their infections most likely pre-dated safe-sex campaigns and they were more likely to live in major urban centers where HIV was most prevalent and opportunity structures for greater numbers of sexual contacts were available to them.

Consider another scenario related to the question of *who* made the changes, with implications for the impact of partner reduction on HIV transmission. If people reduce the number of their partners, this probably will result in being more selective with respect to those with whom they will have sex. It is very doubtful that the selection criteria themselves will change: physical beauty will still be the primary standard. Thus if numbers are reduced, the impact is most likely to be felt at the lower end of the desirability hierarchy; one may have a situation where the most handsome are still having the most partners, and the least attractive being forced to reduce. This could be called the "Gaetan Dugas Effect," i.e., the most attractive being most desired, most sexually active, and as a result most likely to be infected (if engaging in unsafe sex). If there is any tendency to engage in riskier behavior with more attractive than with less attractive partners, the stage is set for a significant increase in transmission associated with a reduction in the number of partners. With a reduction in partners, each new partner counts for more. This effect may have been mitigated to some extent by a countervailing tendency to fear the likelihood that the more handsome would be more likely to be infected, a fairly common supposition in the gay community at least during the early years of the epidemic. We need to know who is reducing and by how much to calculate the real impact of reductions in numbers, but if the most active are the ones available to those reducing, the effect of partner reduction could be just the opposite of what was intended by promoting this message.

Of course, if it was the seropositives who reduced their numbers more significantly than seronegatives, that would have a negative impact on transmission. Seropositives, recall, had higher average numbers of partners than seronegatives. Tindall et al. (1989), however, found no significant differences in the number of partners between seronegatives and seropositives who were aware of their serostatus, which may mean that they had reduced from even higher levels prior to learning their serostatus. Doll et al. (1990b) found no differences between such groups *regardless* of awareness or actual serostatus. But then this factor becomes complicated by the question of which group was more likely to employ protection during anal sex. Doll et al. (1990b) report that reductions in high-risk behaviors were independent of knowledge of HIV status, but van Griensven et al. (1989) reported that seropositives were more likely to continue the same rate of anal intercourse over time, while seronegatives and those untested had significantly decreased passive anal sex with nonsteady partners; however, the former were more likely to employ condoms in their encounters.

Evidence suggests that infectiousness is not constant for HIV-positive individuals over time, and that it may be higher during the earliest and latest phases of infection (May, Anderson, and Johnson 1988). Therefore, even if we knew whether the reduction was more pronounced among seropositives than among seronegatives, we would also need to know if the reduction was uniform for individuals at all phases of infection, which is unlikely. Indeed, it seems reasonable, given what we know already, to hypothesize that the reduction tends to be isomorphic with infectiousness (i.e., greater reductions early and late rather than during the generally long asymptomatic period of the disease).

In addition if partners are reduced, does that mean the total amount of sex is reduced? Does partner reduction mean fewer one-night stands balanced by more two-night stands? If so, how much is gained by this strategy—delaying the likely infection date by one month, six months, perhaps a year? If an individual reduced the number of his partners in a year from 25 to 5, and if 20% of the candidate pool in his locale is infected, and if he has sex 5 times with each of the 5 men in order to retain the same level of sexual activity, what has he gained? The odds are that he will have 5 risky encounters—identical to his odds if he had had sex once with each of the 25. Moreover, if knowing a person produces pressures toward relaxing vigilance, then one sees that this strategy actually augments the risk for most people.

Was there an implicit message to have less sex? Risk-reduction materials never stated this explicitly. Most studies of gay male sexual behavior related to AIDS do not report frequencies of sexual encounters, which is regretable since frequency of sexual contact is probably at least as important as number of different partners. Consider another scenario. If a man has 20 partners but has sex only once with each one, using the same prevalence rate as above, in this case he would have been exposed to an infected person 4 times. But if a man has 5 partners and has sex 10 times with each, he has been exposed 10 times. We know that transmission can occur at a single exposure, but we also know that the risk per exposure is rather low. Accordingly the man who continues to have frequent sex with a small number of partners actually has, on average, a higher exposure rate than the man who has one-fourth as many partners but who has more frequent sex. Indeed, in this case, if knowing one's partner means less likelihood of practicing safe sex, the man with fewer partners is likely to have a much higher risk than the man who continues to have many partners. In short, the total risk is distributed differently in the community, but instead of reducing risk it actually is likely to increase it. In their study McKusick et al. (1985) did find a reduction in total number of times *monogamous* men had sex with their primary partner in the preceding month (10.8, 9.7, and 8.5 times in 1982, 1983, and 1984 respectively)—fear of sex was in the air, but they do not report the actual frequencies of sexual encounters not involving primary partners. The suggested reduction could have been attributed to increasing bouts of illness associated with HIV infection. Thus, reducing number of partners without reducing frequency of sexual encounters is not beneficial: it's either monogamy with testing (and that assumes durability) or safe sex.

Finally, it is an open question whether or not the partner reductions documented above were the result of HIV prevention campaigns. Some evidence would suggest that there was little causal link. Fitzpatrick et al. (1990), McKusick et al. (1985), Valdiserri et al. (1988), Burton et al. (1988[1986]), and others have found that changes in risk behavior, condom use, and partner reduction are related to knowing someone who is seropositive or who has AIDS or to having a visual image of AIDS deterioration. Much of the change that occurred in AIDS epicenters took place before the major prevention campaigns. In areas where HIV is less prevalent, the changes in high-risk behavior patterns have been less substantial than in AIDS epicenters (St. Lawrence et al. 1989; Stall, Coates, and Hoff 1988). Bell (1991) reports that rates of high-risk sexual behavior are two to three times higher in three southern cities than in San Francisco in spite of high levels of AIDS knowledge in those cities (see also Kelly et al. 1990). Change in epicenters tended to be most dramatic before 1985 and to have levelled off since then, which is when the campaigns themselves intensified (Patton 1990). It is not inconceivable that the campaigns may have backfired, decelerating change in some places. The reasons for this suggestion are discussed below.

Heterosexual Behavior Change.   Despite predictions that AIDS spelled the end of the sexual revolution, evidence for major changes in patterns of sexual behavior among heterosexuals is scanty; media hype does not correspond to reality. There is no true counterrevolution in sexual behavior, and to the extent that there is some modification in the rhetoric of sexual freedom in recent years, the change is not due to AIDS nor to the moralistic sex-negative campaigns unleashed by the coalition between conservative politicians and religious traditionalists. Instead, any retrenchment that has taken place has been the result of dissatisfaction with some of the complications inherent in sexual freedom (Rubin 1991).

There has been much less research on changes in heterosexual behavior than on changes in gay male behavior, due largely to the existence of several large cohorts of gay men who were recruited early in the epidemic to participate in longitudinal research designed to elucidate the natural history of the disease. Among heterosexuals the research has concentrated more on attitudes than on behavior changes, although there exists an array of studies on adolescents and on condom use.

A recently-released study done in Los Angeles County found that 21% of heterosexuals claim to have reduced the number of their sex partners, 8% stopped seeing prostitutes, and 3% became abstinent; approximately half of these reductions were said to be because of AIDS (Spiegel 1991). Skurnick et al. (1991) found among high school students in New Jersey that 42% of the nonvirgins claimed to have changed their behavior in response to AIDS and 69% of these claimed they had reduced the number of their partners while 64% said they had become monogamous. Of those who formerly were sexually active, 18% claimed to have become abstinent. Another study of teenagers found that 15% had changed sexual behaviors because of AIDS, and of these 10% abstained and 35% were more selective of partners (Strunin and Hingson 1987).

Baldwin, Whiteley, and Baldwin (1990) found that college students did not change the number of their sexual partners following a course in which they received information on AIDS; for vaginal intercourse the average remained approximately 1.5 partners during a 3-month period. This conclusion that college students are not modifying their behavior is echoed by De Buono et al. (1990) who found little change in sexual practices.

Hingson et al. (1990) found that condoms were used least consistently by adolescents with more than 10 partners, but in general condom use was positively associated with number of partners; the percentages of those who used condoms at least some of the time was as follows: 55%, 1 partner; 71%, 2–4 partners; 78%, 5–9 partners; and 92%, 10 or more partners. Thus there appears to be a positive correlation between condom use and promiscuity (cf. Biglan et al. 1990). Freudenberg (1990:592) has concluded that young adult heterosexuals have made the least changes of any group and that "very few adolescents, whether high-school students, dropouts, or college students, are protecting themselves against HIV." He notes further that when they do use condoms they generally stop doing so when they enter a relationship.

In the Netherlands, de Vroome et al. (1990) found a greater increase in monogamy and having fewer partners than in condom use among heterosexuals, but still condom use was higher in percentage than having fewer partners or becoming monogamous as a response to AIDS: 54.2%, 5.9%, and 35.8%, respectively. Only 17.1% of their respondents said that they had made changes in their behavior (total sample); among adolescents the figures were 69.2%, 5.6% and 24.3%, with 24.2% of adolescents claiming to have made some change in behavior due to AIDS. In addition they found that those with casual partners were much more likely to indicate that they intended to use condoms in the future: those with steady partners: 50.3% probably not, 33.2% probably yes; those with casual partners: 14.5% probably not, 78.9% probably yes. Asked whether they had used condoms in the past 6 months, 69.5% of the total sample said "never," whereas of those who engaged in casual sex, only 17.3% never used them. In the Los Angeles study cited above, 16% said they were using condoms more often now than they did before AIDS.

The weight of the evidence for heterosexuals is that the impact of AIDS on number of partners and on safe-sex practices has been weak at best. "The specter of AIDS has not stopped teens from engaging in unprotected sexual intercourse," according to Miller, Turner, and Moses (1990:182). In view of the fact that sex-positive campaigns have been less prevalent among heterosexuals, that the cam-paigns have been fear-based, that abstinence has been the dominant message to teenagers, and that condoms alone have been stressed as the answer for adult heterosexuals, this relative lack of change in behavior should not be surprising. These factors plus the distance that has existed between most heterosexuals and experience with AIDS in their immediate environment may account for the modest changes made in this population.

Misinterpreting the Promiscuity Message.   The emphasis on promiscuity during the first decade of AIDS gave rise to a series of misinterpretations that had a negative impact on the primary mechanism by which transmission of HIV could be prevented, i.e., unsafe sex. One woman, for example, is reported to have denied having multiple partners because, as she said, "I only have sex with one person at a time" (Citizens Commission on AIDS 1989:29). She was not alone in misinterpret-ing the meaning of "multiple partners." Or take the case of the fourteen-year-old girl who responded to the question of whether or not she was "sexually active" as follows: "No, I just lie there" (p. 29). "Casual sex" is another term easily misin-terpreted; for most people sex is not "casual" no matter how many partners they have—it involves emotions and seriousness, not casualness.

Perhaps worse than these mistakes in comprehension of the language of promis-cuity researchers was the fact that an emphasis on promiscuity allowed individuals to compare themselves with the extremely promiscuous and decide they them-selves were not promiscuous because they did not have hundreds of partners annually as did those with AIDS and, therefore, they were not at risk. This gave most people, both gay and straight, the illusion of relative invulnerability (Fisher and Misovich 1990). Only the outliers on a promiscuity scale were seen as people at risk; this permitted people to continue unsafe sex. If risk perception is a significant determinant of whether people will make changes, this stress on not having multiple partners works against risk-reduction messages (O'Brien 1989). Percep-tion of self as promiscuous may result in loss of self-esteem and so there will be a tendency not to identify self with this trait, and that will have a major impact on risk assessment (Weinstein 1984).

Additional Observations.   Did the public believe that the official policy or chastity and monogamy would provide the solution to the AIDS crisis? Apparently not. The results of a National Roper Poll indicated that only "15% believe unmarried adults abstaining from sexual contact is likely to happen as a way to fight HIV/AIDS" and only 26% feel that monogamy is likely to happen (Anonymous 1991:20). In contrast, 81% agreed that explicit sexual material is likely to be needed to educate teenagers about the risks of HIV/AIDS. Evidently, the American public by a wide margin did not believe in the efficacy of the erotophobic agenda emanating from Washington and permeating most HIV-prevention programs.

Hyperbole is characteristic of the biomedical establishment in relation to AIDS; repeated like a mantra, we hear, "we have learned more about this disease in a shorter time than about any other disease in history." And we all recall the prediction made in 1984 by Margaret Heckler, Secretary of Health and Human Services, that there would be an "AIDS vaccine" ready for testing in two years. But hyperbole is evident also in the behavioral realm. Curran claimed that the changes in gay men's sexual behavior was "the most dramatic sexual revolution since the

1960s" (Helquist 1986:65). Ekstrand and Coates (1990:975) state that "these changes may represent the most profound behavior changes ever observed in the literature on health behavior change." This is repeated by the Citizens Commission on AIDS (1989:22): "In what is perhaps the most dramatic health behavior change in recent history, gay men have adopted 'safer sex' practices, with a resulting sharp decrease in the incidence of new infections." And Becker and Joseph (1988:407) state that "this may be the most rapid and profound response to a health threat which has ever been documented."

While I do not wish to detract from the credit that gay men deserve for the responsible changes that have been made and in which they can take pride (the changes are impressive and go beyond what anyone could have anticipated *a priori*), this claim must be tempered if it is not to become a dangerous invitation to complacency and neglect. The bottom line is that 10 years into the epidemic heterosexuals have changed their behavior very little, and among gay men perhaps as many as 50% to 70% or more are still placing themselves at risk because of incomplete adherence to safe-sex guidelines (Siegel et al. 1989). Martin (1986) found that for 40% of the men he studied, the changes did not include absolute elimination of sexual behaviors deemed risky—"risk reduction has tended to occur more in terms of gradations, not absolutes." He notes that intensive change by the few is not occurring but that many men are adopting some measures and not others, i.e., reducing number of partners, reducing extra-domestic sex, or reducing involvement in high-risk behaviors, the smorgasbord approach. What this means is that for those who took all but the last-mentioned course, the change was not very helpful. Change in numbers of partners without reduction in high-risk behavior at best buys a little time; this is not the solution to halting HIV transmission. Thanks to the advice of health experts, e.g., Curran and others at the CDC, they were given a menu and they made the wrong changes. Patton (1990:47) sums it up well: "What was actually achieved by the shift to an emphasis on reducing the number of partners was not so much behavior change, as a change in the mythology of promiscuity." Serious risk reduction was not a byproduct of this approach.

THE REAL RISKS OF PROMISCUITY IN THE AIDS ERA

Quite clearly, the level of risk of contracting HIV infection and of developing AIDS from promiscuous sexual behavior, from having many sexual partners, is dependent on a number of factors which I wish to discuss next (Anderson and May 1988[1987]). The most salient of these are: 1) the stage of the epidemic in the locale involved, and 2) the type of sexual practices engaged in. Although one must be somewhat skeptical of the accuracy of the data used in the analysis, instructive calculations concerning the probability of becoming infected under different circumstances have been made. These calculations of the odds of becoming infected with HIV from single or multiple sexual contacts, homosexual or heterosexual, do not take into consideration all of the relevant variables, and we need to go beyond condom use or non-use in our assessment of risks. May, Anderson, and Blower (1990) raise the important question of whether 10 acts of unprotected intercourse with one person is more or less likely to transmit the virus than 10 acts with 10 different partners. If indeed the acts involving promiscuity are more likely to lead to transmission, this would be a strong argument against having multiple partners *for unprotected sex*. Unfortunately, adequate evidence on this point is lacking, and the question is moot since safe sex must be recommended for all sexual contact except when reproduction is intended.

Theoretically at least, the person who follows safe-sex guidelines should be at low risk for contracting HIV. He, therefore, could have as many partners as he wanted without danger.[34] But there are some problems he faces with promiscuity that he does not face by being involved with a single partner and vice versa. With a steady partner the problem of negotiating the meaning of safe sex—what is risky and what isn't—is minimal, the solution becomes routinized. However, with each new partner the individual must "negotiate" explicitly or implicitly the limits of the action. For gay men this may have been less problematic than it is for straights, since many gay men were long accustomed to expressing their sexual interests to potential partners in advance. Selection from a behavioral repertoire rather than a predetermined focus on one kind of behavior (i.e., vaginal intercourse) was the norm, and sexual desires were visibly expressed in the dress codes, wearing hankies of a certain color and keys in a certain position. With AIDS, new codes were developed: the safety pin and black-and-white checkered handkerchiefs. The question, "What do you do?," between two gay men meeting in a bar, meant "in bed" not as a line of work.

Still, the negotiations before and during sex can be tricky. For example, it is possible to talk about what is acceptable and unacceptable sexual behavior in advance of sexual activity; in this case the risks are minimized. In many cases, though, partners may place trust in more subtle interactions, giving nonverbal cues as sex proceeds, and in this case the dangers become more salient. For example, a person may consider analingus to be too high risk and yet find himself in a situation in which his new partner has begun to perform analingus. Their assessments of what is and what is not safe may not coincide. The first person then must quickly maneuver himself out of position for analingus to continue or state that he does not want to engage in this behavior; either action carries the attendant risk of interrupting the flow of "erotic reality" with the intrusion of the mundane and anxiety-provoking "everyday reality" of AIDS (Davis 1983). Each encounter will be different, posing a new set of possibilities and potential risks.

It is important to note that these problems are minimized in a community in which safe-sex norms have been more or less standardized and institutionalized; they are exacerbated in places where the epidemic is just beginning and new community norms have not solidified, where most people have not had time to internalize the new behavioral standards regarding safety in sexual interactions; subsequently we may find that they will intensify again as the epidemic wanes and vigilance relaxes.

Thus, for the HIV-negative individual, promiscuity involving low risk behaviors is a viable option posing minimal risk in areas where safe-sex guidelines can be consistently followed. But an individual's commitment to the guidelines can be overridden under certain circumstances, too. For example, if the new partner is especially attractive, indeed if it is someone he might like to snare as a permanent partner, he may go beyond his normal safety limits; he is less likely to be able or to want to control the forms of behavior he engages in. He may not normally engage in receptive anal intercourse, for instance, but to please this special partner, he may relax that standard and take his chances. Though research on this point is scant, what one does in bed with a partner surely depends in part on one's appreciation of the qualities of the partner. One may French kiss with some partners and not others, perform fellatio on some partners but only receive fellatio from others, and so forth. Which behaviors one performs are influenced by the context (person, place).

If the search for anonymous or new partners leads to engaging in behaviors that enhance risk-taking, then having multiple partners could become risky. For example, it has been widely claimed that alcohol and drugs increase risk-taking; if seeking partners is likely to increase alcohol or drug use because one looks for partners in bars, then clearly there is a problem. Bolton et al. (1992, this issue) have reviewed the research and criticized the conventional wisdom on this topic, but if indeed there are any concomitants of promiscuity which do increase risk-taking, then being promiscuous could be dangerous. (At this point I am not aware of the existence of such concomitants for which there is convincing evidence, with the possible exception of recreational drugs [Siegel et al. 1989], and even in this case it is not clear that the association is not spurious, i.e., both behaviors caused by an underlying common third factors such as a risk-taking pre-disposition.)

The individual's personality may significantly affect the extent to which he can successfully cope with the process of negotiations associated with having multiple sexual partners. It is reasonable to assume that an individual who has high self-esteem, a high sense of control or personal efficacy, a moderate level of AIDS fear, may be better situated to stick to safe-sex guidelines when faced with demands for unsafe behaviors or desires to engage in same (Siegal et al. 1989). McKusick et al. (1990), for example, found that less personal efficacy was characteristic of those who in 1984 practiced unprotected anal intercourse, and Brendstrup and Schmidt (1990) have proposed, on the basis of qualitative data, the hypothesis that unsatisfactorily treated traumatic events may impede a person's ability to adopt safe sex. Emmons et al. (1986) found that few men in their study perceived difficulties with sexual impulse control, and impulse control was associated only with avoidance of anonymous sex (i.e., inability to control having anonymous sex); importantly, it was not associated with inability to avoid receptive anal intercourse. What this suggests is that men may have a better capacity to avoid risky behaviors than to avoid anonymous sex, which is consistent with the findings that changing specific practices was a more popular strategy for most men than reducing partners or becoming monogamous.

Recent research shows that age is an important predictor of high-risk behavior. Hays, Kegeles, and Coates 1990 found younger men more likely to engage in risky sex. Reasons for this are unclear and probably multiple, but it is possible that younger gay men have poorer communication skills and less experience in negotiating safe sex and therefore are more likely to place themselves at risk in sexual encounters. However, Siegel et al. (1989) found a positive association between risk-taking and the number of years the subject had been engaging in sex with other males, which would seem inconsistent with the experience hypothesis. The interactions of age, length of sexual career, and risk-taking remain to be clarified.

The argument against bathhouses was that they promoted multiple unsafe sex acts because of the setup which permitted them to occur (Siegel and Siegel 1983). But analogues have been invented in the gay community in response to AIDS which are as highly eroticized environments as bathhouses, but restricted to safe sex. I refer to the international phenomenon of JO Clubs, established in major cities in North America and Europe, where parties in which dozens or even hundreds of men (and in the case of Jack-and-Jill-Off Parties, both men and women, gay and straight) may spend hours having sex with many partners in a public setting, but with action restricted to mutual masturbation or S/M. "Body fluids" are not exchanged, there is no oral or anal sex, but sexual activity is intense. Such encounters, occurring with monitoring (generally not required) by those in charge to prevent violations of the rules, are quite safe despite the high level of promiscuity (see Taylor and Lourea 1991, this issue).

Promiscuity poses other dangers for the person who is HIV-positive (Nichols 1986:4). If he fails to follow safe-sex guidelines, of course, there is a chance for re-infection, as well as a danger to his partner. Furthermore, as noted earlier, semen may have a detrimental effect on the immune system and therefore exposure to semen could lead to a more rapid decline in immune system functioning (Connor and Kingman 1989). Since the virus mutates rapidly and has many forms, a re-infection could involve a more lethal form of the virus; there is also the possibility of some sort of synergistic effect of multiple re-infections with different variants of the virus. Complying with safe-sex guidelines makes the risk minimal. Safe-sex guidelines also protect the HIV-positive individual with depleted T-4 cells from other venereal infections which are detrimental to him, since progression to full-blown AIDS may be related to subsequent infections due to various pathogens; the findings on this issue, however, are mixed (Hessol et al. 1989; Coates et al. 1990). But safe-sex guidelines do not protect the HIV-positive person from the danger of infection from airborne pathogens. And these dangers may be serious. He may be exposed to flu, colds, and so forth by intimate contact with someone who is contagious. Thus, someone who is HIV-positive may find that promiscuity involves unacceptably high risks for his health, as does associating with people in crowds or gatherings when contagious diseases are widespread, e.g., the flu season. Promiscuous phone sex remains the only completely healthy alternative form of promiscuity for the HIV-positive individual.

The Dangers of Abstinence and Monogamy

Abstinence and monogamy have been promoted as the only safe solutions to the risks of HIV infection. But each of these options carries significant risks as well, and for some individuals the risks of these options may indeed prove more serious than the risks attendant on promiscuity, contrary to the common sense expectations about relative risk. The abstinence solution may work well for individuals with a low sex drive or with rigidly determined patterns of sexual behavior involving high risk. In risk-reduction group sessions it is not rare to hear individuals state that if they cannot engage in their favorite activity, then sex is not worth doing for them, and they prefer to abstain. Such attitudes would seem to be more common among older individuals. They may also be a temporary phenomenon that occurs during the phase of mourning that many men go through as they deal with the loss of a part of their life that was meaningful but which is no longer a viable option since AIDS. Though some may choose abstinence (we've seen that not many actually do), for most the thought of a life (or at least a period of time until a vaccine or cure is available—and that may be for the lifetime of most current adults) with no sex is not a pleasant one. After all, not many people in Western culture, or any culture for that matter, would appear to find life without sex fulfilling, witness the declining numbers of celibate clergy.

For those unsuited to abstinence, the dangers of making this choice are serious. An individual may make a commitment to abstinence, but eventually the desire for sex may become overwhelming; in such instances, the individual may then break the commitment, doing so with a vengeance. Not schooled in safe sex, releasing pent up desire, he may be more willing than others at that point to throw caution to the winds and engage in very high-risk behavior. The process is analogous to binging patterns seen in alcoholics, who may abstain for a long period and then burst loose, with disastrous consequences. A propos the alcoholism analogy, models of HIV prevention that give credence to "loss of control" as a factor in risk behavior (such as while "under the influence of alcohol or drugs"), do not advocate abstinence, but if loss of control over one's sexual actions does take place, it is more likely to do so among those who have been unable to maintain the commitment to abstinence. As Reiss (1991:5) observes, "vows of abstinence break more easily than do condoms."

Monogamy, too, has its special problems, for both gays and straights, perhaps even more for the latter. The most serious of these is that couples are extremely likely to dispense with safe-sex procedures in their relations with one another (Goldsmith 1988[1987]). Consistent with this also is the finding by Hunt et al. (1990) that most unsafe sex takes place within relationships and that those with regular partners are *more* likely to test positive than those without. It is extremely unlikely, indeed, that most couples will maintain safe-sex practices even though they may employ them at the outset of the relationship. Once they have committed to each other they will generally relax their standards and revert to the Old Sexuality, feeling safe in their monogamous haven. There is a myth that love provides protection. Witness the fact that "most women who become infected with HIV heterosexually become infected by a partner with whom they have had a long-term involvement" (Reiss 1991:6). The evidence against the myth is overwhelming, and almost every study supports this claim. Only a few examples are discussed here. Vincke et al. (1991) found that gay men in monogamous relationships were more likely to engage in unprotected anal intercourse than men without such relationships. Hays, Kegeles, and Coates (1990) report that young men in monogamous relationships tend to dispense with safe sex. van Griensven et al. (1989) found no change over time in the proportion of anal sex engaged in by men with steady partners; unless they were HIV-concordant this was risky even if they did use condoms. Fitzpatrick et al. (1989) report that 16.2% of their informants had passive anal sex without a condom with regular partners but only 5.2% had anal sex without a condom with non-regular partners; for insertive anal sex the figures were 16.2% and 2.6%. These same investigators (Fitzpatrick et al. 1990) found that noncondom use was associated with having fewer sexual partners and with a closed monogamous relationship. Doll et al. (1990b) found that the decline in unprotected receptive anal sex with steady partners between 1983–1984 and 1986–1987 was from 42.2% to 12.3% and with non-steady partners from 17% to 2.2%. Research on prostitutes almost invariably finds the prostitutes may have protected sex with clients but they tend not to do so with lovers or partners (Pleak and Meyer-Bahlburg 1990), and this applies to both male and female prostitutes. Similar results are reported by McKusick et al. (1991), Rietmeijer et al. (1989), Bochow (1990), Lifson et al. (1990), and Valdiserri et al. (1988). It appears that men with steady partners are from 3–5 times more likely to have unprotected anal intercourse with steady partners than with nonsteady ones. In short, people who enter relationships tend to give up safe sex, thereby eliminating their protection. Writings as early as 1983 recognized the folly in recommending monogamy as a strategy for gay men in dealing with AIDS (Siegel and Siegel 1983). But the same applies to heterosexuals.

Under certain strict conditions monogamy may be safe, i.e., if both partners have been tested several times over a period of six to twelve months (preferably the latter inasmuch as a significant proportion of individuals do not seroconvert within six months of having been infected) and both are free of HIV antibodies, or better yet, free of virus as determined by a viral culture or antigen test, if neither one uses intravenous drugs, and if they are totally faithful to each other (or use very safe sex practices with other partners). These are big "ifs", of course, and they do not take into consideration the considerable "cheating" that does go on even in committed marital relationships in American culture, as noted above. If they are not engaging in safe sex within the relationship, too, one wonders whether they will be adept at playing safely in any extra-relationship encounters they might have. A repeated finding is that for men who engage in unprotected intercourse this is their favorite activity; will they then forego this activity if they have sex outside the relationship and have not been able to give it up with their regular partner?

Furthermore, it should be noted that for some the continuation of a relationship, either gay or straight, may depend to some extent on the availability of an option for some extra-relationship sexual encounters. Certainly research on gay relationships suggests that less possessive, less exclusive relationships have greater durability than those in which there is an insistence on absolute fidelity (Kurdek and Schmitt 1988; McWhirter and Mattison 1984). Ironically, then, promoting fidelity may undermine the goal of those who argue for a strategy of risk reduction based on the reduction in the number of partners and the formation of long-term bonds. Infidelity contributes to the persistence of gay relationships.

Thus, we see that abstinence, monogamy, and promiscuity all have their risks; the risks differ but no option is risk-free. Promiscuity, in some senses, offers the least risk, providing the individual who chooses this option is capable of maintaining a commitment to safe-sex procedures. The person who chooses promiscuity may continue to enjoy the pleasures of casual sex, to retain his individual freedom, to experience the thrill of the chase, if he relinquishes consistently certain unsafe sexual practices, i.e. unprotected penetrative sex. The person who chooses abstinence, if he is able to maintain a commitment to no interpersonal sex, can reduce his risk to practically zero, but at a loss of the experience of intimacy and physical pleasure. The person who chooses monogamy may guarantee his own safety by always practicing safe sex even within the relationship, and he may gain a deeper sense of connection to another person (Froman 1990), though that is by no means guaranteed as the large number of miserable marriages attest. There are trade-offs in choosing one option over another, but the idea that what one gains by choosing monogamy or abstinence over promiscuity is protection from HIV infection is an illusion, and a very perilous illusion at that.

Partner Reduction Versus Safe Sex

Most cases of the sexual transmission of HIV have been due to unprotected vaginal or anal intercourse. A handful of cases due to oral sex have been documented in the literature, and anecdotal evidence exists for a smattering of transmission by other forms of sexual behavior. If prevention education had concentrated from the beginning on informing people of the dangers of these high-risk behaviors without adulterating their message with recommendations to reduce the number of partners or become monogamous, there is no doubt that more relevant behavioral change would have occurred, and we would not now be faced with the situation in which a significant proportion of gay men and straights are not adhering strictly to safe-sex guidelines, but have opted for a reduction in partners instead.

The message to reduce the number of partners conflicted with the safe-sex message by implying that there is "an *alternative* to Safer Sex" (Watney 1989b:32). By sanctioning various options, the message encouraged people to choose an unsafe method which allowed them to believe that they had lowered their risk and to claim that they had made significant changes in response to AIDS. Martin (1986) noted that the most frequent option chosen by the men in his study was the elimination of sex in extra-domestic sites, which was a clear response to the anti-bathhouse campaign, about which there is general agreement that the symbolism of the campaign was more significant than the impact on transmission. The advice to abstain or become monogamous was ignored by the majority of gay men (Shernoff and Bloom 1991), and this was fortunate because that advice was not mere empty symbolism. Instead, it was the cause of death for many who chose to follow it and who in doing so dispensed with safe-sex precautions. Reduction in partners had the same fatal outcome for many. The data are available in the literature to permit a sophisticated mathematical modeler to estimate the net loss of life that has occurred as an unintended consequence of the dual-pronged strategy that was adopted and which continues in force today in most prevention programs. It is important to understand that not a single life was lost as a result of promiscuity, but many were lost because of anti-promiscuity propaganda. This was an avoidable tragedy.

That safe sex and reduction in partners became conflated is nicely illustrated in a study by de Vroome et al. (1990). They asked informants what "safe sex" meant. They found that 69% thought that safe sex meant using condoms, 30.5% thought it meant reducing the number of partners, and only 5.2% thought it referred to using safe-sex techniques. Ambiguity and lack of focus of prevention messages have been recognized as major obstacles to promoting change (Citizens Commission on AIDS 1989; Stall et al. 1990b). The argument that the emphasis should have remained on safe sex alone is further supported by the work of Leviton et al. (1990) who found that prevention interventions changed attitudes on numerous variables related to safe sex, but produced no change in attitudes toward having sex with many partners, nor on sex with strangers. Also, Emmons et al. (1986) found that people can more readily control their risky behavior than they could limit having encounters with multiple partners. Likewise, Kelly et al. (1989) found no difference between an experimental group and a control group in number of sexual partners following intervention, but they did find differences in frequency of unprotected anal intercourse and use of condoms when intercourse did occur. And, in fact, the control group had greater partner reduction than the intervention group, which suggests that efforts to promote partner reductions may have the opposite effect of the one intended. It certainly demonstrates that safe-sex techniques and partner reduction are viewed as alternatives rather than mutually supportive risk-reduction strategies.

The conflation of safe sex and condoms is also problematic. Condoms do break at times, and more often they are not properly used (Helquist 1986:63). And an emphasis on condoms sends a message that penetrative sex should be part of one's sexual repertoire when, in fact, it is best avoided (Patton 1990). Martin, Garcia, and Beatrice (1989:501) found that while cessation of anal intercourse was associated with HIV-antibody status, "reducing the number of sexual contacts, becoming monogamous, or eliminating other forms of sexual contact were not related to risk of HIV."

From at least the mid-1980s there was some recognition that recommending a reduction in number of partners was problematic (De Gruttola, Mayer, and Bennett 1988[1986]; De Gruttola and Bennet 1988). Attention to the issue is beginning to surface now in the HIV-prevention literature, and an understanding is growing that recommending monogamy or a reduction in partners is a failed strategy and that it has detracted from safe-sex promotion. Coyle, Boruch, and Turner (1991), in discussing how to evaluate prevention programs, point out that information on monogamy and promiscuity is not as useful as direct measures of the basic risk behaviors, nonetheless, they still include monogamy and avoidance of anonymous sex and promiscuity as indicators of a reduction of risk behaviors (which we have seen is fallacious). Stall et al. (1990b:99) state: "some have argued that it is more effective to seek a reduction in the number or type of sexual partners, while others content that campaigns should seek to encourage safe sex without regard to number of kind of sexual partners." Valdiserri (1989:9) says, "Risk reduction for homosexual men lies primarily in avoiding behaviors that are the most dangerous in terms of HIV infection (that is, receptive anal intercourse without condoms), rather than in emphasizing 'promiscuity' as a risk factor." He adds that the recommendation to reduce partner numbers, while not technically incorrect, "probably misrepresents the benefit of reducing the number of partners in many homosexual communities where the prevalence of infection is already extraordinarily high" (see also Valdierri et al. 1987:201). Martin, already in 1986, argued that it is necessary to stress safe sex rather than partner reduction, but he added that monogamy was still to be advised for heterosexuals because the prevalence of HIV was low among them. These statements seem to imply that the partner reduction strategy is still valid where the HIV prevalence is not high yet. If that is the case, they are dangerously misleading. Such advice is not valid; to follow it will be to make the same mistake in other populations, e.g., among heterosexual adolescents, that was made in the case of gay men. Debates over the issue of the content of prevention messages for adolescents are going on (Wagman and Ludlow 1988), but it remains an open question whether or not those who design campaigns for adolescents and adult heterosexuals will learn from rather than repeat the mistakes that were made in attempting to stop HIV transmission among gay men. As Goldsmith (1988[1987]) argues, the goal must be absolute adherence to safe-sex guidelines by all sexually active people.

The most elegant demonstration of the superiority of stressing safe sex and eliminating partner reduction messages is provided by Reiss and Leik (1989) who developed a mathematical model to test the relative effectiveness of partner-reduction versus condom-use strategies for preventing HIV transmission. The variables included in their model were HIV prevalence, infectivity, number of sexual acts, condom effectiveness, and number of partners. They found that the increase in risk of having multiple partners occurs primarily at low numbers, but more importantly they found that under almost all conditions "consistent and careful use of condoms is a far more effective method of reducing the risk of HIV infection" than is a reduction in the number of partners (p. 411). While acknowledging that the safest alternative is to adopt both condoms and fewer partners, they note that this is unlikely to happen. They state: "We believe that it is time to stop giving voice to restrictive sexual attitudes about multiple partners and start protecting young people by giving them a more realistic view of the risks they are taking, and how those risks can be better managed" (p. 433).

Patton (1990:42) has pointed out that "The first safe sex advice was put into circulation by gay men, and was constructed in opposition to the insulting dictates of doctors." Community activists, who knew their community, prove to have been right about how to stop HIV transmission, whereas the moralists and the medical establishment were wrong; their error has been costly. By continuing to recommend a reduction in partners, this error is being compounded. *The only sane course is to eliminate completely all anti-promiscuity messages from all HIV-prevention programs.*

CONCLUSIONS

The goal of this paper has been to examine the concept of promiscuity in the context of the AIDS epidemic, to demonstrate the complexity of the issues surrounding the use of this concept in AIDS discourse, and to suggest that focussing attention on promiscuity in a completely negative light, as has been done throughout the epidemic, is misguided at best and downright dangerous at worst.[36]

Instead of providing a realistic appraisal of the problems, attacks on promiscuity have been orchestrated by sex-negative forces in American culture intent on turning back the clock, by counter-revolutionaries whose agenda is to eliminate the sexual freedoms won through constant struggle over the past two or three decades. "Morality" masquerading as science is more insidious and pernicious than the overt opposition by cultural conservatives to sex-positive approaches to HIV prevention.

To control the discourse on promiscuity is to control the direction that American society takes as it chooses in the coming years between a return to a sex-negative culture and the invention of a New Sexuality that is sex-positive, creative, experimental and liberated, between the myths of monogamy and chastity and the potentials for pleasure. In a brilliant article entitled "How to Have Promiscuity in an Epidemic," Douglas Crimp (1988:253), taking a gay male perspective, wrote the following:

We were able to invent safe sex because we have always known that sex is not, in an epidemic or not, limited to penetrative sex. Our promiscuity taught us many things, not only about the pleasures of sex, but about the great multiplicity of those pleasures. . . . Gay male promiscuity should be seen . . . as a positive model of how sexual pleasures might be pursued by and granted to everyone if those pleasures were not confined within the narrow limits of institutionalized sexuality . . . Indeed it is the lack of promiscuity and its lesson that suggests that many straight people will have a much harder time learning 'how to have sex in an epidemic' than we did . . . it is our promiscuity that will save us.

Holleran (1988:118) said it this way: "Promiscuity gives us something we can acquire no other way: the wisdom of prostitutes."

Unfortunately, AIDS prevention became a hostage in the 1980s in the cultural war between those who sought to return American culture to that of the 1950s and those who sought to preserve the changes wrought by the sexual revolution, feminism, gay liberation, and the civil rights movement, between those who sought to reconstruct a hegemonic mythical paradise in which sex occurred only within marriage, and those who sought to recognize and protect sexual pluralism, choice, and privacy rights, between an erotophobic ideology and behavioral realities (Reiss 1991; Watney 1989b). While conservatives were not reluctant to wield promiscuity and AIDS as weapons in this struggle, liberals, having no neutral term to use, evaded discussion. Failure to confront the issue squarely, has abetted the moralists, to the detriment of AIDS-prevention efforts.

A major mistake that has been made during the first decade of the epidemic has been to rely on inappropriate models in designing HIV-prevention strategies and to accept irrelevant concepts uncritically. These misleading models include the moralistic model, the epidemiologic model, the addiction model, and the health behavior model.

There is evidence everywhere of the intrusion of the moralistic model of AIDS on the design and implementation of HIV-prevention programs (Jakobowits 1988[1986]; Osborn 1988[1987]; Taylor 1990). It is the moralistic model that opposes needle exchange programs, which have a proven track record in reducing HIV transmission among drug users in areas where they have been tried (Singer, Irizarry, and Schensul 1991). Its influence is obvious in the opposition to condom promotion and distribution programs and to sex-positive, safe-sex campaigns. Moralistic considerations are more subtle yet present in educational messages which inadvisedly emphasize alcohol consumption as a cofactor in risky sex (Bolton et al., this issue). Violating the principle that health educators should "not place the value system of the educator above the value system of the client" (Valdiserri 1989:97), many AIDS educators apparently chose to clash head-on with the gay sexual ideology and the behavioral realities of both gays and straights, and even to some extent the dominant sexual values in American culture; in essence, they accepted the morality of a small but powerful and vocal segment of American society. Goldstein (1989:82) has said that "Most of us are rationalists in the streets and moralists in the sheets." But rationality is not a prime characteristic of AIDS discourse, and suspicion arises that acquiescence to the purveyors of a moralistic approach to HIV prevention by AIDS scientists and educators betrays either a "closet moralism" or greed (to call a spade a spade), i.e., allowing their research and prevention agendas to be set by bureaucrats and politicians rather than by the needs of the populations their work should have served. Patton (1990:43) is perhaps being diplomatic when she says: "Under increasing pressure for standardized, clonable, and statistically evaluable short-range projects, even gay health educators became reluctant to take social risks in order to promote sexual safety." But she also notes elsewhere (1989:118–119) that most health education professionals seem to be trained in the "scared straight" style of prevention, and adds that the changes gay men made in their behavior toward safer sex were the product of community activism that antedated the results of prevention research and the sex-negative agenda implicit in the approaches developed by health professionals, whose actions would "displace the authority for understanding and encouraging safe sex standards from those who engage in sex, onto medical experts."

Among the lessons which this analysis underscores is that models based on epidemiological "facts" are also flawed when imported directly into prevention. We have learned this with other concepts during the epidemic, too. "Risk group," for example (Watney 1989a:185), may be useful in epidemiological tracking, and perhaps even in designating specific populations to be targeted for tailored prevention efforts (Krieger and Appleman 1986), but when the term passes into general discourse it confuses the issues related to prevention, and gives people not identified as members of those groups a false reassurance of safety. There is increasing recognition that the term should be abandoned in favor of risk practices (Cohen and Cohen 1991).

Scientific models drawn from other domains of behavior have also proved detrimental. The Health Belief Model, for instance, became the dominant AIDS research paradigm among prevention specialists (Brown, DiClemente, and Reynolds 1991; Kirscht and Joseph 1989; Pollak and Moatti 1990; Vincke et al. 1991). Derived from research on other health behaviors, this model has not performed well with respect to AIDS (Montgomery et al. 1989). Empirical tests invariably produce low explanatory power even when statistically-significant results emerge. Another example, is the addiction model, from which AIDS researchers have imported the concept of "relapse" (Stall et al. 1990a; Ekstrand and Coates 1990; St. Lawrence et al. 1990), with its connotations of illness and sin and individual failing. Webster's New International Dictionary defines relapse as "to become ill again, to revert to evil habits, to fall back into paganism, heresy" and so forth. The term conjures up connections between disease and sin, thereby stigmatizing the "re-lapser" with moral inferiority and weakness.

These approaches, moreover, tend to focus too much on the individual, as Freudenberg (1990) points out, instead of attempting to understand the social, cultural, and political contexts in which people act and which may be the crucial factors in whether or not people adopt sensible risk-reduction measures. The point that seems to escape scientists working from these paradigms is that sexual behavior is qualitatively different from smoking, drinking, and unhealthy eating habits (Frayser 1991), and that the moralistic traditions from which they emerge have *never* worked in reducing problems associated with sexuality, e.g., child sexual abuse, teenage pregnancies, rape, sexually transmitted disease, and pros-titution. In fact, they exacerbate the problems.

These models share a tendency to emphasize prohibitions; the approach is negative and critical rather than empowering. What is needed is a model that reduces to a minimum advising people to give up pleasurable aspects of their lives, one that provides them with the tools for enhancing their pleasures, and one that emphasizes pleasure rather than danger.[36] The model must be based on behavioral realities and realizable possibilities rather than on restrictive ideologies and wish-ful thinking. AIDS has been a terrible destroyer; HIV prevention must aim to enrich the lives of those who have been spared its worst consequences. Shernoff and Bloom (1991) note that prevention programs must avoid moralizing since such messages may have a negative effect, that they must recognize and accept sexual diversity, and that they should teach appropriate skills for negotiating safe sex in all encounters. The approach they outline is positive and effective.

Indeed, even the overemphasis placed on "risk" may be counterproductive. For some people, it is the very appeal of risk-taking that makes sex so attractive. Sex provides an escape from humdrum daily existence. Moreover, the constant barrage of messages about the riskiness of everything from grilled steaks to ozone deple-tion in American society has begun to deaden sensitivity to this kind of paranoia. Once everything becomes "risky," nothing is risky.

Sexual hypocrisy is the worst enemy of AIDS prevention. The threat of AIDS will not reverse the sexual revolution, but it has resurrected traditional fears and guilt surrounding sexuality. Shernoff and Bloom (1991:39–40) argue that we need to support the "right of each person to choose for himself the fullest expression of his needs. This right is at the heart of any healthy community." The response of AIDS educators will be crucial in determining whether the ultimate legacy of the AIDS tragedy, in which so many lives have been sacrificed, will be a revival of a restrictive sexual order in which individual rights are severely circumscribed or the emergence of a new sexual culture (*la nouvelle sexualité*) based on the values of freedom, choice, creativity, honesty, safety, and responsibility.

With a bow to the example of ACT UP's slogan, let me conclude with a set of fundamental equations which should inform AIDS prevention programs:

FUNDAMENTAL EQUATIONS IN HIV PREVENTION

SEX ≠ INTERCOURSE

UNPROTECTED INTERCOURSE = UNSAFE SEX

SAFE SEX = OUTERCOURSE/PROTECTED INTERCOURSE

MONOGAMY ≠ FIDELITY

FIDELITY ≠ SAFE SEX

PROMISCUITY ≠ UNSAFE SEX

SAFE SEX = LIFE

SILENCE = DEATH

Figure 7.

ACKNOWLEDGMENTS

This paper is dedicated to the memory of a friend and dancing partner, Johnny van Laeken. The author wishes to thank Douglas A. Feldman and Merrill Singer for their comments on an earlier draft of this paper, Peter Nardi for discussions on the subject, Gail Orozco for her assistance in preparing the bibliography, Lynn Thomas for preparing the graphics, Patricia Marshall and Norris Lang for their encouragement, and Lawrence Greene for prodding me to complete this manuscript. A much abridged version of this paper was first presented at the annual meeting of the Society for Applied Anthropology, Santa Fe, New Mexico, April 1989.

NOTES

1. Queer Nation has advocated the theory that by appropriating a term of abuse, its targets can destroy its power. On that rationale, I shall use the term promiscuity in this paper without quotation marks, without apology, and without any of the pejorative connotations normally associated with it. As much as possible, I shall avoid the use of euphemisms and neologisms in discussing this phenomenon.
2. William L. Leap (1990) has written an article that explores how people talk about AIDS, but unfortunately he does not cover in his discussion the concept of promiscuity. Nonetheless, some of the rules used in AIDS discourse that he illustrates (e.g., "discuss the issue but avoid the name") are applicable to the discourse on promiscuity.
3. In the AIDS literature, only three pieces of writing provide evidence of serious, sustained, and insightful contemplation of the concept of promiscuity, and only one of these is by social scientists. Murray and Payne (1988) assess the impact of the "promiscuity paradigm" on the handling of the AIDS epidemic. Their article is complementary to the present one. Another piece, by the gay novelist Andrew Holleran (1988), is a brilliant "essay" entitled "Notes on Promiscuity" which captures the meaning of promiscuity through a numbered listing of free associations on the concept. And the third, "How to Have Promiscuity in an Epidemic," by art critic and AIDS activist, Douglas Crimp (1988), is a commentary on the sex-negative elements in AIDS literature and prevention. I am indebted to all three of these pioneering discussions.
4. Of necessity, I confine this discussion of promiscuity largely to American society. Much of the analysis, I suspect, is applicable to promiscuity in other cultures as well, but the implications for HIV prevention will undoubtedly differ depending on the specific situation in any given milieu. Conant (1988) argues that despite differences between societies, what we learn in one is likely to be relevant to others; his discussion of similarities and differences between problems encountered in the U.S. and Africa, including anti-promiscuity campaigns, illustrates this point.
5. "Primitive promiscuity" and "primeval promiscuity" were salient concepts in 19th Century evolutionary theories. For a discussion of these theories in the writings of Bachofen, Frazer, Morgan, McLennan, Westermarck, and Darwin consult Voget (1975).
6. Officially-sanctioned unions between same-sex partners do exist now in Denmark, for example, and similar legislation is close to being enacted in several other Northern European countries. While conveying most of the same rights and obligations as traditional heterosexual marriage, these legal unions approximate but are not identical to marriage. The legal registration of nonmarital partnership agreements (both gay and straight) at the municipal level of government is the closest American institutions have come to sanctioning gay unions; such registration is available at this time in only a few locales (e.g., San Francisco and West Hollywood, California).
7. The textbook by Schultz (1984) is exceptional in this regard, devoting a chapter to cross-cultural variations in sexuality.
8. For a superb discussion of the limits of sexology and a critique of its claims to scientific neutrality, see Weeks (1985:61–95).
9. The first scientific article on AIDS was not the first publication on the epidemic. That honor goes to an article written by Lawrence Mass, published on May 18, 1981 in the New York Native, a gay publication (Kinsella 1989:259).

10. Analyses of interpretations of AIDS among Africans and/or Haitians can be found in Chirimuuta, Harrison, and Gazi (1988[1987]), Farmer (1990), Leibowitch (1985), Patton (1990), Sabatier (1988), Murray and Payne (1988, 1989), Fettner and Check (1984), and Moore and LeBaron (1986).

11. Hemophiliacs, however, are popularly linked with deviant sexuality through the association of this condition with famous cases among European royalty as a result of inbreeding or incest.

12. Another contemporary theory was that AIDS was caused by "poppers." For a fascinating exchange concerning the relative importance of promiscuity versus poppers in the early studies, see Marmor and Dubin (1990), Hessel (1990), and Grimson (1990).

13. Martin and Vance (1984) observed that differences in numbers of partners between AIDS patients and controls may be exaggerated because of a tendency for the former to overstate their promiscuity to rationalize their diagnosis and for the latter to understate their promiscuity in order to convince themselves that they will not get AIDS.

14. The studies which report associations between promiscuity and AIDS/HIV are too numerous to reference here. A few examples will suffice: Winkelstein et al. (1987a), Darrow et al. (1987), Moss et al. (1987), Goedert et al. (1984), Jeffries et al. (1985), Schechter et al. (1986), Stevens et al. (1986), van Griensven et al. (1987), Meyer-Bahlburg et al. (1991), Clumeck and Van de Perre (1988[1985]), Kuiken et al. (1990), Marmor et al. (1990), Friedland and Klein (1987), Haverkos and Edelman (1988), Hunt et al. (1990).

15. The model developed by Perlman et al. (1990) is an exception in this regard inasmuch as their research is intended to show the influence of condom use on projections of HIV infection in the population.

16. The pamphlet defined "high risk" as more than 10 different partners per month, "medium risk" as between 3–10, and "low risk" as less than 3 partners per month; it also indicates that "high risk" involves anonymous encounters, group sex, and one-timers, "medium risk" involves several times with the same person or sex within a group of friends, and "low risk" is monogamy for both partners.

17. Nussbaum (1990:96–100) discusses the outraged reaction within the gay community to the article by Callen and Berkowitz ("We Know Who We Are: Two Gay Men Declare War on Promiscuity") which had appeared in the *New York Native* (Nov. 8–12, 1982).

18. For more information on gay sexual ideologies, see Bronski (1984, 1989), Locke (1987), Patton (1985b, 1990), Segal (1989), Valverde (1987), Kirk and Madsen (1989), Weeks (1985), Altman (1982), and Spada (1979).

19. The phrase "promiscuous sexual practices" is certainly odd. *People* may be "promiscuous," but it is difficult to imagine what a "promiscuous sexual practice" is.

20. Insightful discussions of the conflicts over abstinence and promiscuity in the public policy arena are to be found in Bayer (1989, 1990), Fumento (1989), Nichols (1989), Crimp (1988) and Shilts (1987).

21. Issues related to chastity education in AIDS prevention are discussed in Brooks-Gunn and Furstenberg (1990), Haffner (1988), Quackenbush (1988), Pickerel (1988), Tatum (1988), Quackenbush and Sargent (1988), and Miller, Turner, and Moses (1990).

22. There is a growing tendency in the U.S. to restrict free speech with respect to sexual and reproductive matters, not only in the area of pornography and obscenity, but also in the medical field. For example, restrictions have been imposed on physicians who, if they work for agencies that receive federal funds, are prohibited from discussing certain medical options with their patients (Bullis 1991).

23. Shilts (1987), a strident opponent of the baths, discusses the issue extensively. Bayer (1989) offers a more nonpartisan analysis of the bathhouse controversy. See also Murray and Payne (1988), Kinsella (1989), Perrow and Guillen (1990), Richwald et al. (1988), Rabin (1986), Siegel and Siegel (1983), and Weinberg and Williams (1975).

24. How the American armed forces dealt with earlier epidemics of venereal diseases among servicemen proves instructive. During World War I moralistic approaches to venereal disease control predominated along with punitive policies directed against prostitutes. Learning that this approach was not very effective, during World War II the military eventually turned increasingly to distributing and urging the use of condoms. As one observer wrote: "We cannot stifle the instincts of man, we cannot legislate his appetite. We can only educate him to caution, watchfulness and the perpetual hazards of promiscuous intercourse; and furnish him with adequate preventive measures." (cited in Brandt 1987:164).

25. The role of prostitutes in the AIDS epidemic is covered in Miller, Turner, and Moses (1990), de Zalduondo (1991), Day (1990), Fumento (1989), Pleak and Meyer-Bahlburg (1990), Richardson (1988), Pheterson (1990), Wilson (1990), and Plant (1990). Given the predominance of heterosexual transmission of HIV in Africa, it is not surprising that prostitution has been even more salient as a topic in the AIDS literature on that continent. See, for example, Simonsen et al. (1990) and articles in Koch-Weser and Vanderschmidt (1988).

26. Treatment of AIDS issues in the media is covered in Kinsella (1989), Albert (1986a, 1986b), Baker (1986), Alcorn (1989), Fumento (1989), Shilts (1987), Crimp (1988), Watney (1987), Gever (1988), Gross (1991), Price (1989) and Milavsky (1988).

27. Having discussed promiscuity in gay discourse above, I shall not attempt to cover the gay press's handling of the issue. Needless to say, the role of promiscuity in the epidemic was a subject of serious concern in gay news media. The interested reader should consult such major publications as *The New York Native, The Advocate, Gay Community News, Frontiers, Christopher Street, Washington Blade, Bay Area Reporter*, and *Out/Look*.

28. For discussions of the topic of extramarital sex see Neubeck (1969), Blumstein and Schwartz (1983), Cole (1969), Whitehurst (1969), Ellis (1969), and Cuber (1969).

29. Lesbians have not been included in this analysis for several reasons. From the onset of the epidemic they were known to be at low risk for contracting AIDS. Lesbian cases do exist, though the numbers are small. In most instances, the risk factor associated with AIDS among lesbians has been IV drug use rather than sexual behavior. Unfortunately, the literature on both lesbian sexual behavior and on AIDS among lesbians is sparse.

30. Evidence for the demise of the Jehovanist ideology can be found not only with respect to promiscuity, but also in changes in sexual practices considered taboo in that version of sexuality. Heterosexual anal intercourse, the use of sex toys, having sex with more than one person at the same time or more than one person in a 24-hour period, and other "deviant" behaviors are relatively common. For example, between 5–6% of women report engaging in anal sex at least once a month, and 43% of white women and 21% of black women report having engaged in this form of sexual behavior at some point (Turner, Miller, and Moses 1989:113). For more details, see also Petersen (1983).

31. It is without doubt the large discrepancy between sexual ideology and sexual reality in American society that prompts conservatives to so adamantly oppose research on sexuality, since they are aware that such research would expose the extent to which their views on sexuality constitute a minority position in American culture and undermine the mythology that they have a vested interest in perpetuating.

32. To demonstrate the absurdity of the term "promiscuous," in my human sexuality classes I ask students who are promiscuous to raise their hand. No one ever does, of course, but what is interesting is to observe the amused smiles on students' faces and their discomfort as they deal with the dissonance they experience knowing that many of them have multiple partners but none thinks of himself or herself as promiscuous.

33. To be sure, privileging condoms in safe sex education is another seriously flawed strategy which emanates partly from a heterosexist bias on what constitutes sex and partly from the exaggerated place that anal sex held in the repertoire of sexual techniques among gay men in San Francisco in comparison to gay men in many other locales where a much lower percentage of gay men appear to engage in this practice as standard fare in a sexual encounter. In the absence of serious efforts to extol the joys of nonpenetrative (i.e., safer) forms of sex, promoting condoms promotes the message that sex should involve intercourse rather than other forms of sexual expression. See Patton (1990).

34. Although I have used the masculine pronoun in this discussion, I would emphasize that the same holds true for women as well.

35. It is *not* a goal of this paper either to advocate or denounce promiscuity. The choice on sexual matters involving mutual consent should rest with the individual. It is not the role of either scientists or public policymakers to intrude on those decisions in any way other than to provide information on likely consequences which will enable the individual to make such decisions knowledgably. It *is* a goal of this paper to provide a corrective to the bad advice that scientists and policymakers alike have given the American public during the 1980s with respect to promiscuity.

36. Examples of publications which teach the eroticization of safe sex include Peters (1988) and McIlvenna (1987); see also Shernoff and Bloom (1991) for a discussion of workshops that use such approaches.

REFERENCES CITED

Abramson, P. R.
  1990 Sexual Science: Emerging Discipline or Oxymoron? (Commentary). The Journal of Sex Research 27:147–165.
Adam, B.
  1978 The Survival of Domination: Inferiorization and Everyday Life. New York: Elsevier.
Ahlgren, D. J., M. K. Gorny, and A. C. Stein
  1990 Model-Based Optimization of Infectivity Parameters: A Study of the Early Epidemic in San Francisco. Journal of Acquired Immune Deficiency Syndromes 3:631–643.
Albert, E.
  1986a Acquired Immune Deficiency Syndrome: The Victim and the Press. IN Studies in Communication, Vol. 3. T. McCormack, ed. Greenwich, CT: JAI Press.
  1986b Illness and Deviance: The Responses of the Press to AIDS. IN The Social Dimensions of AIDS: Method and Theory. D. A. Feldman and T. M. Johnson, eds. Pp. 163–178. New York: Praeger.
Alcorn, K.
  1989 AIDS in the Public Sphere: How a Broadcasting System in Crisis Dealt With an Epidemic. IN Taking Liberties: AIDS and Cultural Politics. E. Carter and S. Watney, eds. Pp. 193–212. London: Serpent's Tail.
Allgeier, A. R., and E. R. Allgeier
  1988 Sexual Interactions. 2nd ed. Lexington: D. C. Heath.
Allgeier, E. R., and A. R. Allgeier
  1984 Sexual Interactions. Lexington: D. C. Heath.
  1991 Sexual Interactions. 3rd ed. Lexington: D. C. Heath.
Altman, D.
  1982 The Homosexualization of America. Boston: Beacon.
  1986 AIDS in the Mind of America: The Social, Political, and Psychological Impact of a New Epidemic. Garden City, N.Y.: Anchor/Doubleday.
Anchell, M.
  1988 Sex Education Is Harmful. IN Teenage Sexuality. N. Bernards and L. Hall, eds. Pp. 49–54. Opposing Viewpoints Series. St. Paul, MN: Greenhaven.
Anderson, R. M., and R. M. May
  1988 [1987] The Dynamics of the AIDS Epidemic. IN The AIDS Reader: Documentary History of a Modern Epidemic. L. K. Clarke and M. Potts, eds. Pp. 136–149. Boston: Branden.
Anonymous
  1988 Lies About Sexual History. Los Angeles Times, Aug. 22.
  1990 Survey Measures AIDS Impact on Same-Sex Couples. Nightlife 514 (July 25), p. 29.
  1991 GMHC Conducts National Roper Poll on HIV/AIDS, Public Attitudes, and Education Needs. SIECUS Report 19(5):20.
Antonio, G.
  1986 The AIDS Cover-Up? The Real and Alarming Facts about AIDS. San Francisco: Ignatius.
Baker, A. J.
  1986 The Portrayal of AIDS in the Media: An Analysis of Articles in the New York Times. IN The Social Dimensions of AIDS: Method and Theory. D. A. Feldman and T. M. Johnson, eds. Pp. 179–194. New York: Praeger.
Baldwin, J. I., S. Whiteley, and J. D. Baldwin
  1990 Changing AIDS- and Fertility-Related Behavior: The Effectiveness of Sex Education. The Journal of Sex Research 27(2):245–262.
Bardach, A. L.
  1991 A Fever in the Blood. Vanity Fair (January), Pp. 24–34.
Bauman, L. J., and K. Siegel
  1987 Misperception Among Gay Men of the Risk for AIDS Associated with Their Sexual Behavior. Journal of Applied Social Psychology 17(3):329–350.

Bayer, R.
  1989 Private Acts, Social Consequences: AIDS and the Politics of Public Health. New York: The Free Press.
  1990 AIDS, Privacy, and Responsibility. IN Living with AIDS. S. R. Graubard, ed. Pp. 159–179. Cambridge: The MIT Press.
Becker, M. H., and J. G. Joseph
  1988 AIDS and Behavioral Change to Reduce Risk: A Review. American Journal of Public Health 78(4):394–410.
Bell, A. P., and M. S. Weinberg
  1978 Homosexualities: A Study of Diversity Among Men and Women. New York: Simon and Schuster.
Bell, N. K.
  1991 Social/Sexual Norms and AIDS in the South. AIDS Education and Prevention 3(2)164–180.
Bersani, L.
  1988 Is the Rectum a Grave? IN AIDS: Cultural Analysis/Cultural Activism. D. Crimp, ed. Pp. 197–222. Cambridge: The MIT Press.
Berzon, B.
  1988 Permanent Partners: Building Gay and Lesbian Relationships that Last. New York: E. P. Dutton.
Berube, A.
  1988 Caught in the Storm: AIDS and the Meaning of Natural Disaster. Out/Look, Fall, pp. 8–19.
Biggar, R. J., L. A. Brinton, and M. D. Rosenthal
  1989 Trends in the Number of Sexual Partners among American Women. Journal of Acquired Immune Deficiency Syndromes 2:497–502.
Biglan, A., C. W. Metzler, R. Wirt, D. Ary, J. Noell, L. Ochs, C. French, and D. Hood
  1990 Social and Behavioral Factors Associated with High-Risk Sexual Behavior Among Adolescents. Journal of Behavioral Medicine 13(3):245–261.
Blumstein, P., and P. Schwartz
  1983 American Couples: Money, Work, Sex. New York: William Morrow.
Bochow, M.
  1990 AIDS and Gay Men: Individual Strategies and Collective Coping. A Follow-Up Study of Gay men in the Federal Republic of Germany. European Sociological Review 6(2):181–188.
Bolton, R.
  1992 Mapping Terra Incognita: Sex Research for AIDS Prevention, An Urgent Agenda for the Nineties. IN The Time of AIDS: Social Analysis, Theory, and Method. G. Herdt and S. Lindenbaum, eds. Newbury Park, CA: Sage.
Bolton, R., J. Vincke, R. Mak, and E. Dennehy
  1992 Alcohol and Risky Sex: In Search of an Elusive Connection. Medical Anthropology 14(2,3,4):323–363.
Bongaarts, J.
  1988 Modeling the Demographic Impact of AIDS in Africa. IN AIDS 1988: AAAS Symposia Papers. R. Kulstad, ed. Pp. 85–94. Washington: American Association for the Advancement of Science.
Brandt, A. M.
  1987 No Magic Bullet: A Social History of Venereal Disease in the United States Since 1880. Expanded edition. New York: Oxford University Press.
Brendstrup, E., and K. Schmidt
  1990 Homosexual and Bisexual Men's Coping with the AIDS Epidemic: Qualitative Interviews with 10 Non-HIV-Tested Homosexual and Bisexual Men. Social Science and Medicine 30(6):713–720.
Bronski, M.
  1984 Culture Clash: The Making of Gay Sensibility. Boston: South End Press.
  1989 Death and the Erotic Imagination. IN Taking Liberties: AIDS and Cultural Politics. E. Carter and S. Watney, eds. Pp. 219–228. London: Serpent's Tail.
Brooks-Gunn, J., and F. F. Furstenberg, Jr.
  1990 Coming of Age in the Era of AIDS: Puberty, Sexuality, and Contraception. The Milbank Quarterly 68 (Suppl. 1):59–84.

Brown, L. K., R. J. DiClemente, and L. A. Reynolds
   1991   HIV Prevention for Adolescents: Utility of the Health Belief Model. AIDS Education and
         Prevention 3(1):50–59.
Bullis, R. K.
   1991   "Gag Rules" and Chastity Clauses: Legal and Ethical Consequences of Title X and the AFLA for
         Professionals in Human Sexuality. Journal of Sex Education & Therapy 17(2):91–102.
Burcham, J. L., B. Tindall, M. Marmor, D. A. Cooper, G. Berry, and R. Penny
   1989   Incidence and Risk Factors for Human Immunodeficiency Virus Seroconversion in a Cohort of
         Sydney Homosexual Men. The Medical Journal of Australia 150:634–639.
Burton, S. W., S. B. Burn, D. Harvey, M. Mason, and G. McKerrow
   1988 [1986]   Letter to the editors. IN The AIDS Reader: Documentary History of a Modern Epidemic.
         L. K. Clarke and M. Potts, eds. Pp. 268–269. Boston: Branden. [The Lancet, November].
Byer, C. O., and L. W. Shainberg
   1991   Dimensions of Human Sexuality. 3rd ed. Dubuque, IA: Wm. C. Brown.
Callen, M., and R. Berkowitz
   1988   Excerpts from "How to Have Sex in an Epidemic: One Approach." IN Surviving and Thriving
         with AIDS: Collected Wisdom. Volume 2. M. Callen, ed. New York: People with AIDS
         Coalition, Inc.
Carne, C. A., A. M. Johnson, F. Pearce, A. Smith, R. S. Tedder, I. V. D. Weller, C. Loveday, A. Hawkins,
P. Williams, and M. w. Adler
   1987   Prevalence of Antibodies to Human Immunodeficiency Virus, Gonorrhoea Rates, and
         Changed Sexual Behavior in Homosexual Men in London. Lancet 1:656–658.
Carrier, J., and R. Bolton
   1991   Anthropological Perspective on Sexuality and HIV Prevention. Annual Review of Sex Research
         2:49–75.
Catania, J. A., T. J. Coates, S. M. Kegeles, M. Ekstrand, J. R. Guydish, and L. L. Bye
   1989   Implications of the AIDS Risk-Reduction Model for the Gay Community: The Importance of
         Perceived Sexual Enjoyment and Help-Seeking Behaviors. IN Primary Prevention of AIDS:
         Psychological Approaches. V. M. Mays, G. W. Albee, and S. F. Schneider, eds. Pp. 242–261.
         Newbury Park, CA: Sage.
Catania, J. A., D. R. Gibson, D. D. Chitwood, and T. J. Coates
   1990a Methodological Problems in AIDS Behavioral Research: Influences on Measurement Error and
         Participation Bias in Studies of Sexual Behavior. Psychological Bulletin 108(3):339–362.
Catania, J. A., D. R. Gibson, B. Marin, T. J. Coates, and R. M. Greenblatt
   1990b Response Bias in Assessing Sexual Behaviors Relevant to HIV Transmission. Evaluation and
         Program Planning 13:19–29.
Chesley, R.
   1984   Night Sweat: A Romantic Comedy. San Francisco (Mimeo).
Chirimuuta, R., R. Harrison, and D. Gazi
   1988 [1987]The Spread of Racism. IN The AIDS Reader: Documentary History of a Modern Epidemic.
         L. K. Clarke and M. Potts, eds. Pp. 308–312. Boston: Branden. [West Africa, February 9].
Citizens Commision on AIDS for New York City and Northern New Jersey
   1989   AIDS Prevention and Education: Reframing the Message. Unpublished document. New York
         City.
Clement, U.
   1990   Surveys of Heterosexual Behaviour. IN Annual Review of Sex Research, Vol. 1. J. Bancroft, ed.
         Pp. 45–74. Mt. Vernon, IA: Society for the Scientific Study of Sex.
Clumeck, N., and P. Van de Perre
   1988 [1985]Letter to the editors. IN The AIDS Reader: Documentary History of a Modern Epidemic.
         L. K. Clarke and M. Potts, eds. P. 245. Boston: Branden. [New England Journal of Medicine,
         July 18].
Coates, R. A., V. T. Farewell, J. Raboud, S. E. Read, D. K. MacFadden, L. M. Calzavara, J. K. Johnson, F.
A. Shepherd, and M. M. Fanning
   1990   Cofactors of Progression to Acquired Immunodeficiency Syndrome in a Cohort of Male Sexual
         Contacts of Men with Human Immunodeficiency Virus Disease. American Journal of Epidem-
         iology 132(4):717–722.

Cochran, S. D., and V. M. Mays
  1990 Sex, Lies, and HIV. New England Journal of Medicine 322(11):774–775.
Cohen, M. A. A., and S. C. Cohen
  1991 AIDS Education and a Volunteer Training Program for Medical Students. Psychosomatics
        32(2):187–190.
Cole, W. G.
  1969 Religious Attitudes Toward Extramarital Intercourse. IN Extra-Marital Relations. G. Neubeck,
        ed. Pp. 54–64. Englewood Cliffs, NJ: Prentice-Hall.
Coleman, E.
  1991 Compulsive Sexual Behavior: New Concepts and Treatments. Journal of Psychology and
        Human Sexuality 4(2):37–52.
Conant, F. P.
  1988 Social Consequences of AIDS: Implications for East Africa and the Eastern United States. IN
        AIDS 1988: AAAS Symposia Papers. R. Kulstad, ed. Pp. 147–156. Washington: American
        Association for the Advancement of Science.
Conant, M., D. Hardy, J. Sernatenger, D. Spicer, and J. A. Levy
  1988 [1986]Condoms Prevent Transmission of AIDS-Associated Retrovirus. IN The AIDS Reader:
        Documentary History of a Modern Epidemic. L. K. Clarke, and M. Potts, eds. Pp. 239–240.
        Boston: Branden.
Connor, S., and S. Kingman
  1989 The Search for the Virus. Revised and updated edition. London: Penguin.
Conservative Family Campaign
  1988 [1986–87]Testimony before the Social Services Committee on Problems Associated with AIDS.
        IN The AIDS Reader: Documentary History of a Modern Epidemic. L. K. Clarke and M.
        Potts, eds. Pp. 270–274. Boston: Branden. [House of Commons, London, 1986–1987 ses-
        sion].
Coyle, S. L., R. E. Boruch, and C. F. Turner, eds.
  1991 Evaluating AIDS Prevention Programs. Expanded ed. Washington: National Academy
        Press.
Crimp, D.
  1988 How to Have Promiscuity in an Epidemic. IN AIDS: Cultural Analysis, Cultural Activism. D.
        Crimp, ed. Pp. 236–271. Cambridge: The MIT Press.
Cuber, J. F.
  1969 Adultery: Reality Versus Stereotype. IN Extra-Marital Relations. G. Neubeck, ed. Pp. 190–196.
        Englewood Cliffs, NJ: Prentice-Hall.
Curran, J. W., H. W. Jaffe, A. M. Hardy, W. M. Morgan, R. M. Selik, and T. J. Dondero
  1988 Epidemiology of AIDS and HIV Infection in the United States. IN AIDS 1988: AAAS Symposia
        Papers. R. Kulstad, ed. Pp. 19–34. Washington: American Association for the Advancement of
        Science. [Science, Vol. 239, p. 610].
Curran, J. W., W. M. Morgan, A. M. Hardy, H. W. Jaffe, W. W. Darrow, and W. R. Dowdle
  1985 The Epidemiology of AIDS: Current Status and Future Prospects. Science 229:1352–1357.
Darrow, W. W., D. F. Echenberg, H. W. Jaffe, P. M. O'Malley, R. H. Byers, J. P. Getchell, and J. W. Curran
  1987 Risk Factors for Human Immunodeficiency Virus (HIV) Infections in Homosexual Men.
        American Journal of Public Health 77(4):479–483.
Darrow, W. W., H. W. Jaffe, and J. W. Curran
  1988 Behaviors Associated with HIV-1 Infection and the Development of AIDS. IN AIDS 1988:
        AAAS Symposia Papers. R. Kulstad, ed. Pp. 226–235. Washington: American Association for
        the Advancement of Science.
Davies, P., P. Weatherburn, A. J. Hunt, F. Hickson, T. J. McManus, and A. Coxon
  1991 Young Gay Men in England and Wales: Sexual Behaviour and Implications for the Spread of
        HIV. Unpublished paper.
Davis, M. S.
  1983 Smut: Erotic Reality/Obscene Ideology. Chicago: The University of Chicago Press.
Day, S.
  1990 Prostitute Women and the Ideology of Work in London. IN Culture and AIDS. D. A. Feldman,
        ed. Pp. 93–109. New York: Praeger.

DeBuono, B. A., S. H. Zinner, M. Daamen, and W. M. McCormack
   1990   Sexual Behavior of College Women in 1975, 1986, and 1989. New England Journal of Medicine 322:821–825.
De Cecco, E.
   1988   Gay Relationships. New York: Harrington Park.
de Vroome, E. M. M., M. E. M. Paalman, Th. G. M. Sandfort, M. Sleutjes, K. J. M. de Vries, and R. A. P. Tielman
   1990   AIDS in the Netherlands: The Effects of Several Years of Campaigning. International Journal of STD & AIDS 1:268–275.
D'Emilio, J., and E. B. Freedman
   1988   Intimate Matters: A History of Sexuality in America. New York: Harper & Row.
D'Eramo, J. E.
   1988   Report from Stockholm: The Enemy Within. Christopher Street, Issue 126, pp. 16–29.
De Gruttola, V., and W. Bennett
   1988   Statistical Issues in Assessing the AIDS Epidemic. IN AIDS 1988: AAAS Symposia Papers. R. Kulstad, ed. Pp. 57–65. Washington: American Association for the Advancement of Science.
De Gruttola, V., K. Mayer, and W. Bennett
   1988 [1986]AIDS: Has the Problem Been Adequately Assessed? IN The AIDS Reader: Documentary History of a Modern Epidemic. L. K. Clarke and M. Potts, eds. Pp. 97–107. Boston: Branden. [Reviews of Infectious Diseases, March-April].
Detels, R., P. English, B. R. Visscher, L. Jacobson, L. A. Kingsley, J. S. Chmiel, J. P. Dudley, L. J. Eldred, and H. M. Ginzburg
   1989   Seroconversion, Sexual Activity, and Condom Use Among 2915 HIV Seronegative Men Followed for up to 2 Years. Journal of Acquired Immune Deficiency Syndromes 2:77–83.
de Zalduondo, B. O.
   1991   Prostitution Viewed Cross-Culturally: Toward Recontexualizing Sex Work in AIDS Intervention Research. The Journal of Sex Research 28(2):223–248.
Doll, L. S., F. N. Judson, D. G. Ostrow, P. M. O'Malley, W. W. Darrow, S. C. Hadler, R. H. Byers, K. A. Penley, and N. L. Altman
   1990a Sexual Behavior Before AIDS: The Hepatitis B Studies of Homosexual and Bisexual Men. AIDS 4:1067–1073.
Doll, L. S., P. M. O'Malley, A. L. Pershing, W. W. Darrow, N. A. Hessol, and A. R. Lifson
   1990b High-Risk Sexual Behavior and Knowledge of HIV Antibody Status in the San Francisco City Clinic Cohort. Health Psychology 9(3):253–265.
Dryfoos, J.
   1988   School-Based Clinics Can Control Teenage Pregnancy. IN Teenage Sexuality. N. Bernards and L. Hall, eds. Pp. 107–112. Opposing Viewpoints Series. St. Paul, MN: Greenhaven.
DuBois, E. C., and L. Gordon
   1984   Seeking Ecstasy on the Battlefield: Danger and Pleasure in Nineteenth-Century Feminist Sexual Thought. IN Pleasure and Danger: Exploring Female Sexuality. C. S. Vance, ed. Pp. 31–49. Boston: Routledge & Kegan Paul.
Duesberg, P.
   1987   Retroviruses as Carcinogens and Pathogens. Cancer Research 47:1199–1220.
Earl, W. L.
   1990   Married Men and Same Sex Activity: A Field Study on HIV Risk Among Men Who Do Not Identify as Gay or Bisexual. Journal of Sex & Marital Therapy 16(4):251–257.
Echols, A.
   1984   The Taming of the Id: Feminist Sexual Politics, 1968–83. IN Pleasure and Danger: Exploring Female Sexuality. C. S. Vance, ed. Pp. 50–72. Boston: Routledge & Kegan Paul.
Edelman, M. W.
   1988   Educational Programs Will Curb Teenage Pregnancies. IN Teenage Sexuality. N. Bernards and L. Hall, eds. Pp. 145–150. Opposing Viewpoints Series. St. Paul, MN: Greenhaven.
Ekstrand, M. L., and T. J. Coates
   1990   Maintenance of Safer Sexual Behaviors and Predictors of Risky Sex: The San Francisco Men's Health Study. American Journal of Public Health 80(8):973–977.

Ellis, A.
  1969 Healthy and Disturbed Reasons for Having Extramarital Relations. IN Extra-Marital Relations. G. Neubeck, ed. Pp. 153–161. Englewood Cliffs, NJ: Prentice-Hall.
Emmons, C.-A., J. G. Joseph, R. C. Kessler, C. B. Wortman, S. B. Montgomery, and D. G. Ostrow
  1986 Psychosocial Predictors of Reported Behavior Change in Homosexual Men at Risk for AIDS. Health Education Quarterly 13(4):331–345.
Essex, M.
  1986 [1985] The Etiology of AIDS: Introduction and Overview. IN AIDS: Papers from Science, 1982–1985. R. Kulstad, ed. Pp. 3–7. Washington: American Association for the Advancement of Science.
Fain, N.
  1982 Is Our "Lifestyle" Hazardous to Our Health? Part II. The Advocate, April.
  1984 Gay Physicians Object to Term "Promiscuity." GMHC Health Newsletter. P. 3. New York: Gay Men's Health Crisis.
Farmer, P.
  1990 AIDS and Accusation: Haiti, Haitians, and the Geography of Blame. *In* Culture and AIDS. D. A. Feldman, ed. Pp. 67–91. New York: Praeger.
Fay, R. E., C. F. Turner, A. D. Klassen, and J. H. Gagnon
  1989 Prevalence and Patterns of Same-Gender Sexual Contact Among Men. Science 243:338–348.
Fettner, A. G., and W. A. Check
  1984 The Truth About AIDS: Evolution of an Epidemic. Revised and updated edition. New York: Holt, Rinehart and Winston.
Fisher, J. D., and S. J. Misovich
  1990 Social Influence and AIDS-Preventive Behavior. IN Social Influence Processes and Prevention. J. Edwards, R. S. Tindale, L. Heath, and E. J. Posavad, eds. New York: Plenum.
Fitzpatrick, R., M. Boulton, G. Hart, J. Dawson, and J. McLean
  1989 High Risk Sexual Behavior and Condom Use in a Sample of Homosexual and Bisexual Men. Health Trends 21:76–79.
Fitzpatrick, R., J. McLean, J. Dawson, M. Boulton, and G. Hart
  1990 Factors Influencing Condom Use in a Sample of Homosexually Active Men. Genitourinary Medicine 66:346–350.
Ford, C. S., and F. A. Beach
  1980 [1951] Patterns of Sexual Behavior. Westport, CT: Greenwood Press.
Fox, R.
  1967 Kinship and Marriage. Middlesex: Penguin.
  1983 The Red Lamp of Incest: An Inquiry into the Origins of Mind and Society. Notre Dame: University of Notre Dame Press.
Francis, D. P.
  1983 The Search for the Cause. IN The AIDS Epidemic. K. M. Cahill, ed. Pp. 137–148. New York: St. Martin's.
Franklin II, C. W.
  1988 Men and Society. Chicago: Nelson-Hall.
Frayser, S. G.
  1985 Varieties of Sexual Experience: An Anthropological Perspective on Human Sexuality. New Haven, CT: HRAF Press.
  1991 The Cultural Context of Sex Research and AIDS Prevention. Unpublished manuscript.
Freudenberg, N.
  1990 AIDS Prevention in the United States: Lessons from the First Decade. International Journal of Health Services 20(4):589–599.
Friedland, G. H., and R. S. Klein
  1987 Transmission of the Human Immunodeficiency Virus. New England Journal of Medicine 317(8):1125–1135.
Froman, P. K.
  1990 Pathways to Wellness: Strategies for Self-Empowerment in the Age of AIDS. New York: Penguin.

Fromer, M. J.
 1983   AIDS: Acquired Immune Deficiency Syndrome. New York: Pinnacle Books.
Fumento, M.
 1989   The Myth of Heterosexual AIDS. New York: Basic Books.
Gagnon, J. H.
 1990   Disease and Desire. IN Living with AIDS. S. R. Graubard, ed. Pp. 181–211. Cambridge: The
        MIT Press.
Geer, J., J. Heiman, and H. Leitenberg
 1984   Human Sexuality. Englewood Cliffs, NJ: Prentice-Hall.
Gever, M.
 1988   Pictures of Sickness: Stuart Marshall's "Bright Eyes". IN AIDS: Cultural Analysis/Cultural
        Activism. D. Crimp, ed. Cambridge: The MIT Press.
Glenn, N. D., and C. N. Weaver
 1979   Attitudes Toward Premarital, Extramarital, and Homosexual Relations in the U.S. in the 1970s.
        The Journal of Sex Research 15(2):108–118.
Goedert, J. J., M. G. Sarngadharan, R. J. Biggar, et al.
 1984   Determinants of Retrovirus (HTLV-III) Antibody and Immunodeficiency Conditions in Homo-
        sexual Men. Lancet 1984-II:711–715.
Goldsmith, M. F.
 1988 [1987]   Sex in the Age of AIDS Calls for Common Sense and "Condom Sense." IN The AIDS
        Reader: Documentary History of a Modern Epidemic. L. K. Clarke and M. Potts, eds. Pp. 184–
        190. Boston: Branden. [Journal of the American Medical Association, May 1].
Goldstein, R.
 1989   AIDS and the Social Contract. IN Taking Liberties: AIDS and Cultural Politics. E. Carter and S.
        Watney, eds. Pp. 81–94. London: Serpent's Tail.
Golubjatnikov, R., J. Pfister, and T. Tillotson
 1983   Homosexual Promiscuity and the Fear of AIDS. Lancet 2:681.
Gorman, E. M.
 1986   The AIDS Epidemic in San Francisco: Epidemiological and Anthropological Perspectives. IN
        Anthropology and Epidemiology. C. R. Janes, R. Stall, and S. M. Gifford, eds. Pp. 157–172.
        Dordrecht: D. Reidel.
Gorman, M., and D. Mallon
 1989   The Role of a Community-Based Health Education Program in the Prevention of AIDS. IN The
        AIDS Pandemic: A Global Emergency. R. Bolton, ed. Pp. 67–74. New York: Gordon and Breach.
Gottlieb, M. S., H. M. Schanker, P. T. Fan, A. Saxon, J. D. Weisman, and I. Pozalski
 1988 [1981]   Pneumocystis Pneumonia—Los Angeles. IN The AIDS Reader: Documentary History
        of a Modern Epidemic. L. K. Clarke and M. Potts, eds. Pp. 69–71. Boston: Branden. [Morbidity
        and Mortality Weekly Report, June 5.]
Gough, J.
 1989   Theories of Sexual Identity and the Masculinization of the Gay Man. IN Coming On Strong:
        Gay Politics and Culture. S. Shepherd and M. Wallis, eds. London: Unwin Hyman.
Gregory, S. J., and B. Leonardo
 1986   Conquering AIDS Now! With Natural Treatment a Non-Drug Approach. New York: Warner.
Grimson, Roger C.
 1990   Letter to the editor, Re: "An Autopsy of Epidemiologic Methods: The Case of "Poppers" in the
        Early Epidemic of the Acquired Immunedeficiency Syndrome (AIDS)". American Journal of
        Epidemiology 131(1):198–199.
Grmek, M. D.
 1990   History of AIDS: Emergence and Origin of a Modern Pandemic. Princeton: Princeton Univer-
        sity Press.
Gross, L.
 1991   Television and AIDS: Can a Homophobic Medium Be Part of the Solution? Paper presented at
        the annual meeting of the International Communication Association, Chicago, May 26.
Haffner, D. W.
 1988   Developing Community Support for School-Based AIDS Education. IN the AIDS Challenge:

Prevention Education for Young People. M. Quackenbush and M. Nelson with K. Clark, eds. Pp. 93–103. Santa Cruz, CA: Network.

Handsfield, H. H.
  1988 [1985]   Letter to the editors. IN The AIDS Reader: Documentary History of a Modern Epidemic. L. K. Clarke and M. Potts, eds. Pp. 246–247. Boston: Branden. [American Journal of Public Health, December].

Harry, J.
  1986   Sampling Gay Men. The Journal of Sex Research 22:21–34.

Haverkos, H. W., and R. Edelman
  1988   The Epidemiology of Acquired Immune Deficiency Syndrome among Heterosexuals. Journal of the American Medical Association 260(13):1922–1929.

Hays, R. B., S. M. Kegeles, and T. J. Coates
  1990   High HIV Risk-Taking Among Young Gay Men. AIDS 4(9):901–907.

Helquist, M.
  1986   Safe Sex: Guidelines That Could Save Your Life. IN Gay Life: Leisure, Love, and Living for the Contemporary Gay Male. E. E. Rofes, ed. Pp. 58–68. Garden City, NY: Doubleday.

Herdt, G., and A. M. Boxer
  1991   Ethnographic Issues in the Study of AIDS. The Journal of Sex Research 28(2):171–187.

Hessel, P. A.
  1990   Letter to the editor, Re: "An Autopsy of Epidemiologic Methods: The Case of "Poppers" in the Early Epidemic of the Acquired Immunodeficiency Syndrome (AIDS)". American Journal of Epidemiology 131(1):196–197.

Hessol, N. A., L. Barnhart, P. O'Malley, et al.
  1989   The Natural History of HIV Infection in a Cohort of Homosexual and Bisexual Men: Cofactors for Disease Progression, 1978–1989. Paper presented at the Vth International Conference on AIDS, Montreal, June 3–9.

Hingson, R. W., L. Strunin, B. M. Berlin, and T. Heeren
  1990   Beliefs about AIDS, Use of Alcohol and Drugs, and Unprotected Sex among Massachusetts Adolescents. American Journal of Public Health 80(3):295–299.

Hoffman, W. M.
  1985   As Is. New York: Vintage Books.

Holleran, A.
  1988   Ground Zero. New York: New American Library.

Hrdy, D. B.
  1987   Cultural Practices Contributing to the Transmission of Human Immunodeficiency Virus in Africa. Reviews of Infectious Disease 9(6):1109–1119.

Huggins, J., N. Elman, C. Baker, R. G. Forrester, and D. Lyter
  1991   Affective and Behavioral Responses of Gay and Bisexual Men to HIV Antibody Testing. Social Work 36(1):61–66.

Hunt, A. J., G. Christofinis, A. P. M. Coxon, P. M. Davies, T. J. McManus, S. Sutherland, and P. Weatherburn
  1990   Seroprevalence of HIV-1 Infection in a Cohort of Homosexually Active Men. Genitourinary Medicine 66:423–427.

Hyde, J. S.
  1979   Understanding Human Sexuality. New York: McGraw-Hill.
  1982   Understanding Human Sexuality. 2nd ed. New York: McGraw-Hill.
  1990   Understanding Human Sexuality. 3rd ed. New York: McGraw-Hill.

Institute of Medicine
  1986   Confronting AIDS: Directions for Public Health, Health Care, and Research. Washington: National Academy Press.

Isensee, R.
  1990   Love Between Men: Enhancing Intimacy and Keeping Your Relationship. New York: Prentice-Hall.

Jacquez, J. A., C. P. Simon, J. Koopman, L. Sattenspiel, and T. Perry
  1988   Modelling and Analyzing HIV Transmission: The Effect of Contact Patterns. Mathematical Biosciences 92:119–199.

Jaffe, H. W., K. Choi, P. A. Thomas et al.
  1983   National Case-Control Study of Kaposi's Sarcoma and Pneumocystis Carinii Pneumonia in Homosexual Men: Part 1, Epidemiologic Results. Annals of Internal Medicine 99(2):145–151.
Jakobowitz, I.
  1988 [1986]   Only a Moral Revolution Can Contain this Scourge. IN The AIDS Reader: Documentary History of a Modern Epidemic. L. K. Clarke and M. Potts, eds. Pp. 225–229. Boston: Branden. [The Times (London), December 27].
Jeffries, E., B. Willoughby, W. J. Boyko, et al.
  1985   The Vancouver Lymphadenopathy-AIDS Study: II. Seroepidemiology of HTLV-III Antibody. Canadian Medical Association Journal 132:1373–1377.
Jones, R. E.
  1984   Human Reproduction and Sexual Behavior. Englewood Cliffs, NJ: Prentice-Hall.
Joseph, J. G., S. B. Montgomery, C. A. Emmons, R. C. Kessler, D. G. Ostrow, C. B. Wortman, K. O'Brien, M. Eller, and S. Eshleman
  1987   Magnitude and Determinants of Behavioral Risk Reduction: Longitudinal Analysis of a Cohort at Risk for AIDS. Psychol Health 1:73–96.
Katchadourian, H. A.
  1985   Fundamentals of Human Sexuality. Fourth edition. New York: CBS College Publishing.
Katchadourian, H., and D. T. Lunde
  1972   Fundamentals of Human Sexuality. New York: Holt, Rinehart and Winston.
Kelly, J. A., J. S. St. Lawrence, T. L. Brasfield, L. Y. Stevenson, Y. E. Diaz, and A. C. Hauth
  1990   AIDS Risk Behavior Patterns among Gay Men in Southern Cities. American Journal of Public Health 80(4):416–418.
Kelly, J. A., J. S. St. Lawrence, H. V. Hood, and T. L. Brasfield
  1989   Behavioral Intervention to Reduce AIDS Risk Activities. Journal of Consulting and Clinical Psychology 57:60–67.
Kim, Y. H.
  1969   The Kinsey Findings. IN Extra-Marital Relations. G. Neubeck, ed. Pp. 65–73. Englewood Cliffs, NJ: Prentice-Hall.
Kinsella, J.
  1989   Covering the Plague: AIDS and the American Media. New Brunswick: Rutgers University Press.
Kipke, M. D., D. Futterman, and K. Hein
  1990   HIV Infection and AIDS During Adolescence. Adolescent Medicine 74(5):1149–1167.
Kirk, M., and H. Madsen
  1989   After the Ball. New York: Doubleday.
Kirscht, J. P., and J. G. Joseph
  1989   The Health Belief Model: Some Implications for Behavior Change, with Reference to Homosexual Males. IN Primary Prevention of AIDS: Psychological Approaches. V. M. Mays, G. W. Albee, and S. F. Schneider, eds. Pp. 111–127. Newbury Park: Sage.
Koch-Weser, D., and H. Vanderschmidt, eds.
  1988   The Heterosexual Transmission of AIDS in Africa. Cambridge: Abt Books.
Kolata, G.
  1986 [1983]   Congress, NIH Open Coffers for AIDS. IN AIDS: Papers from Science, 1982–1985. R. Kulstad, ed. Pp. 58–60. Washington: American Association for the Advancement of Science. [Science, News and Comment, 29 July].
Koop, E. C.
  1987   Surgeon General's Report on Acquired Immune Deficiency Syndrome. Washington: U. S. Department of Health and Human Services.
  1988 [1987]   Teaching Children about AIDS. IN The AIDS Reader: Documentary History of a Modern Epidemic. L. K. Clarke and M. Potts, eds. Pp. 202–207. Boston: Branden. [Issues in Science and Technology, Fall].
Koopman, J., C. Simon, J. Jacquez, L. Sattenspiel, and T. Park
  1988   Sexual Partner Selectiveness Effects on Homosexual HIV Transmission Dynamics. Journal of Acquired Immune Deficiency Syndromes 1(5):486–504.

Kopelman, L.
1988 The Punishment Concept of Disease. IN AIDS: Ethics and Public Policy. C. Pierce and D. VanDeVeer, eds. Pp. 49–55. Belmont, CA: Wadsworth.

Kramer, L.
1978 Faggots. New York: Warner.
1985 The Normal Heart. New York: New American Library.
1989 Reports from the Holocaust: The Making of an AIDS Activist. New York: St. Martin's.

Krauthammer, C.
1988 School-Based Clinics Do Not Encourage Promiscuity. In Teenage Sexuality. N. Bernards and L. Hall, eds. Pp. 103–106. Opposing Viewpoints Series. St. Paul, MN: Greenhaven.

Krieger, R., and R. Appleman
1986 The Politics of AIDS. Oakland: Frontline Pamphlets.

Kuharski, M. A.
1988 School-Based Clinics Encourage Promiscuity. IN Teenage Sexuality. N. Bernards and L. Hall, eds. Pp. 100–102. Opposing Viewpoints Series. St. Paul, MN: Greenhaven.

Kuiken, C. L., G. J. P. van Griensven, E. M. M. de Vroome, and R. A. Coutinho
1990 Risk Factors and Changes in Sexual Behavior in Male Homosexuals Who Seroconverted for Human Immunodeficiency Virus Antibodies. American Journal of Epidemiology 132(3):523–530.

Kurdek, L. A., and J. P. Schmitt
1988 Relationship Quality of Gay Men in Closed or Open Relationships. IN Gay Relationships. J. P. De Cecco, ed. Pp. 217–234. New York: Harrington Park.

LaHaye, T.
1988 Sex Education Belongs in the Home. IN Teenage Sexuality. N. Bernards and L. Hall, eds. Pp. 55–60. Opposing Viewpoints Series. St. Paul, MN: Greenhaven

Laner, M. R., and G. W. L. Kamel
1988 Media Mating I: Newspaper "Personals" Ads of Homosexual Men. IN Gay Relationships. J. De Cecco, ed. Pp. 73–89. New York: Harrington Park.

Lang, N. G.
1990 Sex, Politics, and Guilt: A Study of Homophobia and the AIDS Phenomenon. IN Culture and AIDS. D. A. Feldman, ed. Pp. 169–182. New York: Praeger.

Leap, W. L.
1990 Language and AIDS. IN Culture and AIDS. D. A. Feldman, ed. Pp. 137–158. New York: Praeger.

Lee, J. A.
1988 Forbidden Colors of Love: Patterns of Gay Love and Gay Liberation. IN Gay Relationships. J. P. De Cecco, ed. Pp. 11–32. New York: Harrington Park.

Leibowitch, J.
1985 A Strange Virus of Unknown Origin. New York: Ballantine.

Leslie, W. D., and R. C. Brunham
1990 The Dynamics of HIV Spread: A Computer Simulation Model. Computers and Biomedical Research 23:380–401.

Levine, M. P., and R. R. Troiden
1988 The Myth of Sexual Compulsivity. The Journal of Sex Research 25(3):347–363.

Leviton, L. C., R. O. Valdiserri, D. W. Lyter, C. M. Callahan, L. A. Kingsley, J. Huggins, and C. R. Rinaldo
1990 Preventing HIV Infection in Gay and Bisexual Men: Experimental Evaluation of Attitude Change from Two Risk Reduction Interventions. AIDS Education and Prevention 2(2):95–108.

Lifson, A. R., W. W. Darrow, N. A. Hessol, P. M. O'Malley, J. L. Barnhart, H. W. Jaffe, and G. W. Rutherford
1990 Kaposi's Sarcoma in a Cohort of Homosexual and Bisexual Men: Epidemiology and Analysis for Cofactors. American Journal of Epidemiology 131(2):221–231.

Lin, X.
1991 Qualitative Analysis of an HIV Transmission Model. Mathematical Biosciences 104:111–134.

Locke, R.
1987 In the Heat of Passion: How to Have Hotter, Safer Sex. San Francisco: Leyland.

Lumby, M. E.
    1988   Men Who Advertise for Sex. IN Gay Relationships. J. De Cecco, ed. Pp. 61–71. New York: Harrington Park.
Luria, Z., S. Friedman, and M. D. Rose
    1987   Human Sexuality. New York: John Wiley & Sons.
Lynch, F. R.
    1987   Non-Ghetto Gays: A Sociological Study of Suburban Homosexuals. Journal of Homosexuality 13:13–42.
Macdonald, D. I.
    1988   Sex Education Should Emphasize Abstinence. IN Teenage Sexuality. N. Bernards and L. Hall, eds. Pp. 72–77. Opposing Viewpoints Series. St. Paul, MN: Greenhaven.
Mahoney, E. R.
    1983   Human Sexuality. New York: McGraw-Hill.
Marcus, E.
    1988   The Male Couple's Guide to Living Together: What Gay Men Should Know About Living with Each Other and Coping in a Straight World. New York: Harper & Row.
Marmor, M., and N. Dubin
    1990   Letter to the editor, Re: "An Autopsy of Epidemiologic Methods: The Case of "Poppers" in the Early Epidemic of the Acquired Immunodeficiency Syndrome (AIDS)". American Journal of Epidemiology 131(1):195–196.
Marmor, M., K. Krasinski, M. Sanchez, H. Cohen, N. Dubin, L. Weiss, A. Manning, D. Bebenroth, N. Saphier, C. Harrison, and D. J. Ribble
    1990   Sex, Drugs, and HIV Infection in a New York City Hospital Outpatient Population. Journal of Acquired Immune Deficiency Syndromes 3:307–318.
Marmor, M., L. Laubenstein, D. C. William, A. E. Friedman-Kien, R. D. Byrum, S. D'Onofrio, and N. Dubin
    1982   Risk Factors for Kaposi's Sarcoma in Homosexual Men. Lancet 1:1083–1087.
Marotta, T.
    1981   The Politics of Homosexuality: How Lesbians and Gay Men Have Made Themselves a Political and Social Force in Modern America. Boston: Houghton Mifflin.
Marshall, E.
    1991   Sullivan Overrules NIH on Sex Survey. Science 253:502 (2 August).
Martin, J. L.
    1986   AIDS Risk Reduction Recommendations and Sexual Behavior Patterns among Gay Men: A Multifactorial Categorical Approach to Assessing Change. Health Education Quarterly 13(4):347–358.
    1987   The Impact of AIDS on Gay Male Sexual Behavior Patterns in New York City. American Journal of Public Health 77(5):578–581.
Martin, J. L., M. A. Garcia, and S. T. Beatrice
    1989   Sexual Behavior Changes and HIV Antibody in a Cohort of New York City Gay Men. American Journal of Public Health 79(4):501–503.
Martin, J. L., and C. S. Vance
    1984   Behavioral and Psychosocial Factors in AIDS: Methodological and Substantive Issues. American Psychologist 39(11):1303–1308.
Martin, T. C., and L. L. Bumpass
    1989   Recent Trends in Marital Disruption. Demography 26(1):37–51.
Marx, J. L.
    1986a [1983]   Health Officials Seek Ways to Halt AIDS. IN AIDS: Papers from Science, 1982–1985. R. Kulstad, ed. Pp. 22–24. Washington: American Association for the Advancement of Science. [Science, Research News, 21 January].
    1986b [1982]   New Disease Baffles Medical Community. IN AIDS: Papers from Science, 1982–1985. R. Kulstad, ed. Pp. 11–16. Washington: American Association for the Advancement of Science. [Science, Research News, 13 August].
Masters, W. H., V. E. Johnson, and R. C. Kolodny
    1985   Human Sexuality. 2n. ed. Boston: Little, Brown.

1988   Human Sexuality. 3rd ed. Glenview, IL: Scott, Foresman.

May, R. M., R. A. Anderson, and S. M. Blower
   1990   The Epidemiology and Transmission Dynamics of HIV-AIDS. IN Living with AIDS. S. R. Graubard, ed. Pp. 65–103. Cambridge: The MIT Press.

May, R. M., R. M. Anderson, and A. M. Johnson
   1988   Patterns of Infectiousness and the Transmission of HIV-1. IN AIDS 1988: AAAS Symposia Papers. R. Kulstad, ed. Pp. 73–83. Washington: American Association for the Advancement of Science.

McCary, J. L.
   1979   Human Sexuality. 2nd brief ed. New York: D. Van Nostrand.

McCary, J. L., and S. P. McCary
   1982   McCary's Human Sexuality. Belmont, CA: Wadsworth.

McCombie, S. C.
   1990   AIDS in Cultural, Historic, and Epidemiologic Context. IN Culture and AIDS. D. A. Feldman, ed. Pp. 9–27. New York: Praeger.

McCoy, H. V., C. Y. McKay, L. Hermanns, and S. Lai
   1990   Sexual Behavior and the Risk of HIV Infection. American Behavioral Scientist 33(4):432–450.

McIlvenna, T., ed.
   1987   The Complete Guide to Safe Sex. San Francisco: Specific Press.

McKirnan, D. J., and P. L. Peterson
   1989   AIDS-Risk Behavior Among Homosexual Males: The Role of Attitudes and Substance Abuse. Psychology and Health 3:161–171.

McKusick, L., T. J. Coates, S. F. Morin, L. Pollack, and C. Hoff
   1990   Longitudinal Predictors of Reductions in Unprotected Anal Intercourse among Gay Men in San Francisco: The AIDS Behavioral Research Project. American Journal of Public Health 80(8):978–983.

McKusick, L., C. C. Hoff, R. Stall, and T. J. Coates
   1991   Tailoring AIDS Prevention: Differences in Behavioral Strategies among Heterosexual and Gay Bar Patrons in San Francisco. AIDS Education and Prevention 3(1):1–9.

McKusick, L., J. A. Wiley, T. J. Coates, R. Stall, G. Saika, S. Morin, K. Charles, W. Horstman, and M. A. Conant
   1985   Reported Changes in the Sexual Behavior of Men at Risk for AIDS, San Francisco, 1982–84: The AIDS Behavioral Research Project. Public Health Report 100(6):622–629.

McLaws, M.-L., B. Oldenburg, M. W. Ross, and D. A. Cooper
   1990   Sexual Behaviour in AIDS-Related Research: Reliability and Validity of Recall and Diary Measures. The Journal of Sex Research 27(2):265–281.

McWhirter, D. P., and A. M. Mattison
   1984   The Male Couple: How Relationships Develop. Englewood Cliffs, NJ: Prentice-Hall.

Melbye, M., R. J. Biggar, P. Ebbesen, M. G. Sarngadharan S. H. Weiss, R. C. Gallo, and W. A. Blattner
   1984   Seroepidemiology of HTLV-III Antibody in Danish Homosexual Men: Prevalence, Transmission, and Disease Outcome. British Medical Journal 289:573–575.

Merino, N., R. L. Sanchez, A. Munoz, G. Prada, C. F. Garcia, and B. F. Polk
   1990   HIV-1, Sexual Practices, and Contact with Foreigners in Homosexual Men in Colombia, South America. Journal of Acquired Immune Deficiency Syndromes 3(4):330–334.

Meyer-Bahlburg, H. F. L., T. M. Exner, G. Lorenz, R. S. Gruen, J. M. Gorman, and A. A. Ehrhardt
   1991   Sexual Risk Behavior, Sexual Functioning, and HIV-Disease Progression in Gay Men. The Journal of Sex Research 28(1):3–27.

Milavsky, R.
   1988   AIDS and the Media. Paper presented at the annual meeting of the American Psychological Association, Atlanta, August 15.

Miller, H. G., C. F. Turner, and L. E. Moses, eds.
   1990   AIDS: The Second Decade. Washington: National Academy Press.

Montgomery, S. B., J. G. Joseph, M. H. Becker, D. G. Ostrow, R. C. Kessler, and J. P. Kirscht
   1989   The Health Belief Model in Understanding Compliance with Preventive Recommendations for AIDS: How Useful? AIDS Education and Prevention 1(4):303–323.

Moore, A., and R. D. LeBaron
    The Case for a Haitian Origin of the AIDS Epidemic. *In* The Social Dimensions of AIDS:
    Method and Theory. D. A. Feldman and T. M. Johnson, eds. Pp. 77–93. New York: Praeger.
Moran, J. S., H. R. Janes, T. A. Peterman, and K. M. Stone
    1990   Increase in Condom Sales following AIDS Education and Publicity, United States. American
            Journal of Public Health 80(5):607–608.
Moss, A. R., D. Osmond, P. Bacchetti, et al.
    1987   Risk Factors for AIDS and HIV Seropositivity in Homosexual Men. American Journal of
            Epidemiology 125:1035–1047.
Murdock, G. P.
    1949   Social Structure. New York: The Free Press.
Murray, S. O., and K. W. Payne
    1988   Medical Policy without Scientific Evidence: The Promiscuity Paradigm and AIDS. California
            Sociologist 11(1–2):13–54.
    1989   The Social Classification of AIDS in American Epidemiology. IN The AIDS Pandemic: A Global
            Emergency. R. Bolton, ed. Pp. 23–36. New York: Gordon and Breach.
Nardi, P., and R. Bolton
    1991   Gay Bashing: Violence and Aggression Against Gay Men and Lesbians. IN Targets of Violence
            and Aggression. R. Baenninger, ed. Pp. 349–400. Amsterdam: Elsevier.
Neubeck, G.
    1969   The Dimensions of the "Extra" in Extramarital Relations. IN Extra-Marital Relations. G.
            Neubeck, ed. Pp. 12–24. Englewood Cliffs, NJ: Prentice-Hall.
Nichols, Eve K.
    1986   Mobilizing Against AIDS. Cambridge: Harvard University Press.
    1989   Mobilizing Against AIDS. Rev. ed. Cambridge: Harvard University Press.
Nussbaum, B.
    1990   Good Intentions: How Big Business and the Medical Establishment Are Corrupting the Fight
            Against AIDS. New York: The Atlantic Monthly Press.
O'Brien, B. J.
    1989   AIDS and the Subjective Risk Assessment: A Critical Review. Health Policy 13:213–224.
Office of Science and Technology Policy
    1988   A National Effort to Model AIDS Epidemiology. Report of a Workshop held at Leesburg,
            Virginia, July 25–29, 1988. Washington, D.C.
Oppenheimer, G. M.
    1988   In the Eye of the Storm: The Epidemiological Construction of AIDS. IN AIDS: The Burden of
            History. E. Fox and D. M. Fox, eds. Pp. 267–300. Berkeley: University of California Press.
Osborn, J. E.
    1988 [1987]   AIDS and the Communities. IN The AIDS Reader: Documentary History of a Modern
            Epidemic. L. K. Clarke and M. Potts, eds. Pp. 194–201. Boston: Branden. [Congressional
            Record, November 19].
    1989   Public Health and the Politics of Prevention. IN Living With AIDS. S. R. Graubard, ed. Pp. 401–
            422. Cambridge: The MIT Press.
Padian, N., L. Marquis, D. P. Francis, R. E. Anderson, G. W. Rutherford, P. M. O'Malley, and W.
Winkelstein
    1987   Male to Female Transmission of Human Immunodeficiency Virus. Journal of the American
            Medical Association 258(6):788–790.
Patton, C.
    1985a   Heterosexual AIDS Panic. Gay Community News, February 9. [Reprinted in Human Sexu-
            ality: Vol. 1. Opposing Viewpoints Series. Pp. 179–182. St. Paul, MN: Greenhaven].
    1985b   Sex and Germs: The Politics of AIDS. Boston: South End.
    1989   The AIDS Industry: Construction of "Victims," "Volunteers," and "Experts". IN Taking
            Liberties: AIDS and Cultural Politics. E. Carter and S. Watney, eds. Pp. 113–125. London:
            Serpent's Tail.
    1990   Inventing AIDS. New York: Routledge.

Peplau, L. A.
   1988   Research on Homosexual Couples: An Overview. IN Gay Relationships. J. P. De Cecco, ed. Pp. 33–40. New York: Harrington Park.
Peplau, L. A., and S. D. Cochran
   1988   Value Orientations in the Intimate Relationships of Gay Men. IN Gay Relationships. J. P. De Cecco, ed. Pp. 195–216. New York: Harrington Park.
Perlman, J. A., J. Kelaghan, P. H. Wolf, W. Baldwin, A. Coulson, and A. Novello
   1990   HIV Risk Difference Between Condom Users and Nonusers Among U. S. Heterosexual Women. Journal of Acquired Immune Deficiency Syndromes 3:155–165.
Perrow, C., and M. F. Guillen
   1990   The AIDS Disaster: The Failure of Organizations in New York and the Nation. New Haven: Yale University Press.
Peters, B.
   1988   Terrific Sex in Fearful Times. New York: St. Martin's.
Petersen, J. R.
   1983   The Playboy Readers' Sex Survey. Playboy, Vol. 30, January and March.
Peto, J.
   1988 [1986]Letter to the editors. IN The AIDS Reader: Documentary History of a Modern Epidemic. L. K. Clarke and M. Potts, eds. Pp. 263–265. Boston: Branden. [The Lancet, October 25].
Petrow, S.
   1990   Dancing Against the Darkness: A Journey through America in the Age of AIDS. Lexington, Mass.: Lexington Books.
Pheterson, G.
   1990   The Category "Prostitute" in Scientific Inquiry. The Journal of Sex Research 27(3):397–407.
Pickerel, C.
   1988   AIDS Education in Religious Settings—A Catholic Response. IN The AIDS Challenge: Prevention Education for Young People. M. Quackenbush and M. Nelson with K. Clark, eds. Pp. 211–218. Santa Cruz, CA: Network.
Piot, P., F. A. Plummer, F. S. Mhalu, J.-L. Lamboray, J. Chin, and J. M. Mann
   1988   An International Perspective on AIDS. IN AIDS 1988: AAAS Symposia Papers. R. Kulstad, ed. Pp. 3–18. Washington: American Association for the Advancement of Science.
Plant, M., ed.
   1990   AIDS, Drugs, and Prostitution. London: Tavistock/Routledge.
Pleak, R. R., and H. F. L. Meyer-Bahlburg
   1990   Sexual Behavior and AIDS Knowledge of Young Male Prostitutes in Manhattan. The Journal of Sex Research 27(4):557–587.
Pollak, M., and J.-P. Moatti
   1990   HIV Risk Perception and Determinants of Sexual Behaviour. IN Sexual Behaviour and Risks of HIV Infection. M. Hubert, ed. Pp. 17–44. Brussels: Facultés Universitaire Saint-Louis.
Potts, M.
   1988   Introduction: The Most Presumptuous Pox. IN The AIDS Reader: Documentary History of a Modern Epidemic. L. K. Clarke and M. Potts, eds. Pp. 1–12. Boston: Branden.
Presidential Commission on the Human Immunodeficiency Virus Epidemic
   1988   Report of the Presidential Commission on the Human Immunodeficiency Virus Epidemic. Washington, D.C.
Price, M. E.
   1989   Shattered Mirrors: Our Search for Identity and Community in the AIDS Era. Cambridge: Harvard University Press.
Quackenbush, M.
   1988   AIDS Education in School Settings: Grades 10–12. IN The AIDS Challenge: Prevention Education for Young People. M. Quackenbush and M. Nelson with K. Clark, eds. Pp. 195–203. Santa Cruz, CA: Network.
Quackenbush, M., and M. Nelson with K. Clark, eds.
   1988   CDC Guidelines for Effective School Health Education to Prevent the Spread of AIDS

(Appendix A). IN The AIDS Challenge: Prevention Education for Young People. M. Quacken-bush and M. Nelson with K. Clark, eds. Pp. 433–446. Santa Cruz, CA: Network.

Quackenbush, M., and P. Sargent
  1988 The Issue of Abstinence (Appendix E) IN The AIDS Challenge: Prevention Education for Young People. M. Quackenbush and M. Nelson with K. Clark, eds. Pp. 479–481. Santa Cruz, CA: Network.

Quadland, M. C., and W. D. Shattls
  1987 AIDS, Sexuality, and Sexual Control. Journal of Homosexuality 14(1–2):277–298.

Quam, M. D.
  1990 The Sick Role, Stigma, and Pollution: The Case of AIDS. IN Culture and AIDS. D. A. Feldman, ed. Pp. 29–44. New York: Praeger.

Rabin, J. A.
  1986 The AIDS Epidemic and Gay Bathhouses: A Constitutional Analysis. Journal of Health Politics, Policy and Law 10:729–747.

Rechy, J.
  1967 Numbers. New York: Grove Press.

Rappoport, J.
  1988 AIDS, Inc.: Scandal of the Century. San Bruno, CA: Human Energy.

Reece, R., and A. E. Segrist
  1988 The Association of Selected "Masculine" Sex-Role Variables with Length of Relationship in Gay Male Couples. IN Gay Relationships. J. P. De Cecco, ed. Pp. 177–194. New York: Harrington Park.

Reinisch, J. M., S. A. Sanders, and M. Ziemba-Davis
  1988 The Study of Sexual Behavior in Relation to the Transmission of Human Immunodeficiency Virus: Caveats and Recommendations. American Psychologist 43(11):921–927.

Reiss, I. L.
  1991 Sexual Pluralism: Ending America's Sexual Crisis. SIECUS Report, February/March.

Reiss, I. L., and R. K. Leik
  1989 Evaluating Strategies to Avoid AIDS: Number of Partners vs. Use of Condoms. The Journal of Sex Research 26(4):411–433.

Rice, F. P.
  1989 Human Sexuality. Dubuque, IA: Wm. C. Brown.

Richards, J. M., J. M. Bedford, and S. S. Witkin
  1986 [1984] Rectal Insemination Modifies Immune Responses in Rabbits. IN AIDS: Papers from Science, 1982–1985. R. Kulstad, ed. Pp. 142–146. Washington: The American Association for the Advancement of Science. [Science, Report, 27 April].

Richardson, D.
  1988 Women and AIDS. New York: Methuen.

Richwald, G. A., D. E. Morisky, G. R. Kyle, A. R. Kristal, M. M. Gerber, and J. M. Friedland
  1988 Sexual Activities in Bathhouses in Los Angeles County: Implications for AIDS Prevention Education. Journal of Sex Research 25(2):169–180.

Rietmeijer, C. A. M., K. A. Penley, D. L. Cohn, A. J. Davidson, C. R. Horsburgh, and F. N. Judson
  1989 Factors Influencing the Risk of Infection with Human Immunodeficiency Virus in Homosexual Men, Denver 1982–1985. Sexually Transmitted Diseases April-June.

Rodman, H., S. H. Lewis, and S. B. Griffith
  1988 Sex Education Belongs in the Schools. IN Teenage Sexuality. N. Bernards and L. Hall, eds. Pp. 66–71. Opposing Viewpoints Series. St. Paul, MN: Greenhaven.

Roffman, D. M.
  1991 The Power of Language: Baseball as a Sexual Metaphor in American Culture. SIECUS Report 19(5):1–6.

Ross, J. W.
  1988 Ethics and the Language of AIDS. IN AIDS: Ethics and Public Policy. C. Pierce and D. VanDeVeer, eds. Pp. 39–48. Belmont, CA: Wadsworth.

Rubin, G.
   1984   Thinking Sex: Notes for Radical Theory of the Politics of Sexuality. IN Pleasure and Danger: Exploring Female Sexuality. C. S. Vance, ed. Pp. 267–319. Boston: Routledge & Kegan Paul.
Rubin, L. B.
   1991   Erotic Wars: What Happened to the Sexual Revolution? New York: Harper Perennial.
Rubinson, L., and L. De Rubertis
   1991   Trends in Sexual Attitudes and Behaviors of a College Population Over a 15-Year Period. Journal of Sex Education and Therapy 17(1):32–41.
Rutten, T.
   1991   One Congressman's Fight Against a Sexual 'Conspiracy'. Los Angeles Times, pp. B1,6. August 9.
Sabatier, R.
   1988   Blaming Others: Prejudice, Race and Worldwide AIDS. Washington: The Panos Institute.
Sack, A. R., J. F. Keller, and D. E. Hinkle
   1984   Premarital Sexual Intercourse: A Test of the Effects of Peer Group, Religiosity, and Sexual Guilt. The Journal of Sex Research 20(2):168–185.
Sanderson, C. A., and S. N. Wilson
   1991   Desperately Seeking Abstinence. SIECUS Report 19:28–29.
Sattenspiel, L., and C. Castillo-Chavez
   1990   Environmental Context, Social Interactions, and the Spread of AIDS. American Journal of Human Biology 2:397–417.
Sattenspiel, L., J. Koopman, C. Simon, and J. A. Jacquez
   1990   The Effects of Population Structure on the Spread of the HIV Infection. American Journal of Physical Anthropology 82:421–429.
Schechter, M. T., W. j. Boyko, B. Douglas, et al.
   1986   The Vancouver Lymphadenopathy-AIDS Study, 6: HIV Seroconversion in a Cohort of Homosexual Men. Canadian Medical Association Journal 135:1355–1360.
Schechter, M. T., K. J. P. Craib, T. N. Le, B. Willoughby, B. Douglas, P. Sestak, J. S. G. Montaner, M. S. Weaver, K. D. Elmslie, and M. V. O'Oshaughnessy
   1989   Progression to AIDS and Predictors of AIDS in Seroprevalent and Seroincident Cohorts of Homosexual Men. AIDS 3:347–353.
Schneider, B. E.
   1988   Gender and AIDS. IN AIDS 1988: AAAS Symposia Papers. R. Kulstad, ed. Pp. 97–106. Washington: American Association for the Advancement of Science.
Schultz, D. A.
   1984   Human Sexuality. 2nd ed. Englewood Cliffs: Prentice-Hall.
Segal, L.
   1989   Lessons from the Past: Feminism, Sexual Politics and the Challenge of AIDS. IN Taking Liberties: AIDS and Cultural Politics. E. Carter and S. Watney, eds. Pp. 131–145. London: Serpent's Tail.
Sergios, P., and J. Cody
   1988   Importance of Physical Attractiveness and Social Assertiveness Skills in Male Homosexual Dating Behavior and Partner Selection. IN Gay Relationships. J. P. De Cecco, ed. Pp. 95–109. New York: Harrington Park.
Shernoff, M., and D. J. Bloom
   1991   Perspectives: Designing Effective AIDS Prevention Workshops for Gay and Bisexual Men. AIDS Education and Prevention 3(1):31–46.
Shilts, R.
   1987   And the Band Played On: Politics, People, and the AIDS Epidemic. New York: St. Martin's.
Siegel, F. P., and M. Siegel
   1983   AIDS: The Medical Mystery. New York: Grove.
Siegel, K., L. J. Bauman, G. H. Christ, and S. Krown
   1988   Patterns of Change in Sexual Behavior Among Gay Men in New York City. Archives of Sexual Behavior 17(6):481–497.

Siegel, K., F. P. Mesagno, J.-Y. Chen, and G. Christ
    1989   Factors Distinguishing Homosexual Males Practicing Risky and Safer Sex. Social Science and
           Medicine 28(6):561–569.
Simonsen, J. N., F. A. Plummer, E. N. Ngugi, C. Black, J. K. Kreiss, M. N. Gakinya, P. Waiyaki, L. J.
D'Acosta, J. O. Ndinya-Achola, P. Piot, and A. Ronald
    1990   HIV Infection among Lower Socioeconomic Strata Prostitutes in Nairobi. AIDS 4(2):139–144.
Singer, M., R. Irizarry, and J. J. Schensul
    1991   Needle Access as an AIDS Prevention Strategy for IV Drug Users: A Research Perspective.
           Human Organization 50(2):142–153.
Skurnick, J. H., R. L. Johnson, M. A. Quinones, J. D. Foster, and D. B. Louria
    1991   New Jersey High School Students' Knowledge, Attitudes, and Behavior Regarding AIDS.
           AIDS Education and Prevention 3(1):21–30.
Spada, J.
    1979   The Spada Report: The Newest Survey of Gay Male Sexuality. New York: New American
           Library.
Spanier, G. B., and R. L. Margolis
    1983   Marital Separation and Extramarital Sexual Behavior. The Journal of Sex Research 19(1):23–48.
Spiegel, C.
    1991   Study Shows AIDS Changing Sexual Behavior. Los Angeles Times, August 17.
Sprecher, S.
    1989   Premarital Sexual Standards for Different Categories of Individuals. The Journal of Sex
           Research 26(2):232–248.
St. Lawrence, J., T. L. Brasfield, and J. A. Kelly
    1990   Factors Which Predict Relapse to Unsafe Sex by Gay Men. Poster presented at the VI
           International AIDS Conference, San Francisco, Abstract F. C. 725.
St. Lawrence, J. S., H. V. Hood, T. Brasfield, and J. A. Kelly
    1989   Differences in Gay Men's AIDS Risk Knowledge and Behavior Patterns in High and Low AIDS
           Prevalence Cities. Public Health Reports 104(4):391–395.
Stall, R., T. J. Coates, and C. Hoff
    1988   Behavioral Risk Reduction for HIV Infection among Gay and Bisexual Men: A Review of
           Results from the United States. American Psychologist 43(11)878–885.
Stall, R., M. Ekstrand, L. Pollack, L. McKusick, and T. J. Coates
    1990a Relapse from Safer Sex: The Next Challenge for AIDS Prevention Efforts. Journal of Acquired
           Immune Deficiency Syndromes 3(12):1181–1187.
Stall, R., C. Frutchey, M. T. Fullilove, and P. Christen
    1990b Lessons from San Francisco: Principles of Program Design. IN Ending the HIV Epidemic:
           Community Strategies in Disease Prevention and Health Promotion. Pp. 98–110. S. Petrow,
           ed. Santa Cruz, CA: Network.
Stevens, C. E., P. E. Taylor, E. A. Zang, et al.
    1986   Human T-Cell Lymphotropic Virus Type III Infection in a Cohort of Homosexual Men in New
           York City. Journal of the American Medical Association 255:2167–2172.
Strunin, L., and R. Hingson
    1987   Acquired Immunodeficiency Syndrome and Adolescents: Knowledge, Beliefs, Attitudes, and
           Behavior. Pediatrics 85:24–29.
Symons, D.
    1979   The Evolution of Human Sexuality. New York: Oxford University Press.
Tatum, M. L.
    1988   Controversial Issues in the Classroom. IN The AIDS Challenge: Prevention Education for
           Young People. M. Quackenbush and M. Nelson with K. Clark, eds. Pp. 243–253. Santa Cruz,
           CA: Network.
Taylor, C. C.
    1990   AIDS and the Pathogenesis of Metaphor. IN Culture and AIDS. D. A. Feldman, ed. Pp. 55–65.
           New York: Praeger.
Taylor, C. L., and D. Lourea
    1992   HIV Prevention: A Dramaturgical Analysis and Practical Guide to Creating Safer Sex Interven-
           tions. Medical Anthropology 14(2,3,4):243–284.

Thompson, A. P.
   1983   Extramarital Sex: A Review of the Literature. The Journal of Sex Research 19(1):1–22.
Tindall, B., C. Swanson, B. Donovan, and D. A. Cooper
   1989   Sexual Practices and Condom Usage in a Cohort of Homosexual Men in Relation to Human
          Immunodeficiency Virus Status. The Medical Journal of Australia 151:318–322.
Tovey, S. J.
   1988 [1987]Letter to the editors. IN The AIDS Reader: Documentary History of a Modern Epidemic.
          L. K. Clarke and M. Potts, eds. Pp. 236–237. Boston: Branden. [The Lancet, March 7].
Troiden, R. R., and M. P. Jendrek
   1987   Does Sexual Ideology Correlate with Level of Sexual Experience? Assessing the Construct
          Validity of the SAS. The Journal of Sex Research 23(2):256–261.
Trudell, B., and M. Whatley
   1991   Sex Respect: A Problematic Public School Sexuality Curriculum. Journal of Sex Education &
          Therapy 17(2):125–140.
Tuller, N. R.
   1988   Couples: The Hidden Segment of the Gay World. IN Gay Relationships. J. P. De Cecco, ed. Pp.
          45–60. New York: Harrington Park.
Turner, C. F.
   1989   Research on Sexual Behaviors That Transmit HIV: Progress and Problems. AIDS 3(suppl):S63–
          S69.
Turner, C. F., H. G. Miller, and L. F. Barker
   1988   AIDS Research and the Behavioral and Social Sciences. IN AIDS 1988: AAAS Symposia
          Papers. R. Kulstad, ed.. Pp. 251–267. Washington: American Association for the Advancement
          of Science.
Turner, C. F., H. G. Miller, and L. E. Moses
   1989   AIDS, Sexual Behavior and Intravenous Drug Use. Washington: National Academy Press.
Ulene, A.
   1987   Safe Sex in a Dangerous World. New York: Vintage.
Valdiserri, R. O.
   1989   Preventing AIDS: The Design of Effective Programs. New Brunswick: Rutgers University
          Press.
Valdiserri, R. O., D. W. Lyter, L. C. Leviton, K. Stoner, and A. Silvestre
   1987   Applying the Criteria for the Development of Health Promotion and Education Programs to
          AIDS Risk Reduction Programs for Gay Men. Journal of Community Health 12(4):199–212.
Valdiserri, R. O., D. W. Lyter, L. C. Leviton, C. M. Callahan, L. A. Kingsley, and C. R. Rinaldo
   1988   Variables Influencing Condom Use in a Cohort of Gay and Bisexual Men. American Journal of
          Public Health 78(7):801–803.
   1989   AIDS Prevention in Homosexual and Bisexual Men: Results of a Randomized Trial Evaluating
          Two Risk Reduction Interventions. AIDS 3:21–26.
Valverde, M.
   1987   Sex, Power and Pleasure. Philadelphia: New Society.
Vance, C. S.
   1984   Pleasure and Danger: Toward a Politics of Sexuality. IN Pleasure and Danger: Exploring Female
          Sexuality. C. S. Vance, ed. Pp. 1–27. Boston: Routledge & Kegan Paul.
van Griensven, G. J. P., E. M. de Vroome, R. A. P. Tielman, J. Goudsmit, F. de Wolf, J. van der Noordaa,
and R. A. Coutinho
   1989   Effect of Human Immunodeficiency Virus (HIV) Antibody Knowledge on High-Risk Sexual
          Behavior with Steady and Nonsteady Sexual Partners Among Homosexual Men. American
          Journal of Epidemiology 129(3):596–603.
van Griensven, G. J. P., E. M. M. de Vroome, F. de Wolf, J. Goudsmit, M. Roos, and R. A. Coutinho
   1990   Risk Factors for Progression of Human Immunodeficiency Virus (HIV) Infection Among
          Seroconverted and Seropositive Homosexual Men. American Journal of Epidemiology
          132(2):203–210.
van Griensven, G. J. P., R. A. P. Tielman, J. Goudsmit et al.
   1987   Risk Factors and Prevalence of HIV Antibodies in Homosexual Men in the Netherlands.
          American Journal of Epidemiology 125:1048–1057.

Vaughan, M. A., and J. T. C. Li
    1988 [1986]Letter to the editors. IN The AIDS Reader: Documentary History of a Modern Epidemic.
        L. K. Clarke and M. Potts, eds. Pp. 266–268. Boston: Branden. [The New England Journal of
        Medicine, June 12].

Vincke, J., R. Mak, R. Bolton, and P. Jurica
    1991 Factors Affecting AIDS-Related Sexual Behavior Change Among Flemish Gay Men. Unpub-
        lished manuscript.

Voget, F. W.
    1975 A History of Ethnology. New York: Holt, Rinehart and Winston.

Volberding, P. A.
    1988 The AIDS Epidemic: Problems in Limiting Its Impact. IN The AIDS Challenge: Prevention
        Education for Young People. M. Quackenbush and M. Nelson with K. Clark, eds. Pp. 13–35.
        Santa Cruz, CA: Network.

Wagman, E., and S. O. Ludlow
    1988 Teacher Training for AIDS Education. IN The AIDS Challenge: Prevention Education for Young
        People. M. Quackenbush and M. Nelson with K. Clark, eds. Pp. 111–125. Santa Cruz, CA:
        Network.

Watney, S.
    1987 Policing Desire: Pornography, AIDS and the Media. Minneapolis: University of Minnesota
        Press.
    1989a AIDS, Language and the Third World. IN Taking Liberties: AIDS and Cultural Politics. E.
        Carter and S. Watney, eds. Pp. 183–192. London: Serpent's Tail.
    1989b Taking Liberties: An Introduction. IN Taking Liberties: AIDS and Cultural Politics. E. Carter
        and S. Watney, eds. Pp. 11–57. London: Serpent's Tail.

Weeks, J.
    1985 Sexuality and Its Discontents: Meanings, Myths & Modern Sexualities. New York: Routledge
        & Kegan Paul.

Weinberg, M. S., and C. J. Williams
    1974 Male Homosexuals: Their Problems and Adaptations. New York: Penguin.
    1975 Gay Baths and the Social Organization of Impersonal Sex. Social Problems 23:124–136.

Weinstein, N. D.
    1984 Why It Won't Happen to Me: Perceptions of Risk Factors and Susceptibility. Health Psychology
        3(5):431–457.

Weyer, J., and H. J. Eggers
    1990 On the Structure of the Epidemic Spread of AIDS: The Influence of an Infectious Coagent.
        Zentralblatt fur Bakteriologie 273:52–67.

Whitehurst, R. N.
    1969 Extramarital Sex: Alienation or Extension of Normal Behavior. IN Extra-Marital Relations. G.
        Neubeck, ed. Pp. 129–145. Englewood Cliffs, NJ: Prentice-Hall.

Wiktor, S. Z., R. J. Biggar, M. Melbye, P. Ebbesen, G. Colclough, R. DiGioia, W. C. Sanchez, R. J.
Grossman, and J. J. Goedert
    1990 Effect of Knowledge of Human Immunodeficiency Virus Infection Status on Sexual Activity
        Among Homosexual Men. Journal of Acquired Immune Deficiency Syndromes 3:62–68.

Williamson, J.
    1989 Every Virus Tells A Story: The Meanings of HIV and AIDS. IN Taking Liberties: AIDS and
        Cultural Politics. E. Carter and S. Watney, eds. Pp. 69–80. London: Serpent's Tail.

Willis, E.
    1988 Teenagers Have a Right To Express Their Sexuality. IN Teenage Sexuality. N. Bernards and L.
        Hall, eds. Pp. 175–179. Opposing Viewpoints Series. St. Paul, MN: Greenhaven.

Wilson, D. S.
    1990 Think No Evil: Male Prostitution and AIDS in the U.S. Paper presented at the annual meeting
        of the American Anthropological Association, New Orleans, Louisiana.

Winkelstein, W., D. M. Lyman, N. Padian, R. Grant, M. Samuel, J. A. Wiley, R. E. Anderson, W. Lang, J.
Riggs, and J. A. Levy
    1987a Sexual Practices and Risk of Infection by the Human Immunodeficiency Virus: The San
        Francisco Men's Health Study. Journal of the American Medical Association 257(3):321–325.

Winkelstein, W. M. Samuel, and N. S. Padian et al.
  1987b The San Francisco Men's Health Study: III. Reduction in Human Immunodeficiency Virus Transmission among Homosexual/Bisexual Men, 1982–1986. American Journal of Public Health 77:685–689.
Worth, D.
  1990 Minority Women and AIDS: Culture, Race, and Gender. IN Culture and AIDS. D. A. Feldman, ed. Pp. 111–135. New York: Praeger.
Zierler, S., L. Feingold, D. Laufer, P. Velentgas,
I. Kantrowitz-Gordon, and K. Mayer
  1991 Adult Survivors of Childhood Sexual Abuse and Subsequent Risk of HIV Infection. American Journal of Public Health 81(5):572–575.

Medical Anthropology, Vol. 14, pp. 225–242
Reprints available directly from the publisher
Photocopying permitted by license only

AIDS, Sex and Condoms: African Healers and the Reinvention of Tradition in Zaire

Brooke Grundfest Schoepf

Condoms offer considerable protection against sexual transmission of AIDS. Yet many Africans who are at risk of infection reject condoms as "unnatural." Data from Zaire have been used to examine this culturally constructed category in relation to sexuality, procreation, gender roles, class formation and international health and development policy. Much more than a simple transfer of biomedical technology is involved. Condom use with regular partners raises issues of cultural politics at many levels.

"Traditional" African healers represent important social networks with considerable authority in poor urban communities. They are able to reinterpret cultural categories and endow behavior with new meanings. Action-research in Kinshasa was used to explore roles that healers might play in promoting change to safer sex practices.

Key words: AIDS education, traditional healers, Zaire, ethnology

INTRODUCTION

This contribution addresses issues of cultural politics that have arisen in the context of AIDS prevention in Africa, where heterosexual transmission accounts for about eighty per cent of HIV infection. As many women as men are infected, and 30 to 40 per cent of infants born to seropositive women develop AIDS. From 35 to more than 90 per cent of poor commercial sex workers sampled in the cities of Central and East Africa are seropositive. Other young, sexually active women are at high risk, especially—but not only—those with multiple partners. Seroprevalence among urban parturient mothers—most of whom are married—ranges from 6 to 40 per cent. Among men, seroprevalence is highest in samples of high-income managers, the military, long distance traders and truck drivers. Co-factors which increase risk include other sexually transmitted diseases, unprotected sex with multiple partners, cervical ectopia and perhaps, lack of circumcision in men. Regular partners of infected persons are at risk, especially as immunosuppression progresses.[2]

Gender relations and sexual meanings are crucial to understanding HIV transmission and to developing effective disease control strategies (Schoepf, Payanzo, Rukarangira et al. 1988; Schoepf, Rukarangira, Schoepf et al. 1988; Schoepf, Walu, Rukarangira et al. 1988, 1991, in press). Since prevention depends upon behavior

BROOKE GRUNDFEST SCHOEPF, *13 Spencer Baird Rd., Woods Hole, MA 02543, is a medical and economic anthropologist and human relations trainer who has conducted research in eight African countries. In 1989 she organized the Pan-African Action-Research Network for Community-Based HIV/AIDS Prevention. She is currently a consultant to UNICEF on AIDS prevention.*

change, lack of attention to socioeconomic and cultural issues may contribute to the spread of HIV (cf contributors to Miller and Rockwell 1988; Schoepf 1988a,b,c). At the same time, there is a danger that cultural explanations may serve to excuse failures by policy makers in the international health arena to support effective prevention strategies (Schoepf 1991a).

Condoms offer considerable protection against sexual transmission of AIDS. Yet the argument has been made that many Africans who are at risk of infection reject condoms as "unnatural" and particularly inappropriate for use in regularly constituted partnerships.[3] Ethnographic data from Zaire have been used to explore these culturally constructed categories in relation to sexuality, procreation, gender identity, class formation and international health and development policy. Since much more than a simple transfer of biomedical technology is involved in advising people to use condoms, narrow technocratic approaches will have limited effectiveness. When programs fail, the victims, rather than the planners, may be blamed. Anthropological research that illuminates the context of these cultural issues may be used to help people reshape society as they institute and support protective behavior changes (Schoepf 1990f, 1991d). The case study reported here is one such learning-by-doing approach.

Earlier papers have described medical anthropology research conducted by the CONNAISSIDA Project in Zaire from 1985 to 1990. Constructed from the French word *connaissance* (knowledge) and *SIDA*, the acronym for AIDS, the project's name has a double signification. CONNAISSIDA means knowledge of AIDS (a passive form) and also knowing, or getting to know about AIDS (conceived as an active, participatory process). The collaborative project sought to develop a broad understanding of the spread of infection and the ways that AIDS is perceived and reacted to by the population—the cultural construction of AIDS—as well as to work with informants to develop culturally appropriate means of limiting the epidemic (Schoepf, Rukarangira and Matumona 1986; Schoepf 1986c). Methods included participant-observation, depth interviews with key informants, surveys, group interviews and action-research by a team of experienced investigators at home in the culture(s) of Zaire's two largest cities, Kinshasa and Lubumbashi, with a combined population of approximately 4 million.

Zaire is the second largest and the third most populous nation of sub-Saharan Africa, with an estimated 35 million people. Nearly 40 per cent live in urban areas. Zaire borders on nine other countries located in the high prevalence "AIDS Belt" stretching across Central Africa. This was the first epicenter of HIV infection in Africa. Some of CONNAISSIDA's findings are relevant for cultures and societies throughout the area (Obbo 1989; SWAA 1989; Bassett and Mhloyi 1991; Schoepf 1991e). They highlight the conjunction of the AIDS pandemic, economic crisis and gender roles (Schoepf, Payanzo et al. 1988; Schoepf, Rukarangira et al. 1988; Schoepf 1988a,b, 1989a,b; Rukarangira and Schoepf 1991).

CONNAISSIDA has argued that AIDS should be viewed as a "disease of development" (cf Hugues and Hunter 1970) and of "underdevelopment." That is, while AIDS is caused by a virus and biological co-factors enhance transmission of infection, the spread of the HIV is determined by socioeconomic processes set in motion by political and economic relations between Africa and the West. A number of studies have focused on probable impacts of HIV morbidity and mortality; others have identified cultural and behavioral risk factors in need of change.

However, relatively few scholars have turned their gaze toward the socioeconomic production of AIDS in Africa. Without understanding the social forces at work, it is unlikely that the HIV pandemic can be halted. In contrast, viewing AIDS as a development issue can open the way to community-based approaches to primary health care and HIV prevention (Schoepf, Rukarangira, Schoepf et al. 1988; Schoepf 1988b).

Disease epidemics often erupt in times of crisis. Zaire, like most other sub-Saharan nations and much of the Third World, is in the throes of a downward economic spiral (Young and Turner 1985; Nzongola-Ntaladja 1986). Propelled by declining terms of trade and burdensome debt service, the contradictions of distorted peripheral economies with rapid class-formation have created what appears to be permanent, deepening crisis (UNECA 1989; Adedeji 1990). Longitudinal family studies, life histories and household budgets show how the crisis affects women differently from men and how class and gender intersect (Schoepf and Walu 1987, 1991; Walu 1989; Schoepf 1992). Throughout Zaire, as in much of Africa, the crisis has been exacerbated by structural adjustment policies with especially deleterious effects on poor women and children (Schoepf 1988; 1990f; Newbury and Schoepf 1989; Adedeji 1990; Mbilinyi 1990; Seidman 1990; contributors to Gladwin 1991; Schoepf, Walu, Russell and Schoepf 1991). Linking macrolevel political economy to microlevel sociocultural analysis shows how sexual survival strategies used by poor women, in the presence of HIV have turned into death strategies. Action-research employing culturally informed participatory methods was used to study sexual behavior, to design community-based health promotion and to support preventive health action in different social settings (Schoepf, Walu, Rukarangira et al. 1988, 1991, in press). At the same time that the results indicate the potential for socially empowering community mobilization, they also point to the limitations of strategies that focus on individual behavior change.

The next section describes some of the action-research initiated by the CONNAISSIDA Project in Kinshasa, a city of 3.5 million people, in 1987. Some obstacles to change are noted. In the third section another form of alternative community-based prevention is described. "Traditional" healers were enlisted in reinterpreting cosmological elements in a way that may help to maximize condom use among couples at risk. The discussion explores advantages and disadvantages of enlisting healers in AIDS prevention.

ANTHROPOLOGY AND AIDS PREVENTION IN AFRICA

Early in 1985, as we learned of cases of heterosexually transmitted AIDS in Zaire, my colleagues and I proposed that understanding the cultural construction of this new disease would be crucial to slowing the spread of infection (Schoepf, Rukarangira, and Matumona 1986). We assumed that it would be necessary to address sensitive issues of sexuality and reproduction in their specific social contexts. In addition to innovative mass media communications, we suggested other culturally appropriate interventions that could be useful (Schoepf 1986c, 1987a). Rather than collecting questionnaire data on attitudes or sexual networks, we decided to look for naturally occurring interpersonal communication situations that could help people to assess their own risks and those of people close to them.[4]

We proposed that participatory anthropological research could be used to foster social empowerment leading to AIDS prevention and generate social support for change.

We adopted a team approach. Beginning in our own social networks, we listened to people in order to understand constraints to change. This yielded a non-random, snowballing sample which eventually included more than 1,200 interviews with people from many ethnic groups and from every socioeconomic level. Findings were discussed at weekly team meetings. Then we set out to find ways to disseminate information to people with limited literacy and little access to the mass media.[5] Using participatory non-formal education methods we sought ways to make complex biological knowledge understandable and to reduce mis-understandings among people with quite different concepts of health and illness than those of cosmopolitan biomedicine. We invited participants in these work-shops to join with us in devising ways to overcome constraints to change. These are things which our community-based pilot workshops have been extremely successful in doing. We also undertook a series of training workshops for BA-level social science graduates working as assistants in various government research units and selected several participants to conduct action-research with the team.[6]

The goal of finding appropriate forms of social support throughout the society to generate the impetus for behavior change met with rather less success. We had intended to conduct workshops with high level decision-makers as well as with ordinary people. The National AIDS Campaign, begun in mid-1987 with technical and financial support from the World Health Organization's Global Programme on AIDS (WHO/GPA), rapidly became a centralized bureaucratic affair which, predic-tably, stifled local initiatives such as ours (Schoepf, in press a).[7]

Nevertheless, we were able to conduct experimental risk-reduction workshops, first with women in a low-income neighborhood (Schoepf, Walu, Rukarangira, et al. 1988, 1991, in press) and subsequently with various other groups. Experiential training using structured exercises and other group dynamics techniques helped people to make their own risk assessments.[8] A combination of cognitive, emotional and social processes created a supportive environment in which many people were able to surmount the avoidance and denial stratagems which give rise to non-adaptive behavioral responses. Evaluation of these efforts showed that information and the desire to avoid infection are not sufficient to reduce situations of risk. For the vast majority of women at all socioeconomic levels, as well as for teen-age girls who will be at risk as soon as they become sexually active, the crucial issues are gender and class differences in economic and social power (Schoepf 1988a,b, 1989c; Schoepf and Walu, 1987, 1990, 1991; Schoepf, Walu, Rukarangira, et al. 1991, in press).[9] Many women, regardless of their age and socioeconomic circumstances, are not in a position to say "No" to sex or to negotiate the use of condoms.

Given these circumstances, personal empowerment and self-assertiveness train-ing may not be sufficient to change behavior. Commercial sex workers who as a result of the workshops began to introduce condoms to their clients, were stymied when university students "learned" from a European media source that condoms are "useless." When a group of churchwomen decided to discuss risk assessment and condoms with husbands whom they knew or suspected had outside partners, some angry husbands retaliated with threats; one withheld housekeeping money.

Women informants told us that change must begin with men, a conclusion shared by the pan-African Society of Women Against AIDS in Africa (SWAA 1989).

These difficulties notwithstanding, the women's groups have effectively supported members' efforts to change their children's behavior. Evaluation in December, 1989 found that the group had decided that the AIDS crisis is a new situation calling for new solutions. Some mothers had broken the taboo which constrains discussion of sexual subjects with unmarried children in order to help them understand the need for condom protection (Schoepf and Walu 1990). Several had supplied teens with condoms. They reported that husbands, while not taking similar action, tended to approve of the mothers' initiatives in this respect. However, most men still rejected dialogue with wives on the subject of personal risk assessment.

Because plural marriages are frequent and some sex occurs outside of marriage, many women feel vulnerable to HIV infection.[10] Some people (mainly but not exclusively women) adhere to precepts of marital fidelity and premarital abstinence which were present in some, but not all pre-colonial cultures and have been part of Christian teachings. However, cultural resistance to lifetime monogamy and Western-inspired views of sexuality is strong (especially, but not exclusively, among men). Peer pressures among men serve to maintain the "bar culture" (Schoepf 1987b), in which drinking leads to sexual adventures. Wives who attempted to raise the issue of extra-marital relations were rebuffed for their "atteinte aux Droits de l'Homme" (attack on The Rights of Man).

Sex also is part of the expected exchanges in various forms of patron-client relationships. Sexual harassment of schoolgirls and women in formal employment is reported widespread (cf Schoepf 1978). Personal identity, self-worth confirmed by others and social power are at stake for men. Complementing our analysis of linkages between sex and trade (Schoepf, Walu, Rukarangira et al. 1988; Rukarangira and Schoepf 1991), numerous informants point to links between sex and politics that have become institutionalized during the past twenty-five years of state-society conflict. These issues are explored in other work (Schoepf 1990d, in preparation).

Another goal developed during the course of research: to assess the impact of the national AIDS control campaign which began in 1987, using both survey and ethnographic methods.[11] Mass media campaigns stressed marital fidelity, avoidance of prostitutes and "sexual vagabondage," as well as clean injection syringes and blood transfusions. Condom protection was not vigorously pursued either in the media, or through leaflets and posters until 1990.[12] Many men, including some in official positions, attributed this avoidance to "traditional" norms of public discourse. However, since both Kenya and Uganda, with broadly similar "traditional" norms of polite speech have instituted poster campaigns, the "cultural" explanation may be specious. Media campaigns can use popularly understood circumlocutions—including those invented by the people themselves (Schoepf 1990c). It appears more likely that fear of offending religious leaders—many of whom are particularly conservative (Yates 1982)—coupled with the desire to control women's sexuality, contributed to muting the condom message.[13]

Focusing on prostitution, the campaign failed to convey explicit advice to all those who have had numerous partners in the past and those unable to limit their sexual relations to a single monogamous lifetime partner known to be infection-free. Although HIV infection is not confined to any particular risk group, many persons at risk continue to be unaware that they should use condoms for all sexual encounters *including* relations with regular partners. While one-fourth of single men sampled in 1988 reported that they had used condoms with casual partners (Bertrand, et al. 1991) and condom use is gaining favor (Mivumbi 1988; Harris 1990; Payanzo, Mivumbi, and Kakera 1990; Payanzo, Kakera, and Walmeier 1990), most contacts with regular partners continue to be unprotected even among those whose risk is quite high (Rukarangira and Schoepf 1989; Rukarangira et al. 1990).[14]

Other changes also are taking place. Some married men among our informants report that they have become faithful to their current partners. However, many more men report that although they have not limited their sexual activity to one partner, they have become more selective in their choice of partners. Selection criteria include:

choosing very young girls—to which commercial sex workers have responded by donning school uniforms;

choosing plump women, since weight loss is perceived as a sign of AIDS;

choosing women from the outlying neighborhoods, since women in the central city are perceived as a high-risk group;

restricting sexual relations to women they already know.

This partial list indicates that the National AIDS Committee's advice has been reinterpreted in light of popular assumptions about behavioral risk (Schoepf 1991b). In fact, many men who are at risk apparently have not yet come to terms with the full extent of the behavioral changes needed to prevent AIDS. Social legitimation of regular condom use is likely to be more effective than restrictive moralistic exhortation.

In view of widespread denial and avoidance, the urgent question is how to encourage people to make more realistic risk assessments without arousing so much fear that they "turn off" and become "fatalistic." Both of these dangers are immanent. For example, in early 1987 when the media reported as fact a U.S. physician's speculation that mosquitoes transmit AIDS, many people reasoned that since mosquitoes are ubiquitous, there is no escaping infection and therefore "we might as well enjoy life while we can." Early in 1988 a rumor that condoms do not protect from sexual transmission had a similar effect (Schoepf, Walu, Rukarangira et al. 1988). Reports of cures and vaccines offer false reassurance, diminishing people's perceived need for protective sexual behavior change.

Some cultural norms can be used to provoke preventive measures. Children are highly valued and constitute the *sine qua non* of most enduring unions. The news that children of infected mothers can be born with the infection is a powerful incentive for change. Some wives have urged husbands to join religious groups to help support their resolve to remain faithful. Young women from elite families in ethnic groups in which pre-marital virginity was highly valued, have sought to legitimate a "return to tradition" as a means to resist male pressure to have sex. A group of married blue-collar workers decided that, with discreet language, they could use their positions as clan elders to introduce the subject of protection of future generations. Nevertheless, they were dubious about the success of this initiative.

An interrelated set of constraints creates obstacles to condom use among stable couples (Schoepf 1988a, 1989a,b).[15] These include partners' inability to discuss their sexual histories or share realistic risk assessments, the desire for children, and cosmological concepts.

The first objection stated by many people is that condoms are "not natural." This appears to be a metaphor for the widespread belief that repeated contributions of semen are needed to form or "ripen" the growing fetus.[16] For those who believe thus, condoms are not merely "unnatural" in the Western sense of a pleasure-inhibiting technological intrusion. They also impede the natural human development process as this is culturally construed. Many believe that semen is a vital force, bringing "vitamins" necessary to women's continued physical and mental health, beauty and future fertility. Moreover, since condoms have been associated with prostitution and disease, proposing a condom signifies mistrust of the partner and is experienced as insulting. These are matters that extend beyond sexual partners to their respective families, which means that without a change in value consensus, "using condoms could cause endless complications," to quote one informant (Schoepf 1988a).

CULTURALLY APPROPRIATE CHANGE AGENTS

Given these beliefs, action-patterns, and social structures, who might be appropriate change agents? Social scientists have advised that in Africa "traditional" healers have an important role to play in caring for persons with AIDS (Good 1988). In addition, some have suggested that healers' knowledge of medicinals might be useful (G. Bibeau, personal communication, July 1986). Zairian scientists and WHO/GPA are evaluating natural substances used by traditional healers as potential anti-viral agents. The GPA also is interested in ". . . the utilization of traditional healers in the provision of social/medical support to AIDS patients. . . " (J. Esparza, personal communication, May 1989). Rather than relying on healers solely for treatment, I wished to discover if some might play a role in prevention (cf Good 1989), particularly in counselling risk reduction assessment and condom use.

An opportunity arose in February 1989 when I met Muganga Ilanga, who in addition to his duties as President of the Zairian Traditional Healers Association, also directs an experimental treatment center which combines "traditional" and biomedical therapies. One of several such facilities in Kinshasa, this one is patroned by the President's wife. Several AIDS patients had been referred to the Muganga's care by physicians. There are some special prevention issues which healers appear to be well-situated to address. The belief in the role of semen in fetal development, noted above, is one of these. I asked Muganga Ilanga if this might be interpreted metaphorically. My question was based on a suggestion by a nurse with three years of post-primary education who had reasoned thus in a workshop held with her Church Mothers' Club:

When the mother knows she is pregnant, the baby is already on its way to growing. The ancient ones meant that the husband should take an interest in his wife and not run around with other women while she awaits the child.

I suggested that while the ancestors were correct in stressing the health value of frequent sexual intercourse, they were not confronted by an AIDS epidemic which makes infected semen dangerous. The Muganga stated that "Of course it is love that grows the child and not the actual semen." He agreed to take up the challenge of AIDS prevention and invited me to hold a workshop with a group of his colleagues.

During the workshop an animated discussion on the meaning of semen and its role in procreation ensued. The healers' professional role became clearer in the process (cf Last and Chavunduka 1986). The group decided that they could tell people that semen is a metaphor for repeated intercourse. In other words, parents' frequent sexual relations foster the mutual love and understanding needed to provide a favorable nurturing environment for fetal growth. Thus actual semen is not needed and condoms can be used following conception to reduce risks of HIV infection to partners of people who do not know their serostatus. Since, like their predecessors, today's healers also are concerned with family and cultural survival, they are able to interpret cosmology in ways that facilitate condom use.

By asking about the possibility of such an alternative explanation, I had obliquely suggested a way for the healers to reshape cosmology in the context of a new situation. However, like their President, the healers' group opted for a view in which this interpretation, adapted to preserving health in the new context, always had been present in "traditional" cosmology. While none made explicit mention of it, this strategy enables them to claim that they are merely providing an explanation of an immanent principle rather than introducing change. To the anthropologist participant-observer, however, it is clear that the healers are reinventing tradition (cf Hobsbawm and Ranger 1984). Moreover, they are doing so in a way that demonstrates to biomedical practitioners that they are in possession of knowledge which is unassailable by "modern," i.e. biomedical, criteria.[17] The term "traditional" healers has been used with quotation marks due to the confusion it encapsulates (Schoepf 1986b). African healing methods and theory have not remained frozen in a timeless ethnographic present, but have changed and adapted with the times.

I emphasize this because the outworn notion of social versus biological causality is still applied with respect to AIDS. A discussant of my paper on AIDS research and ethics (Schoepf 1988c) declared that since Africans do not believe in the germ theory of disease causation, they cannot understand the need for protection from the HIV virus. Thus, by implication, efforts to promote behavior change are destined to fail. This sort of spurious cultural explanation also has been used by some physicians, in the U.S. as in Africa, to excuse their profession for its failures to respond to the sociocultural dimensions of disease (Schoepf 1975, 1988c, in press). However, while healers and their clients may attribute life-threatening and chronic conditions to social or supernatural etiology, the germ theory has also been accepted on a pragmatic basis. As elsewhere in Africa (Frankenberg and Leeson 1976; Gillies 1976; Ngubane 1977; Chavunduka 1978; Janzen 1978) urban healers in Kinshasa and Lubumbashi and many lay people, as well, employ pluralistic explanations (Schoepf 1976, 1982, in press a).

Studies of African healing practices show that pre-colonial traditions have been reinvented by incorporating symbols and practices from biomedicine (which healers may view as an invented, rigid tradition). In Zaire the new elements include white coats, the red cross, stethoscopes, examining tables and medicine cabinets and facsimiles of laboratory instruments. Occasionally one also sees elements from European folk healing traditions incorporated, for example a cat's skin formerly used in France and Belgium to cure chest ailments.

Nevertheless, change does not occur instantaneously. Although a consensus appeared to have emerged from the first workshop, several healers had reservations about using condoms. A second, impromptu, workshop took place when I visited the treatment center the following week. The healers, who had no further patient visits scheduled that afternoon, ushered me into the President's office. A woman who had not participated in the first session was brought up to date by her colleagues. They used the opportunity to pose questions which had occurred to them during the interval. The discussion indicated that they were engaged in making their own personal risk assessments and weighing the constraints which would impede behavior change. When discussion got blocked, role plays devised on the spot, helped the healers to re-center attention on finding solutions.

Arriving one hour into this discussion, the President took a seat behind his desk, extracted a condom from his pocket and tossed it across the room to me. He said: "We need to talk about this thing. A physician friend gave this to me." His gesture legitimated a demonstration of condom use which he understood that I had been reluctant to perform with this group of elder men and women. The eldest of the healers, a man in his fifties, expressed his own continuing reluctance to use the protective technology. He shook his head slowly:

I want to have another child. Since my wife is too old, I am going to take a "free woman" whose past, I have no doubt, places her at high risk. But since I want to procreate, I cannot use one of those things.

Instead of trying to dissuade him from a course of behavior upon which he evidently already had embarked, his colleagues explained how he could increase his chances of protection.

You can still protect yourself. When you want your wife to conceive, you don't use condoms. Then when you discover she is pregnant, you begin using the *Prudence*. You use them all the time that she is pregnant and while she is nursing the baby.

Prudence is the brand name for the condom distributed by a USAID-funded social marketing project. The package is printed with a leaping leopard, widely understood as a symbol of power and virility. The brand name has become synonymous with the prophylactic and is used as a euphemism by those who are reluctant to use the word condom (Rukarangira and Schoepf 1989). This solution is admittedly imperfect but more realistic than advising people to abstain from procreation. It would reduce the risk of partner infection and perinatal transmission in stable relationships.[18]

Continuing the healers' discussion, a woman colleague added:

That way the baby can nurse longer and the mother can have a rest. Then when you want another child, once again you stop using the condoms. You know how our grandmothers had children every three or four years. . .

Her contribution touched on another major issue involved in condom promotion. One aspect of the construction of condoms as "unnatural" is linked to its promotion as a population control technology by Western donor agencies. Many ordinary Zairians and officials reject this as an imperialist design (Schoepf et al. 1988a; Schoepf 1988b). While fertility continues to be highly valued, many people accept the idea of birth spacing and maternal protection (Schoepf 1983). This subject, dealt with obliquely by the healers, is one more example of the complex culturally sensitive issues involved in AIDS prevention. It indicates that the process of coming to terms with AIDS risk has both personal and political dimensions.

DISCUSSION

The two workshops held with leaders of Zaire's Traditional Healers' Association are an example of action-research which combines research and intervention. It is a form of learning-by-doing that engages researchers and key informants in dialogue, problem-posing and a search for solutions based on culturally-specific knowledge and pooled experience. The example shows how culture can be mobilized as a resource for overcoming constraints to change and illustrates one type of contribution anthropologists can make to AIDS prevention.

While their potential role merits further investigation, healers may be appropriate sexual behavior change agents for a number of reasons. First, they are an authoritative presence to many in the popular quarters and often are consulted by patients and families seeking treatment for sexual and reproductive health disorders. Healers legitimately give advice to people of all ages and both sexes. They have a ready-made lexicon for discussing sexual organs and acts not available in most polite discourse. This is important where cultural proscriptions tend to circumscribe ordinary conversation. Healers are more likely than many biomedical health workers to feel comfortable talking to people about sex. Perhaps most important, some healers are able to address men of high social status on the subject in ways that others cannot.

Second, as legitimate interpreters of customary rules of conduct, healers often are involved in reshaping or inventing "tradition" to meet changing circumstances. Third, while many healers today are Christians, they appear to have come to terms with religious, as well as medical, pluralism. Their discourse, while heavily seasoned with Christian belief, is nowhere near as moralizing as that of many university-trained men who have expressed opposition to educating the general public about condoms.

Fourth, African healing traditions involve patients' families not only as "therapy managers" (Janzen 1978), but as advisors and decision-makers in relations between sexual partners. Healers can legitimately address advice to senior members of kin groups to relax their objections to condoms. Since numerous informants cited elders' objections as a factor preventing dialogue between partners about AIDS prevention, removing this constraint might prove significant.

As we explore the potential of healers as change agents in AIDS prevention, a few words of caution are in order. Healers do not simply treat sickness with herbal preparations and other empirical methods, for which by biomedical evaluation might provide assessments of efficacy and safety. Many are also charismatic ritual specialists whose treatment of psychogenic disorders is probably the least controversial of their interventions. Closely associated with these activities is the use of charisma and power for social control (Schoepf 1981, 1982; Janzen 1982; Feierman 1985). Some are expert poisoners (Mudimbe 1981); this knowledge may be called upon to speed release from suffering.

The system rests upon etiological assumptions which many of us would not wish to bolster, particularly since women and the elderly often tend to be blamed for "causing" illness and death (Schoepf 1976, 1982, 1986b, 1989c).[19] Healers and politicians sometimes seek to enhance their social power by claiming to have caused death by sorcery. Alternatively, accusations may be made against political opponents in order to reduce their effectiveness. As AIDS deaths mount, the danger of scapegoating increases (Schoepf 1990a, 1991a). Anthropologists need to recognize and avoid providing legitimation for these processes.[20]

Additional questions arise with respect to other types of advice. A number of healers in Kinshasa and elsewhere believe that AIDS is an old African disease, for which some claim to have cures and vaccines. Most are likely to share popular misconceptions about transmission, as well. Some have advised patients to rid themselves of AIDS by transmitting it to others, an extension of an old, widespread belief. Elsewhere, this advice has been transformed into having sex with a virgin to rid men of AIDS; one consequence is increasing rape of young girls.

Without on-going collaboration and training, healers will act with their customary charisma and authority, rather than offering empowering dialogue effective for lasting behavior change. In view of these considerations, creating a new role for healers—who already provide much of the primary health care for poor rural and urban Africans—should be carefully planned and supported selectively. The effectiveness of this strategy should be assessed by means of participant-observation and user-focused impact evaluation as well as by controlled comparisons (Schoepf 1986c; Schoepf and Rukarangira 1989; Schoepf, Walu, Rukarangira et al. in press).

CONNAISSIDA has sought various ways to reach "hard-to-reach" groups with culturally appropriate non-formal adult education methods. There are many other organizations apart from churches that reach into the popular quarters of the city (Payanzo 1987).[21] Although they tend to be invisible to health agency officials, some, including the national trade union, taxi drivers', artisans', craft apprentices' and market women's associations and local elders' councils, could designate AIDS outreach workers to be trained and supported (Schoepf 1987a; Schoepf and Rukarangira 1989).

However, during CONNAISSIDA's lifetime, these were government organizations. Specialized units of the still-dominant, and until mid-1990, only, national political party, they were part of a corporatist state apparatus. As political changes begin to free these associations from such constraints, their new leaders may become more accountable to and trusted by their members. Such organizations might then be more amenable to HIV risk-reduction using social empowerment strategies. In the event, AIDS prevention could become part of a process of genuine (in contrast to formal) democratisation.

CONCLUSION

Condoms offer considerable protection against sexual transmission of AIDS, yet many who are at risk of infection reject them as "unnatural." Data from Zaire have been used to explore this culturally constructed category in relation to sexuality, procreation, gender roles, class formation and international health and development policy. Since much more than a simple transfer of biomedical technology is involved in condom adoption, ethnographic studies are needed to understand both resistance to change and the changes that are taking place. Such understanding can orient further prevention efforts.

Community-based AIDS prevention is needed to develop inter-personal methods of AIDS education and risk reduction support which complement mass media communications. The latter increase people's knowledge, but do not lead to rapid, widespread behavior change among many of those who are at risk in high-prevalence areas. Serious efforts to develop community-based strategies will have to move out of the health departments and look beyond the churches. There is a need to de-medicalize AIDS prevention without allowing it to be captured by a set of competing moralist discourses, to support the effort with funds and qualified professional collaborators.

"Traditional" African healers constitute important social networks with considerable authority in poor urban communities. Action-research in Kinshasa has been used to illustrate the role "traditional" healers might play in promoting change to safer sex practices. The healers' pragmatism contrasts with the moralistic stance of many intellectuals outside the health field. It indicates the extent of the healers' professionalism, and demonstrates that "traditionalism" is not necessarily an obstacle to change when cultural survival is understood to be at stake. This needs to be emphasized because "culture" is sometimes assumed to be the major obstacle to change despite anthropological research demonstrating dynamic interrelations of culture, social structure and human agency.[22]

The cultural construction of AIDS is complex, as are the social forces shaping the sexual relations that have led to the virus' spread. The latter include the region's historical political economy, and rapid class formation following independence, with their special gendered aspects. Because AIDS is a disease of development and underdevelopment, a product of the societies that have resulted from relations between Africa and the West, narrowly focused prevention strategies addressed to individuals are bound to fail.

Responsible anthropologists who grasp the nature of cultural reinterpretation processes taking place in a wide variety of milieux can do more than serve as adjuncts to the biomedical profession. The challenge to Western scholars with deep knowledge of African societies to collaborate with African colleagues will have to be met by a substantial resource commitment to theory-driven, anthropologically informed action-research on AIDS. Community-based reduction strategies using empowerment methods can help many people to protect themselves and others from HIV infection. However, broader societal change is needed to reverse the tide of deepening economic and social crisis which continues to reproduce risky behavior.

NOTES

1. Revised version of a paper presented at the 88th annual meeting of the American Anthropological Association, Washington DC, November 18, 1989. Submitted March 1, 1990; accepted November 20, 1990.

    Research was funded in part by the Rockefeller Foundation, Health Sciences Division and the Wenner-Gren Foundation for Anthropological Research. The article was written in 1989–90, while the author was an Evelyn Green Davis Fellow in the Social Sciences at the Bunting Institute of Radcliffe College. Grateful acknowledgement of this support and that of colleagues in Projet CONNAISSIDA, including Walu Engundu, Rukarangira wa Nkera, Payanzo Ntsomo and Claude Schoepf, does not imply their endorsement of findings. These remain the sole responsibility of the author.

2. References cited in Schoepf, Rukarangira, Schoepf et al. (1988) and new data summarized from Abstracts of the VI International AIDS Conference, San Francisco, June 20-24, 1990, 3 vols.

3. Numerous Western and African physicians and social scientists encountered at professional meetings between 1986 and 1990 expressed the view that African men (or men and women) would not accept condoms even though most are aware that AIDS is fatal and sexually transmitted.

4. A bilateral agency which received our proposals offered instead to fund a questionnaire survey of knowledge, attitudes and practices (KAP) by CONNAISSIDA's Zairian members under the direction of a physician. The offer was refused. USAID had already funded a large population-based KAP survey in Kinshasa (Bertrand et al. 1991).

5. Only 36 percent of households sampled in Kinshasa in 1986 had radios and the majority did not read newspapers (Houyoux et al. 1986).

6. These workshops received additional funding from OXFAM/UK.

7. The phenomenon is known locally as *"lourdeur administrative,"* a euphemism for bureaucratic corruption. It is part of the class formation process, with both political and economic aspects.

8. The workshop design was adapted by the author from experiential management training used previously in Zaire. It is similar to the participatory community development strategy based on Freirian pedagogy elaborated by Hope, Timmel, and Hodzi (1984).

9. Contemporary urban teenagers go to school when they can and look for income-earning opportunities when they cannot. Both women and men in cities rarely marry before age twenty and many do not marry until they are thirty or older. Teen sexuality is a delicate subject, particularly in the case of unmarried females, for whom it may not be considered legitimate (Schoepf 1988a).

10. Two-thirds of married women informants said that they knew or suspected that husbands had other partners.

11. Dr. Rukarangira (1990, in preparation) led a team surveying knowledge, attitudes and reported behavior in Lubumbashi early in 1987 and again in mid-1988. Two other projects have conducted large KABP surveys; CONNAISSIDA also made small KABP surveys with convenience samples of students and other respondents.

12. Other cited papers describe Zaire's AIDS control campaign.

13. Scripts for controlling women's sexuality have limited men's acceptance of family planning technology. For example, Professor Buakasa (in a 1985 paper for which I have lost the reference) opines that women who do not fear pregnancy will be prone to commit adultery. Despite lack of empirical evidence, this belief is widely shared.

    The Zaire Association of Moralists focused on "sexual discipline" as the way to prevent AIDS (cf Mvumbi 1987); its leaders opposed condom distribution to sex workers. In mid-1989, however, Professor Mvumbi withdrew his opposition (E. Walu, personal communication, January 1990).

14. An anonymous reviewer asks if the concept of adolescence is "appropriate for Zaire where not so

long ago, a woman could be married and have the full responsibility of adulthood once menses occurred. They were and still are considered young women, not adolescent girls." The reviewer conflates the cultures of some groups with all of Zaire and collapses time into an ethnographic present. Adolescence has existed in the Western sense at least since secondary school education became available to and sought-after by girls. Elsewhere, I argue that methodological and theoretical concerns are better served by historical specificity with respect to sexuality and marriage, as well as with respect to the status of women and gender relations (Schoepf 1985, 1987, 1989b,d,e, 1990c,d,f).

15. Abstracts of the Fifth International Conference on AIDS in Africa (10-12 October, 1990) indicate that the problem is common across the continent, but do not identify its causes.

16. The belief has been reported among the Zulu in South Africa (Ngubane 1977) and among the Kpelle in Liberia (Dr. Caroline Bledsoe, personal communication, January 1989). However, the Baganda do not share it (Dr. Christine Obbo, personal communication, November 1989; Dr. Mere Kisekka, personal communication, April 1990), nor do Tanzanian groups such as the Chagga and the Shambaa (interviews, August-October,1991).

17. Ranger (cf Hobsbawm and Ranger 1984) proposes that newly invented traditions (such as those made up by colonial officials to facilitate their rule) are more resistant to change than are "authentic" traditions which are continually being adapted, hence "re-invented."

18. Recent papers report that 50 percent of seropositive mothers whose infants were HIV infected continued to have children despite counselling (Abstracts, VI International AIDS Conference 1990).

19. An anonymous reviewer, who apparently ignored these concerns, advises that

. . . the author should emphasize the importance of the anthropologist-stranger in legitimizing the 'real' values of neo-colonial societies . . . those values that exists [sic] but the importance of which are often denied by those in positions of authority . . . [who are] often unwilling to acknowledge the authority of the precolonial world, traditional doctors, elders, etc.

The anthropologist then forms an interesting bridge in societies like Zaire where leaders feel impelled to appear Westernized . . . [despite anthropologists] collecting salaries associated with Western lifestyles. . .

Several of this reviewer's assumptions are mistaken. First, Zairian leaders and biomedically trained physicians acknowledge the role of "traditional" healers in several ways, some of which are indicated in this paper and in others cited. "Traditional" medicine is relied upon to provide health care to those who cannot obtain biomedical services or whom biomedicine fails. Many leaders retain diviners to enhance their political and business success, as well as to protect them from poisoning, sorcery and plotting by their enemies. CONNAISSIDA did not seek to legitimate the authority of healers or to enhance their power. In our view, to do so would be irresponsible (Schoepf 1981, 1982).

Second, contemporary urban culture is not merely an extension of pre-colonial cultures overlain by Western "accoutrements;" neither do elites automatically reject what the reviewer terms "real" values integral to earlier civilizations. Today's reality is extremely complex and diversely perceived by actors variously situated within a rapidly changing society.

Third, "the anthropologist" should not be assumed to be a Westerner; three of CONNAISSIDA's leaders are Zairian. Nor is the Western anthropologist in this case the beneficiary of "salaries associated with Western lifestyles." Both Claude Schoepf and I contributed our labor and knowledge *gratis* to this project. The "bridging" role involved obtaining U.S.-based resources, including grant funds and current international scientific literature.

20. A symposium of Traditional Healers at the VI International Conference on AIDS rejected this view.

21. Professor Payanzo, a founding member of CONNAISSIDA, was President of Kinshasa Region's parliamentary caucus in the National Legislative Council from 1984 to 1987. In 1989-1990 he was consultant to the USAID-funded Social Marketing Project; in 1991 he became Minister for Higher Education and Scientific Research.

22. See, for example, the debates which raged in the U.S. in an earlier period over the "culture of poverty" notion and cultural constraints to Third World development proposed by "modernization" writers.

REFERENCES CITED

Adedeji, A.
  1990   Development and Ethics: Can Africa Put Itself on the Road to Self-Reliant and Self-Sustaining Process of Development? Plenary Address, annual meeting of the African Studies Association. Baltimore, November 1-4.
Bassett, M.T., and M. Mhloyi
  1991   Women and AIDS in Zimbabwe: The Making of an Epidemic. International Journal of Health Services 21(1):143–146.
Bertrand, J.T., B. Makani, S.E. Hassig, et al.
  1991   AIDS-related Knowledge, Sexual Behavior and Condom Use Among Men and Women in Kinshasa, Zaire. American Journal of Public Health 81(1):53–58.
Chavunduka, G.
  1978   Traditional Healers and the Shona Patient. Gweru, Zimbabwe: Mambo Press.
Feierman, S.
  1985   Struggles for Control: The Social Roots of Health and Healing in Modern Africa. African Studies Review 28(2/3):73–147.
Frankenberg, R., and J. Leeson
  1976   Disease, Illness and Sickness: Social Aspects of the Choice of a Healer in a Lusaka Suburb. In Social Anthropology and Medicine. J. Loudon, ed. Pp.223–258. London: Academic Press.
Gillies, E.
  1976   Causal Criteria in African Classification of Disease. In Social Anthropology and Medicine. J. Loudon, ed. Pp. 358–395. London: Academic Press.
Gladwin, C., ed.
  1991   Structural Adjustment and African Women Farmers. Gainesville, FL: University of Florida Press.
Good, C.
  1988   Traditional Healers and AIDS Management. In AIDS in Africa: Social and Policy Impact. N. Miller and R. Rockwell, eds. Pp.97–113. Lewiston, NY: Edwin Mellen Press.
  1989   The Community in African Primary Health Care. Lewiston, NY: Edwin Mellen Press.
Harris, J.
  1990   USAID's Strategy for AIDS Prevention in Africa. Presentation at Roundtable on AIDS Research and Ethical Issues. Annual meeting of African Studies Association, Baltimore, November 1-4.
Hobsbawm, E., and T. Ranger, eds.
  1984   The Invention of Tradition. New York: Cambridge University Press.
Hope, A., S. Timmel, and P. Hodzi.
  1984   Training for Transformation: A Handbook for Community Workers (3 vols.) Gweru, Zimbabwe: Mambo Press.
Houyoux, J., N. Kinyavwidi, and O. Okita
  1986   Budgets ménagers à Kinshasa, Zaire. Kinshasa: Département du Plan.
Hughes, C., and J. Hunter
  1970   Disease and 'Development' in Tropical Africa. Social Science and Medicine 3:443–493.
Janzen, J.
  1978   The Quest for Therapy in Lower Zaire. Los Angeles, CA: University of California Press.
  1982   Lemba 1650-1930: A Drum of Affliction in Africa and the New World. New York: Garland Press.
Last, M., and G.L. Chavunduka, eds.
  1986   The Professionalisation of African Medicine. Manchester: Manchester University Press with International African Institute.
Miller, N., and R. Rockwell, eds.
  1988   AIDS in Africa: Social and Policy Impact. Lewiston, NY: Edwin Mellen Press.
Mivumbi, N.
  1988   Le marketing social comme un des moyens de lutte contre le SIDA. Paper presented at N'sele Condom Conference, Kinshasa, October.
Mudimbe, V.Y.
  1981   Signes thérapeutiques et prose de la vie en Afrique Noire. Social Science and Medicine 15B(3):195–211.

Mvumbi, N.
  1987   Anarchie sexuelle, SIDA et discipline de l'instinct sexuel. USAWA, Revue Africaine de Morale
         (Kinshasa) 2:27–36.
Newbury, C., and B.G. Schoepf
  1989   State, Peasantry and Agrarian Crisis in Zaire: Does Gender Make a Difference? In Women and
         the State in Africa. J.L. Parpart and K.A. Staudt, eds. Pp. 91–110. Boulder, CO: Lynne Reinner.
Ngubane, H.S.
  1977   Body and Mind in Zulu Medicine. London: Academic Press.
Nzongola-Ntaladja, ed.
  1986   The Crisis in Zaire: Myths and Realities. Trenton, NJ: Africa World Press.
Obbo, C.
  1989   AIDS, Women and Children in Uganda. Paper presented at the annual meeting of the African
         Studies Association, Atlanta, November 5.
Payanzo, N.
  1987   Structure et organisation de la ville de Kinshasa: Relevance pour la lutte contre le SIDA.
         Presented at CONNAISSIDA Training Workshop, CRSH, Kinshasa, July 15.
Payanzo, N., N. Mivumbi, and L. Kakera
  1990a AIDS, STDs and Condom Acceptability in High Risk Groups in Matadi, Zaire. Abstract Th D
         782. VI International AIDS Conference. San Francisco, June 20–24.
Payanzo, N., L. Kakera, and G. Wahlmeier
  1990b Condom Usage and Demand Among Zaire River Boat Travelers. Abstract Th D 783. VI
         International AIDS Conference. San Francisco, June 20-24.
Rukarangira, wN.
  in prep. Response to AIDS in Lubumbashi, Zaire. Takemi Program in International Health.
         Cambridge, MA: Harvard School of Public Health.
Rukarangira, wN., K. Ngirabakunzi, Y. Bihini, and K. Mpala
  1990   Evaluation of the AIDS Information Program Using Mass Media Campaign in Lubumbashi,
         Zaire. Abstract FD 844, VI International AIDS Conference. San Francisco, June 20-24.
Rukarangira, wN., and B.G. Schoepf
  1989   Social Marketing of Condoms in Zaire. WHO AIDS Health Promotion Exchange 3:2–4.
  1991   Unrecorded Trade in Shaba and Across Zaire's Southern Borders. In The Real Economy in
         Zaire. J. MacGaffey, ed. Pp. 72–96. London: James Currey; Philadelphia: University of
         Pennsylvania Press.
Schoepf, B.G.
  1975   Human Relations versus Social Relations in Medical Care. In Topias and Utopias in Health:
         Policy Studies. S.R. Ingman and A.E. Thomas, eds. Pp.99–120. The Hague: Mouton.
  1976   Recherches en anthropologie médicale: Théorie et perspectives méthodologiques. Bulletin
         d'Anthropologie Médicale (Lubumbashi) I:2 (Aout):20–36.
  1978   Les femmes dans l'economie informelle de Lubumbashi. Paper presented at IV International
         Congress of African Studies, Kinshasa, December 12–16.
  1981   Responsible Anthropology in Health Planning: Rethinking the Traditional-Modern Interface in
         Health Care Systems. Paper presented at the 80th annual meeting of the American Anthro-
         pological Association, Los Angeles, December.
  1982   Technology Transfer, Values and Social Relations in Health. In Proceedings of the Tuskegee
         Institute Inaugural Symposium. P. Wall, ed. Tuskegee Institute: Carver Research Foundation.
  1986a Out of Africa? Sociocultural Aspects of International AIDS Research. Colloquium, Depart-
         ment of Urban Studies, Public Health Program, Rutgers University, February 5.
  1986b Primary Health Care in Zaire. Review of African Political Economy 35:54–58.
  1986c CONNAISSIDA: AIDS Control Research and Interventions in Zaire. Proposal submitted to
         Rockefeller Foundation, November 12.
  1987a Community-Based Primary Prevention of AIDS in Zaire. Proposal submitted to USAID/
         Washington, Science and Technology/Health and Population, January 16.
  1987b Social Structure, Women's Status and Sex Differential Nutrition in the Zairian Copperbelt.
         Urban Anthropology 16 (1)73–102.
  1988a Women, AIDS and Economic Crisis in Zaire. Canadian Journal of African Studies 22 (3):625–
         644.

1988b Political Economy, Culture and AIDS Control. Paper presented at the International Union of Anthropological and Ethnological Sciences, Zagreb, July 26.

1988c Methodology, Ethics and Politics: AIDS Research in Africa for Whom? Paper presented at annual meeting of the American Anthropological Association, Invited Symposium on Ethics in AIDS Research, Phoenix, November.

1989a The Social Production of Heterosexual AIDS in Africa. Lecture in Medical Science and Moral Values. History of Science seminar series, Marine Biological Laboratory, Woods Hole, MA. July 20.

1989b Women and Children at Risk: An Update on AIDS in Zaire. Paper presented at the annual meeting of the African Studies Association, Atlanta, November 5.

1989c That Ethereal Light. . . The Invention of Marx in Africa. Paper presented at the annual meeting of the U.S. African Studies Association, Atlanta, November 5. To appear in Public Culture.

1989d At Risk for AIDS: Women's Lives in Zaire. Colloquium, Murray Research Center, Radcliffe College. December 12.

1989e Sex, Gender and Society in Zaire: The Sociocultural Production of AIDS. Bunting Lecture, Radcliffe College, December 13.

1990a AIDS in Eriaz. *In* AIDS on the Planet: The Plural View of Anthropology. G. Herdt, ed. Anthropology Today 6 (3):13–14.

1990b Theory and Practice in Anthropological Research with African Women. Paper prepared for Wenner-Gren symposium No.III, AIDS Research: Issues for Anthropological Theory, Method and Practice. Estes Park, CO. June 25-July 1.

1990c Sex, Gender and Society in Zaire. Paper prepared for IUSSP Seminar on Anthropological Studies Relevant to the Sexual Transmission of HIV. Sonderborg, Denmark, November 19-22.

1990d Political Economy, Culture and Meanings of AIDS in Zaire. Paper prepared for Symposium on Cultural Studies of Disease Epidemics, Massachusetts Institute of Technology, October, 19-20.

1990e Widening the Gaze: Empowerment Strategies for AIDS Prevention. Presentation at Roundtable on AIDS Research and Ethical Issues. 33rd annual meeting of African Studies Association, Baltimore, November 1-4.

1990f Gender Relations in Development: Political Economy and Culture. Review paper commissioned by the ASA Task Force on Sustainable Development in Africa, Workshop on Gender and Households. 33rd annual meeting of African Studies Association, Baltimore, November 1-4.

1991a Ethical, Methodological and Political Issues of AIDS Research in Central Africa. Social Science and Medicine 33(7):749–763.

1991b Connaissances du SIDA: Représentations et pratiques populaires à Kinshasa. Anthropologie et Sociétés 15,2-3

1991c Comments on Packard and Epstein. Social Science Medicine 33(7):791–793.

1991d HIV/AIDS Draft Strategy Statement, UNICEF, Tanzania.

1992 Women at Risk: Case Studies From Zaire. *In* Social Analysis in the Time of AIDS. G. Herdt and S. Lindebaum, eds. Pp.259–286. Newbury Park, CA: Sage Publications.

in press a Political Economy and Cultural Logics: A View From Zaire. African Urban Quarterly.

in press b Knowledge of Women, Women's Knowledge: Texts of 'Tradition' and 'Modernity' in Zaire. *In* The Transfer of Knowledge From Europe to Africa. B. Jewsiewicki, ed.

in prep. Women, Sex and Power: Zaire in the AIDS Era.

Schoepf, B.G., N. Payanzo, wN. Rukarangira, E. Walu, and C.Schoepf
1988 AIDS, Women and Society in Central Africa. *In* AIDS 1988: AAAS Symposium Papers, R. Kulstad, ed. Pp.175–181. Washington, DC: AAAS.

Schoepf, B.G., and wN. Rukarangira
1989 CONNAISSIDA: Community-Based HIV Risk Reduction Support in Zaire. Proposal submitted to USAID/Washington, HAPA Grants Program for Africa, March.

Schoepf, B.G., wN Rukarangira, and M.M. Matumona
1986 Etude des Réactions à une nouvelle maladie transmissible (SIDA) et des possibilités de démarrage d'un programme d'education populaire. Research Proposal to Government of Zaire and USAID, August.

Schoepf, B.G., wN. Rukarangira, N. Payanzo, C. Schoepf, and E. Walu
1988 AIDS and Society in Central Africa: A View From Zaire. *In* N. Miller and R. Rockwell, eds. Pp.

211–235. Reprinted in The Heterosexual Transmission of AIDS in Africa, D. Koch-Weser and H. Vanderschmidt, eds. Pp. 265–280. Boston: Abt.

Schoepf, B.G., and E. Walu
  1987   Women's Survival Strategies and AIDS in Kinshasa. Colloquium, Columbia University, Institute of African Studies, December 4.
  1990   CONNAISSIDA: Community-Participation in AIDS Research. Worshop on AIDS Research Methodologies, Siavonga, Zambia, April 16-22.
  1991   Women's Trade and Contribution to Household Budgets in Kinshasa. *In* The Real Economy in Zaire, J. MacGaffey, ed. Pp. 124–151. London: James Currey; Philadelphia: University of Pennsylvania Press.

Schoepf, B.G., E. Walu, wN Rukarangira, N. Payanzo, and C. Schoepf
  1988   Community-Based Risk Reduction Support in Zaire. Paper presented at 1st SIECS meeting Ixtapa, Mexico, October 10-15. Revised version forthcoming in AIDS Prevention Through Health Promotion: Changing Behaviour. R. Birkvens, ed. Geneva, WHO.
  1991   Gender, Power and Risk of AIDS in Central Africa. *In* Women and Health in Africa, M. Turshen, ed. Pp 184–203. Trenton, NJ: Africa World Press.
  in press   Action-Research on AIDS with Women in Kinshasa. Social Science and Medicine.

Schoepf, B.G., E. Walu, D. Russell, and C. Schoepf
  1991   Women and Structural Adjustment in Zaire. *In* Structural Adjustment and African Women Farmers. C. Gladwin, ed. Pp. 151–168. Gainesville, FL: University of Florida Press.

Seidman, A.
  1990   Africa: Development and Ethics. Presidential address, 33rd annual meeting of the African Studies Association, Baltimore, MD, November 1-4.

Society for Women and AIDS in Africa (SWAA)
  1989   Report of the 1st International Workshop on Women and AIDS in Africa. Harare, May 10-12.

United Nations Economic Commission for Africa (UNECA)
  1989   African Alternative to Structural Adjustment Programmes: A Framework for Transformation and Recovery. Addis Ababa: UNECA.

Walu, E.
  1987   Stratégies de survie des kinoises face à la crise economique. Seminar, Center for International Studies, University of North Carolina, Chapel Hill, November 17.
  1989   SIDA et sociètè: Histoires à vie des kinoises. Paper presented at AIDS and Society Workshop, Centre de Recherches en Sciences Humaines, Kinsha, July 15.

Yates, B.
  1982   Colonialism, Education, and Work: Sex Differentiation in Colonial Zaire. *In* Women and Work in Africa. E.G.Bay, ed. Pp. 127–152. Boulder, CO: Westview Press.

Young, M.C., and T. Turner
  1985   The Rise and Decline of the Zairian State. Madison, WI: University of Wisconsin Press.

Medical Anthropology, Vol. 14, pp. 243–284
Reprints available directly from the publisher
Photocopying permitted by license only

HIV Prevention: A Dramaturgical Analysis and Practical Guide to Creating Safer Sex Interventions

Clark L. Taylor and David Lourea

Safer sex is currently a major strategy for preventing HIV transmission. We examine safer sex interventions using an interactionist form of dramaturgical analysis. This approach yields a dynamic model with which to generate novel safer sex interventions highly sensitive to changing individual, cultural, and social variables. Our goal is to help medical anthropologists, applied social scientists, health educators, community outreach specialists, and those who are sexually active apply safer sex strategies more effectively.

Key words: HIV, prevention, education, intervention

INTRODUCTION

In this article, we first discuss safer sex as an approach to preventing HIV transmission. Then we examine the structure and content of selected safer sex interventions using dramaturgical analysis.[1] This analysis allows us to organize and compare a wide range of safer sex techniques and to construct a dynamic model of safer sex interventions. The usefulness of the model lies in its ability to help integrate general safer sex principles into the changing matrix of individual, cultural, and social variables encountered in prevention contexts.

The interventions chosen for analysis draw heavily upon our personal experience as sexologists with training in applied medical anthropology, sex education, and sex therapy. Many of the safer sex strategies sexologists use are shared with other professions and grassroots groups. However, applying an anthropological analysis to sexological perspectives helps focus attention directly upon sexual well-being and the purposeful construction of safer sex subcultures.

Like many other professionals working in HIV prevention, we as sexologists use qualitative ethnographic methodologies and applied social science techniques to

CLARK L. TAYLOR *is a medical anthropologist and sexologist at The Institute For Advanced Study Of Human Sexuality in San Francisco, California. He is also Director of The AIDS/STD Prevention Applied Research and Education Project of The Center for Research and Education in Sexuality (CERES), San Francisco State University, 1600 Holloway Avenue, Psychology Bldg. Rm. 502, San Francisco, CA 94132 . His research interests include sexual health, behavioral modification and culture change.*

DAVID LOUREA *is a sex therapist and senior faculty member of The Institute For Advanced Study Of Human Sexuality, 1523 Franklin Street, San Francisco, CA 94109. He co-founded and directs the Bisexual Counseling Services, one of the first agencies for bisexuals in the United States. His special research interests are sexual health, HIV prevention and bisexuality.*

learn the sexual culture of the communities we serve and to integrate community sexual strengths and weaknesses into our interventions. Further, we recruit sexual community members to help in intervention design and the creation of culturally specific materials, and to participate in actual presentations. Unmarried or non-monogamous sexually active people and members of many sexual subcultures have a long history of being abused by sex negative elements of the formal social structure. Participation in the educational process helps to develop trust in professional safer sex interventions. Inclusion also helps turn the populations served into active participants in the solution to prevention problems. It turns participants in the intervention process into community resources, leaders and safer sex advocates.

Our major objective in writing this article is to help medical anthropologists, applied social scientists, health educators, community outreach specialists, and sexually active readers use safer sex strategies more effectively.[2]

SAFER SEX AND THE SAFER SEX MOVEMENT

"Safer sex" is a supportive approach to preventing HIV transmission. It seeks to bring sexual patterns into agreement with medically sound AIDS prevention guidelines. Since 1981 safer sex has emerged as a grassroots social movement and major epidemiological strategy. Indeed, programs using safer sex techniques are currently implemented throughout the world (Cassidy and Porter 1988).[3]

The safer sex movement is based upon cultural values of the first U.S. sexual communities ravaged by AIDS and the humanistic orientation of many in the professions who came to their assistance—the health field, sexology, social work, education, and the social sciences. The sexual communities first affected were primarily gay and bisexual males, their female partners, and S&M subcultures. Many (but certainly not all) of the early professionals working to develop safer sex were also respected members of the communities served.

As its origins might imply, safer sex is a practical application of intellectual, social, and political worldviews which emerged from the sexual revolution of the 1950s and the sexual liberation movements of the 1960s and 1970s. Indeed, some look at AIDS as both a challenge and an opportunity to move the sexual revolution forward by purposefully incorporating sexually transmitted disease prevention into our personal lives and cultural institutions (McIlvenna 1987:1–23).[4]

The safer sex movement views sexuality as a positive aspect of life. A basic tenet is that most individuals find their sexual lifestyles enjoyable, but that AIDS makes changes in many activities, customs, and attitudes necessary. The movement seeks to help people modify sexual behavior associated with transmission in order to eliminate or reduce potential danger. It works to expand the range of health supportive sexual options people can enjoy and to maximize the erotic appeal of HIV prevention. Guidelines couched in desexualized academic jargon are translated into the language of intimacy, passion, and sex: physical barrier prophylactics, condoms, are transformed into healthy sex toys, accessories for increased sexual enjoyment.

The movement approaches safer sex as fun. Before AIDS, members of sexual communities forever were exploring new forms of sexual enjoyment. Safer sex is a purposeful continuation of this process. Sexologists find it is much easier for people to increase sexual options than to extinguish established patterns, make unfamiliar substitutions, or achieve abstinence. When people have many low risk techniques for achieving sexual satisfaction, it is less burdensome to let go of unsafe sex. Psychologically, having as a goal a richer, healthier, more satisfying sexlife is easier to work toward than trying to resist temptation, failing, and relapsing or maintaining a low level of sexual functioning (McIlvenna 1987:6).

To help the most people, the safer sex movement focuses upon personal empowerment and social transformation. Ten years into the AIDS epidemic our experience is that given sex-positive, non-judgmental information in a supportive environment, most people create the safer sex lifestyles and cultural forms that best express who they are and meet their personal needs. A basic strategy of safer sex is to validate the strength individuals have and help people use the knowledge learned during interventions to empower the sexual communities in which they participate. In transforming their personal lives and working within their sexual communities, people impact not only their own subcultural values, norms, and expression, but also the total culture of sex. Reviews of safer sex and behavioral change support the view that safer sex is significantly impacting HIV transmission (Becker 1978:394–411; Stall and Coates 1988:878–885). And popular response to the safer sex movement indicates that not only do millions of people want sex positive healthy lifestyles, they also are willing to give money to promote them.

The safer sex movement attempts to articulate prevention strategies within the total context of the subcultures being addressed. It recognizes that issues such as: racism, sexism, ethnocentrism, the economics of everyday life, religious values, addiction, other health issues, and ethnic survival in a pluralistic society, may be more important to the groups served than HIV prevention.

The safer sex movement brings balance and contrast to approaches which regard *unsafe sex* as a manifestation or cofactor of mental illness, low self esteem, lack of reason, sexual obsession, drug and alcohol addiction, poverty, prostitution, homelessness, and so forth. Medical and social problems contribute to unsafe sex, and programs to alleviate these conditions are extremely important. However, as a general approach, traditional "medical" or "welfare" models tend to: a) look at personal dysfunction or inadequacy as the main cause of unsafe sex; b) neglect the difficulties ordinary people often have in coping with HIV prevention guidelines and; c) ignore non-pathological factors embedded in the culture of sex which can aid or impede prevention.[5]

Mental health, high self-esteem, reason, continence, temperance, financial security, and virtue are highly desirable, but as the lists of those with HIV disease or who have died of AIDS prove, these qualities do not assure compliance with HIV guidelines. When people are not having sex, reason can convince them safer sex is wise and necessary. However, actual sexual encounters are rarely exercises in meditation and reason. In the heat of passion and other powerful emotions, choosing prevention often depends more on physical pleasure, habit, meaning, acceptability, and excitement than on information, logic, and virtue. Prevention must be compelling and seductive on all levels to prevail when circumstances make compliance most difficult. This is why the safer sex movement concentrates both upon maximizing the physical, emotional enjoyment of sexual health strategies and developing an exuberant, erotic culture of safer sex contexts, meanings, customs, folkways, patterns, and institutions. These approaches are equally appropriate to the general public as well as those who are receiving rehabilitative assistance.[6]

SAFER SEX AND DRAMATURGICAL ANALYSIS

The form of dramaturgical analysis used in this paper is derived from social interactionist approaches to understanding human behavior. Interactionist perspectives in general strive to compare discrete but cognitively related social interactions and to describe the rules governing the dynamics of such behavior. For example, in the following analysis, we integrate and provide a structural framework for such diverse safer sex interventions as workshops, community outreach, training programs, and actual safer sex encounters.

Those who take an interactionist perspective often use analytical frames drawn from the artificially constructed worlds of games, ritual, and drama to aid in creating dynamic models of "everyday" social behavior. We have chosen a theatrical frame of analysis because the major form of interventions studied here *are* conscious performances, scripted and presented much like theater. Our model equally applies, however, to more spontaneous interventions (such as actual safer sex encounters) and these are also included in our analysis.

As an adjunct to the theatrical frame, we look at safer sex interactions as a form of play or love games.[7] Sex usually takes place during play or leisure time, and we want our educational interventions to parallel or simulate sexual reality as often as possible. As a caution, "play" and "games" should not imply that safer sex interventions are simply an exercise in frivolity. There are serious, frivolous, educational, romantic, comical, mundane, and many other kinds of safer sex interventions.

When we think of the real world in terms of theater or games, we are able to remove ourselves somewhat from everyday existence. This makes it easier to reflect on regularities, patterns, and relationships that exist in the continuously flowing, unfolding experience of life. It also provides a rich variety of tools and concepts with which to study these structural components, identify ordinary problems, or create novel variations.

We construct a model of safer sex interventions somewhat as a critic employs dramatic concepts to study a genre of plays. Just as a critic picks and chooses from the conventions of theater to find what best fits the task, we carefully select the concepts which help us analyze safer sex interventions as accurately as possible. The theatrical frame furnishes conceptual tools such as audiences, players, rehearsals, plots, dialogues, and action. The framework of games supplies teams, moves, winning, losing, et cetera.

TITLES AVAILABLE—A SAFER SEX PERFORMANCE REPERTOIRE

We open our analysis with a catalogue of safer sex interventions amenable to dramaturgical analysis. There is a bewildering variety of safer sex interventions from the individual steps people take to elaborate, coordinated international programs. A first step in organizing these myriad activities is to divide them into discrete units. This we do in the present context by defining each safer sex intervention, no matter how small or large, as a "dramatic scripting" or simply a "performance" (Goffman 1974:124–125). Thus, for example, "entering a store and buying condoms" would be one dramatic scripting or performance; "creating a safer sex program for the deaf" another; and "attending a safer sex party" still another. Dramatic scriptings often overlap, are disconnected or form part of larger safer sex performances on life's stage. Thus the following repertoire is merely suggestive of the interventions available for analysis.

Pure Performances and Cheap Spectacles

Dramatic scriptings, nightclub acts, personal appearances of various sorts, the ballet, and much of orchestral music are pure. No audience, no performance. [Goffman 1974:24]

*   Safer sex lectures, workshops, erotic non-sexual demonstrations, theatrical productions, and live safer sex explicit entertainment.
*   Training and certification programs for health professionals, educators and others who work in safer sex.
*   Periodic safer sex events such as National Condom Week and National AIDS Day.
*   Safer sex "house parties" or "fuckerware parties" where friendship networks or members of special ethnic or sexual groups get together in a home to learn safer sex techniques and technology.
*   All male (Jack), all female (Jill) and heterogeneous (Jack and Jill) group masturbation club events and parties.
*   Private condom testing parties using low risk sexual activities to become adept at condom use before future employment in penetration sex.
*   Cooperative ventures between AIDS prevention agencies and sexual communities to provide guided, concrete safer sex experiences and create community support.

Daily Dramas, Serials and Tableaux

*   The ongoing creation, marketing and distribution of a large array of safer sex materials including (but not limited to) training manuals for experts, self help books, condom sampler kits, erotic safer sex short stories, cartoon strips, comic books, safer sex billboard ads, phone sex lines, computer networks, novels, explicit and non-explicit educational videos, explicit safer sex entertainment videos, calen-

dars, posters, lapel buttons, condom key chains and "Safe Sox" (socks with side pockets that hold condoms).[8]

* The distribution of free or low cost condoms, dental dams, latex gloves, lubricants and spermicides.

* Safer sex fashion shows and home demonstrations of novel accessories such as condoms that are extra stretchy, scented, or glow in the dark and condom compatible flavored lubricants; latex fantasy clothes, pelvic harnesses for dental dams, and latex shorts with built-in condoms and/or dildos.

* The recruitment, participation and varied display of attractive, famous or appropriate role models to serve as "Rubbermen," "Poster Puppies," and "Safe Sex Playmates."

* The regular appearance of safer sex "want ads" and advice columns in local, national and international publications.

Improvisation and Command Performances

* Safer sex encounters in bedrooms, bathrooms, kitchens, parks, beaches, theaters, laundromats, elevators, alleys, cars, vans et cetera.
* Safer sex surprise performances in new or ongoing relationships.
* Premier condom debuts of virgins, rakes, porno stars and spouses.
* Home video documentaries of outstanding safer sex performances.

Within the vast range of safer sex interventions we will concentrate primarily upon the more formal or "pure" type performances with occasional references to other types of scriptings. Since our model is constructed to fit all types of safer sex interventions, we have included an abbreviated script of an eight-day training workshop as Appendix A to help unfamiliar readers visualize how a finished product using this type of model might look.

THEATERS, STAGES, PLAYERS AND AUDIENCES

All the world *is* like a stage, we *do* strut and fret our hour on it, and that is all the time we have. But what's the stage like, and what are those figures that people it? [Goffman 1974:124]

Having reviewed the repertoire of performances, let us look briefly at the theaters where these dramatic scriptings take place, the repertoire companies which enact them and the audiences for whom they are performed. To use the following model for actual safer sex encounters, specific outreach educational interactions and other less formal scriptings simply modify the scope, variables and scenario to fit the particular occasion. Add or discard dramaturgical and gaming concepts as appropriate to meet the requirements of specific interventions.

Theaters

Safer sex theaters and stages are any place safer sex dramatic scriptings can occur. This may be actual theaters or auditoriums, but more often they are classrooms, club houses, churches, cafeterias, community centers, bars, bath houses, schools, brothels, night clubs, convention halls, barracks, dormitories and lounges. For less formal scriptings such as outreach work in sexual locales, the theaters of action are streets, alleys, parks, beaches, rest stops, bathrooms, bedrooms, hotel rooms— anywhere educational performances are possible. And of course, explicit safer sex encounters take place anywhere people can find enough safety and privacy. As we will see, every safer sex theater has its advantages and limitations.

Players, Audiences, and Interactional Theater

We often think of players and audiences as distinct groups separated from each other physically and by convention. As Goffman points out:

A line is ordinarily maintained between a staging area where the performance proper occurs and an audience region where the watchers are located. The central understanding is that the audience neither has the right nor the obligation to participate directly in the dramatic action occurring on the stage. . . . [Goffman 1974:124]

From this perspective, it is very easy to tell who the actors and audience are; the actors are those who impart safer sex interventions and the audiences are those who receive them. Highly staged safer sex performances sometimes follow these conventions. However, more often dramatic scriptings use a technique which dramatists call "interactional theater." In interactional theater, the traditional line between audience and players shifts, becomes indefinite and sometimes vanishes. The technique is commonly used in night club acts, TV talk shows, magic acts and improvisational skits. Members of an audience are brought onto the stage to take part in a production; actors leave the stage and go into the audience and talk with the spectators or watch the audience become the show (here, the audience area becomes the stage). Sometimes actors and audiences collude to make the stage disappear entirely—they play as though a performance were not taking place at all.

The use of interactional theater in staged safer sex performances is perhaps most clear in participatory exercises such as psychodrama, discussion groups, condom team relay games and communication exercises. In public outreach and sponta- neous interventions, interactional theater is usually the norm. To illustrate chang- ing roles and stages consider a hypothetical safer sex outreach worker: first s/he is in role performing safer sex dramatic scriptings for audiences of clients; then the worker might become part of an audience being taught safer sex by the clients themselves (who have become the performers); next, perhaps the worker becomes involved in a "play within a play"—being watched by an audience of interested bystanders while engaged in a dramatic scripting with clients.

While interactional theater is useful for describing the ever changing nature of safer sex theater, actors and audience, it has other important functions. We can use interactional theater to help modulate and predict the amount of information an audience will learn and be able to translate into behavior in their sexlives. An important learning principle, supported by extensive research, is that persons learn best when they are actively involved in the learning process. The most abstract and distant information is from the learner, the less a person learns; and the more concrete a learning experience is (the closer it duplicates or simulates reality), the greater the learning and transferability become (Dale 1954:42–56; Stewart 1969:134–171). From this perspective, the greater the amount of interactional theater used in safer sex interventions, the more effective the intervention will be.

Thus, performances which use a strict division between audience and actors provide a low amount of learning and transferability while scriptings which employ a high degree of interaction between players and audience create an environment for high learning and transferability. Performances in which the audience become the actors stimulate the highest degree of learning and transferability. As a pioneer in learning systems theory, Egar Dale, once wrote "Direct reality itself as we experience it firsthand. . . is the rich full-bodied experience that is the bedrock of all education" (1954:43). From this perspective, actual guided safer *sex* is potentially the best form of risk reduction education a person can receive.

There are examples of such interventions in our safer sex performance repertoire. However, explicit safer sex performances obviously are not possible in most formal educational contexts. In addition, audiences must be viewed from the perspective of how they best access information. For since safer sex performances are embedded in social context, the effectiveness and desirability of concrete interventions is mediated by factors such as the motivation and ability of an audience to accept such performances and the suitability of the theatrical locale to support them. But the continuum—abstract instruction to simulated and concrete experience—provides a highly useful measurement of program effectiveness. Based upon Dale's Cone of Learning (1954:42) and Stewart's learning systems concept simulation protocol (1969:161), safer sex strategists can anticipate that people will remember and be able to transfer to real life situations approximately:

   a) 10% of what they *read*
   b) 20% of what they *hear*
   c) 30% of what they *see*
   d) 50% of what they *hear* and *see*
   e) 70% of what they *say or write*
   f) 90% of what they *say as they do a thing*

In learning systems theory, all of the modalities listed above should be built into educational modules to take advantage of the ways in which individual members learn best and to fit the learning technique to the material being presented. In planning safer sex interventions, first look at the nature of the information to be imparted, then decide the type and amount of interactional theater to use taking into account the nature of the locale, and receptivity of the audience.

Safer sex performances are only as good as the accuracy of the medical guidelines presented. It is by far best as a strategy to discuss the range of medical opinion accurately and encourage the participants to decide what is most appropriate to their particular life circumstances. Players who facilitate erotic safer sex presentations must have a low burden of guilt and shame about their own sexuality and an accepting attitude about the sexuality of others to work effectively. Facilitators without these qualities sabotage and destroy performances.[9]

MAGIC TIME AND SPACE

As an altered state of consciousness, sex occurs in a magic time and place. Theatrical performances and games also share this important quality. In educational safer sex performances this similarity can be used to great advantage. Presenters and audience alike can *"take time out"* from *"real life"* to create *"play"* or *"make believe"* worlds in which the ordinary rules of social life are temporarily suspended.[10] Safely removed from ordinary time and space, people are much more open to learning and/or trying out new safer sex possibilities. When the "play" is over, and "real life" resumes, participants are free to discard or incorporate elements of their safer sex "stage persona" into their "real selves." Whether the audience consists of educators in training or ordinary people, the participants have rehearsed and learned healthy scripts for the roles they play in the sexual dramas of everyday life.

To make the greatest use of this quality, the performance space must be emotionally and physically safe. Emotionally, space can be made safe by assuring confidentiality, anonymity and non-judgmental support for the questions and behavior participants need to discuss and rehearse. Physical safety is achieved in workshops and trainings by the use of enclosed structures such as rooms or auditoriums with closed doors. But in outreach situations when performances take place in locales such as streets, bars, hotel lobbies, bathrooms, parks and beaches, safety often requires improvisation.

In open spaces hills, clumps of bushes, automobiles or areas where "outsiders" can be safely monitored offer security. In public areas where safer sex dramatic scriptings are not considered a proper type of involvement, it often is necessary to employ "involvement shields." These are areas and activities which serve as barriers to outsiders' perception and "behind which individuals can safely do the kind of things that ordinarily result in negative sanctions" (Goffman 1963:38–42).

A few examples of involvement shields commonly used by outreach workers to distribute condoms and explicit safer sex information under difficult conditions include:

* **[involvement shield]** "Social work." Helping outreach populations solve any immediate or ongoing crisis. **[primary involvement]** Creating good will and being useful so that target population will look to outreach workers for safer sex information.

* **[involvement shield]** "Just relaxing or cruising." Apparently relaxing or maybe looking for sex (in the park, bushes, behind the highway rest stop). **[primary involvements]** Flirting with men who are looking for sex in order to get to talk with them about AIDS and offer them safer sex guidelines, condoms, lubricants and advice (without offending them or destroying the ongoing sexual games and thus losing the opportunity to work with others later).

* **[involvement shield]** "Hanging out." Appearing to be just another member of the friendly neighborhood street corner gang, drop in center regulars, student lounge group, etc. **[primary involvement]** Getting accepted by the outreach populations in order to assess their specific safer sex needs and become a trusted resource.

Sometimes outreach workers drop involvement shields and perform a highly visible dramatic scripting instead. For example, one night on a busy street in a high crime area, outreach workers and sexologists created a magic time and space by blowing up condoms over their heads. This risked social disapproval from passers-by and unwanted attention from the police. However, the intended audience was a gang of street youths, and the purpose was to increase interest in condoms and demonstrate how strong they are. The show was successful and increased the demand for condoms. Some no doubt simply were used over the adolescents' heads. But for this population, risk taking and condom use in a context of humor and harmless street antics increased the cultural acceptability of condoms and popularity of the outreach workers as well.[11]

DRAMATIC TENSION

The greatest problem faced in creating and controlling the magic world of safer sex theater is embedded in a paradox of social life. The rules of public and private behavior are frequently reverse images of one another. That which is offensive and polluting in public is often the very essence of intimacy in private.[12] Explicit, illustrated, erotic interactions usually are defined as private matters.

In ordinary public contexts, vivid details of sexual conduct and explicit STD information are strictly avoided: but in private life with sexual partners, intimate friends, and professionals, these areas are often appropriate and highly valued subjects for exploration. Inverting the rules of public and private domains to create an erotic world of public safer sex education potentially generates tremendous dramatic tension. But to increase learning safer sex in ways that translate into actual behavior, this is exactly what performers and audiences do.

During performances, audiences are helped to transform the pollution associated in public places with sex, bodily excreta and prophylactics into a public acknowledgment and tribute to their high status during sexual intimacy. Semen, vaginal fluids, saliva, urine, and fecal matter have their hour of public glory while topics such as fucking, sucking and ass play take over the center stage.

The audience must also focus its attention upon symptoms and transmission of disease and the emotions these involve. This is often as difficult as coping with sex and the details of prevention. But fevers, chills, blindness, painful sores, diarrhea, pus, life long infections, defective/infected babies, and death must be squarely faced when dealing with AIDS and other STDs.

Further, ordinary people often come to performances with feelings of deep grief and sorrow over the need to change or give up cherished sexual activities, and with the knowledge that they may be at risk for HIV infection or have HIV disease. The closer that AIDS is, and the more empathetic an audience is, the greater their distress seems to be. These feelings must be dissipated in order to make way for the joys of safer sex. Processes for letting go of these emotions often induce highly dramatic cathartic states.

The dramatic tension resulting from such extreme deviations and transformations of the ordinary world can cause audiences to experience strong reactions. These sometimes require additional coping since many of the feelings are usually reserved for private. Experienced directors and performers working with sex positive, determined audiences often find controlling dramatic tension relatively easy and enjoyable. But under ordinary circumstances the problems can become formidable. We discuss ways to work successfully with these problems throughout the article. But for now the most important technique to know is progressive desensitization:

Begin with the least threatening information, presentations, requests and as the audience becomes comfortable, progress to more challenging levels.

Ironically, while dramatic tension is problematic, it is also a potent adjunct to learning and even culture change. For the essential delving into the forbidden, taking chances with others in a public place is in part what makes safer sex education effective and exciting. This is a particularly important quality for helping members of an audience mold and impact the sexual communities to which they return after a presentation. As Huizinga states:

A play-community generally tends to become permanent even after the game is over. Of course, not every game of marbles or every bridge-party leads to the founding of a club. But the feeling of being "apart together" in an exceptional situation, of sharing something important, of mutually withdrawing from the world and rejecting the usual norms, retains its magic beyond the duration of the individual game. [Huizinga 1964:12]

AUDIENCE MANAGEMENT

Practical tasks for successful safer sex performances are:
1. Carefully selecting and managing audiences;
2. Ascertaining the potential comfort level of participants; and
3. Modifying dramatic scriptings to fit within each audience's capacity.
Different audiences have distinct comfort levels regarding erotic or sexually explicit information and materials. Audiences of fundamentalist clergy and of workers in the sex industry provide examples of the extremes. Presentations which are very erotic to one audience can be inflammatory or dull to another. When groups of high vulnerability are segregated from those of substantial tolerance it is much easier to avoid embarrassment, boredom, fights, and other problems among participants.

To separate audiences, presentations should be carefully named and advertised. For example, events entitled "What Every Parent and Concerned Adult Needs to Know About Safe Sex" draw not only those concerned about the health of young people, but also the shy and closeted. Presentations advertised as "A Hot And Healthy Playshop" attract people who are ready for education with an erotic sizzle or who might be put off by a dry, sexless performance. The phrase "safer sex" is enough to prepare timid audiences to expect a sex-supportive presentation in the first example, and the terms "hot" (erotic, arousing) and "playshop" assure sex positive audiences that they will not be assailed with calls to moral rearmament, sexual purity and work.

In planning performances, we sometimes offer one kind of event for those who are interested primarily in building safer sexual relationships and another for those who simply want to enjoy sex safely. Advertisements such as "Sex and Love in the

Age of AIDS" versus "Explore The *SEX* In Safe Sex" will usually accomplish the task. When audiences have different or opposite interests in this regard, it is useful to explain before beginning that sexuality *and* relationships will be thoroughly addressed during the safer sex process. Otherwise people at the extremes in interest begin to feel left out and sometimes leave before they can be helped.

Ethnic factors also must be considered in selecting and preparing an audience. A monograph entitled "Ethnographic Perspectives on Nonpenetrative Sexual Behavior" (Cassiday and Porter 1988) is an excellent source for culturally specific material. To give an example of ethnic factors here, working with Mexican sexologists to create a workshop for Latin American psychologists, we decided that the term "erotic life" (*vida erotica*) was preferable to "sexlife." "Erotic life" is a more inclusive phrase and is more in tune with Latin sensibilities while "sexlife" (though narrow) is direct, focused and typical of cultures of Northern European derivation.

Sexual variations and associated lifestyles are important considerations in constituting an audience. Homosexuality, bisexuality, heterosexuality, and family life are all acceptable topics for many audiences. However, each of these subjects is capable of creating negative reactions when presented to the wrong audience or an audience which has not been properly prepared. In private life S&M, voyeurism, exhibitionism, transvestism, and fetishism are normal, joyous aspects of many peoples' sexlives (McIlvenna 1987:73–81, 174–178). But in the public sphere they quite often are labeled as sexual deviations and mental disorders.[13]

Regardless of one's position on such matters, the audience must not be kept ignorant. Excluding information on these topics dooms many participants to possible infection. Yet full disclosure to the "uninitiated" can be so overpowering that the basic information is lost and the prevention messages totally eclipsed. A fairly acceptable solution in a general group is to acknowledge different sexual lifestyles, present any important special risk reduction guidelines necessary, and invite members who have more questions to approach the presenters after the event. This must be augmented, of course, with separate presentations and special outreach to minority sexual subcultures.

EFFECTIVE STAGING

As we have noted, safer sex presentations are given in an enormous variety of settings: each has its potential strengths and weaknesses as a stage. Formal public locales such as high schools and churches demand more careful attention to audience and administrators' sensitivity and can seriously limit the amount of explicit information presented. For example, Catholic schools and universities often prohibit discussion of condoms and limit acknowledgment of sexual behavior so stringently that only abstract scriptings are possible. However, such locales also encourage wider attendance and give some reassurance to squeamish audiences that they will be inspired but not overwhelmed. Once prepared, those who were reluctant at first may wish to attend more complete performances in other types of social settings. Thus an important tactic is to inform the audience where clearer more informative performances are playing.

Audiences with low levels of tolerance for sexual information are potentially at higher risk than those who are comfortable with sex. People with minimal information and the lowest comfort level are often the least prepared to reduce risk when opportunity and an overpowering desire for sex occur. Frequently they have not developed negotiating skills, do not have condoms and spermicides available or even know how to use them.[14]

In sensuous and potentially erotic locales such as discos, bars, and singles parties, if presentations are too formal and non-sexual the audience may feel turned off, deceived, and betrayed. On the positive side, those attending such places are often looking for sexual partners. Thus spicy risk reduction education provides a positive, supportive context for communication and commitment to safer sex at a very opportune moment.

As we have seen, performances in public spaces where sexual activity is a clandestine but important form of interaction (such as parks, rest stops, shopping malls, and streets) require careful attention to behavior appropriate to the social occasion while imparting prevention information that can be given quickly to those looking for sexual encounters. As Lyman and Scott point out:

Even in those cases in which the weaker party secretly plays a different game with its own risks and stakes, he must take into account the game defined by the more powerful person and in the process mobilize his sign equipment to satisfy the requirements of the dominant game. Thus, while several games may be going on in the same encounter, it is certainly relevant to inquire into the hierarchy of domination that governs the engagement and the modifications on game play imposed by this hierarchy. [Lyman and Scott 1970:66–67]

Education must fit in with the sex games under way lest the educators become intrusive, spoil the action, or be classified as morality enforcers. At the same time, clear lines must be drawn between participants in the sex play and educators, lest police or bashers mistake those taking an AIDS prevention role for members of the sexual dramas in action. An excellent guide to working in such exposed and potentially dangerous locales is "AIDS Prevention in Public Sex Environments: Outreach and Training Manual" (Beckstein 1990).

COSTUMES

Clothes can be used to great advantage in safer sex presentations. In highly formal performances, a suit or business dress creates a type of respectability which allows the educator to say and do many things that otherwise would seem crude or undignified. On the other hand, in erotic locales the costumes of sexual subcultures and leisure worlds create a feeling of solidarity which helps to add credibility to a presentation. Outlandish costumes such as huge body condoms, walking "bleach bottles," masks, wigs, and funny hats create a lighthearted sense of play and adventure. When dramatic scriptings are actual sexual encounters, costuming can help create a playful, exploratory atmosphere for introducing new safer sex techniques more easily.

PROPS AND SCENERY

As mentioned earlier, a major goal of safer sex educators is to turn medical devices and hygienic techniques into sexual toys and play. Seasonally appropriate props full of condoms and spermicides (such as valentines, Christmas stockings, Easter egg baskets and Thanksgiving cornucopias) add a festive, "gift giving" air to presentations. Placing artifacts of sexual health in a general context of sex toys— feather boas, dildos, flavored massage lotions, and lubricants—helps to take away some of the pharmaceutical quality of condoms, spermicides, latex gloves, and dental dams while eroticizing them by association.

Patriotic symbols such as the flag can also be used to reassure people they are in a good place learning important information to assist them in making wise decisions. Sex positive prevention posters and condom balloons displayed early in a presentation help desensitize audiences to seeing and handling condoms or other sexually charged items later.

During performances, explicit safer sex audio-visual materials are extremely important. As we discussed in the section on interactional theater, audio visual aids can be 30% more effective in helping people learn prevention techniques than words alone. Equally important, aside from live sexual demonstrations and direct experimentation, seeing explicit safer sex material is one of the only ways many people can truly begin to appreciate that safer sex can be extremely arousing and satisfying. As pointed out, strong erotic appeal is absolutely essential to widespread use of safer sex when it is needed most.

As much as possible, presentations should use audio-visuals which represent the subcultures of the audiences in attendance. Race, ethnicity, age, economic class, sexual orientation, and lifestyles are all important parameters to consider. As examples, while it is possible for heterosexuals and lesbians to learn safer sex techniques from gay male materials, heterosexual or lesbian examples are more effective; S&M audiences are much more inspired by safer S&M visuals; Asians, Latinos and blacks respond much more to materials which express their culture and background.

As a general rule, begin with soft erotic images and progress to more explicit safer sex materials.[15] When possible, we find it helpful to have erotic slides with safer sex themes flashing on a wall or above the staging area as participants enter. This creates an erotic environment and helps the audience become accustomed to sexual messages in public places.

Most audiences express great pleasure and approval of safer sex media. However, since people sometimes can become upset when they see explicit materials in a public context, it is helpful to remind potentially resistant audiences that: a) educators regularly use such materials in sex education classes to familiarize students with the lifestyles of others and make it easier to talk about sex; and b) therapists use explicit materials to help those who have lost their normal sexual functioning due to accidents or disease to learn new, satisfying ways to express themselves erotically. The loss of cherished options and necessary changes caused by AIDS presents a very similar situation.

It is also useful to point out that the value of visual and simulated instruction in nonsexual contexts is unquestioned. People often watch driver education films and use computer driven demonstrators before actually driving a car. Medical students watch films, videos, live presentations and work on synthetic models before conducting live surgery. In AIDS prevention, another life and death matter, watching explicit media before actually using safer sex techniques in real life is just an extension of this powerful approach to learning.

After showing emotionally charged materials, encourage the audience to express their immediate feelings. Do this without censure or judgment no matter what the audience says. This process allows them to discharge their reactions and go on with the show. Otherwise, they sometimes become stuck and dwell upon their feelings waiting for an opportunity for release.

THE PROLOGUE

In actual theater, when the audience is seated but before the curtain goes up, figures sometimes appear and give a prologue to prepare the audience with special information about the main event. In safer sex presentations, it is also useful to provide information and create some basic rules and understandings before actually beginning. Sexologists have developed the following process as a useful way to begin:

1. **We explain that we do not try to change people or tell them what to do.** Our basic assumption is that given adequate information and a variety of choices, people will create the risk reduction lifestyles which best fit their needs and personalities. This defuses attitudes such as "Nobody is going to tell me how to have sex" and "I already know everything I need to know."

2. **We urge participants to take responsibility for their own sexlives.** Each sexual encounter presents different challenges and opportunities to use risk reduction strategies. Furthermore, AIDS guidelines change as more is learned about transmission. Thus it is imperative that each person take responsibility for being informed and making their own individual choices about sexual behavior.

3. **We acknowledge that people often experience strong emotions when they truly understand their risk of HIV infection or transmission and the need to change cherished sexual behavior.** These include shock, fear, denial, anger, helplessness, numbness, depression, loss of sex drive, increased sex drive, and feelings that their sexlife has been destroyed or that spontaneity in sex is completely over.

4. **We assure people these are normal reactions and provide a way for participants to express their feelings.** If time permits we invite personal sharing. We might ask people to discuss how they feel about AIDS, sex, and prevention. Or we might suggest that participants shout out a word or make a sound that expresses how they feel about having to make changes in their sexlives in order to protect their health.

Overlooking this step sabotages the presentation and invites resistance. As long as people are harboring resentment, grief, and other strong negative feelings it is almost impossible for them to participate fully and enjoy exploring new risk reduction possibilities.

5. **We then point out that while these emotions are normal, only safer sex will reduce the chances of contracting or transmitting AIDS/STDs.** This helps ground and focus the participants back on the main purpose of the presentation.

6. **We stress the importance of suspending judgment of other peoples' sexuality in order to cover all the prevention information necessary.** In addition to the reasons already presented, many people really don't know what others do sexually and sometimes react strongly no matter what kind of sexual behavior is discussed. To avoid embarrassment, hurt feelings, and displays of bigotry, it's important to prepare those attending in advance. The following bit of dialogue will usually do the job:

"What you might think is strange or repulsive may be the cherished activity of those sitting next to you or even a secret desire of your partner. We can all get over our initial embarrassment and shock about sex, but we won't get over a fatal infection. For our own sake, for the sake of others present and to protect those we love, let's make this a safe place to explore the full range of sexual expression and prevention."

7. **We discuss using the language of sex in public gatherings.** In an erotic setting this may not be necessary unless it is to assure the group they will not be turned off to safer sex by desexualized terminology. However, in general public spaces, attending to language issues is extremely important. For as we have noted, the language of sex is customarily forbidden in formal public gatherings just as the desexualized language of polite society and academia is usually forbidden during sex.

The exclusive use of non-sexual language in a scripting makes transferring the knowledge gained from the educational module to actual sexual encounters difficult. Also, many people only know common sexual terms and become lost in discussions of vaginal containment, intercrural penetration, and digital anal compaction. As pointed out in *The Complete Guide To Safe Sex*:

We have learned not to use "dirty" words in polite society. The polite terms . . . can obscure the meaning. For example, the following excerpt from a "trashy" novel, "I fucked her asshole doggie-style while squeezing her tits," loses something in its translation to "I engaged in rear entry anal coitus while applying pressure to her breasts." There is . . power in the ability to use, hear, and understand colloquial terms. [McIlvenna 1987:197]

Explaining the problem usually is sufficient to gain an audience's permission to talk in plain, erotic language. This can be helped along significantly by interspersing terms more appropriate for public gatherings with common sexual words, switching back and forth as necessary to assure audience comfort.

With extremely sensitive audiences it is sometimes helpful at first to resuscitate the language of the ancients. A strong diet of phrases such as "frication of the pudenda," "carnal knowledge," and "that which God and nature in their wisdom tried to hide" will usually cause an audience to crave "masturbation," "fucking," and so forth. Occasionally it may become strategic to step back and employ the linguistic armament of yore, but this necessity seldom lasts for long.

THE PLOT LINE

The script of events or plot line presented here for a safer sex production follows a logical sequence. We move from non-sexual time to vague stirrings, choosing options, fantasy, solitary masturbation (or self pleasuring), dating, touch, physical intimacy with others, sexual intimacy with others, repose, and non-sexual time again. This structural framework is called "The Socio-Sexual Response Cycle" (SARguide 1977:49). With most audiences this sequence of events facilitates a slow process of progressive desensitization in which the audience is exposed to the least threatening sexual scenario and moves on to more potentially challenging activities.

Our plot line has another advantage. It recognizes that everyone has strengths and weaknesses in their personal sexual response cycle. For example, in our general experience, some people are great at dating but terrible at negotiating condom use. Others have wonderful negotiating skills but have a hard time meeting prospective partners. Still others possess an incredible ability to think up safer sex fantasies but difficulty actualizing these fantasies with a partner. By using the socio-sexual response cycle as a model, most areas of potential transmission and prevention are covered.

It must be emphasized, however, that both in educational encounters and in real life, the actual order of events is sometimes mixed, goes back and forth or is random. Furthermore, a person can be at different stages of the response cycle with several different people at the same time. The rule is:

Follow the perceived needs and mind set of the people being educated: accept them where they are and take them as far with risk reduction as they can go.

Any other script courts disaster. For example, early in the AIDS epidemic, a group of sexually active gay men began to walk out of a presentation which started with fantasies, sensuous bathing, and erotic massage. Feeling "real sex" (penetration) was so risky it could never freely be engaged in again, the audience was overwhelmed with grief and depression. Progressive desensitization was achieved by starting over with how to correctly use and enjoy barrier protection and *then* moving on to other possibilities.

Our experience also has shown that some groups are so unprepared for discussion of anal, vaginal and oral intercourse that progressive desensitization is extremely hard to achieve. An adequate comfort level at which to teach methods of barrier protection is reached sometimes only after huge amounts of instruction in "the joys of outercourse." Groups which define acceptable eroticism very narrowly can deal with safer sex in only the most general and abstract terms.[16]

Presenters sometimes feel very frustrated knowing that the range of information they can provide is inadequate and that lives will be lost as a result. However, audiences (and administrators) often consider limited presentations a thrilling breakthrough. It is better to accept such audiences where they are philosophically and emotionally and give them a positive orientation to prevention than to challenge their position and possibly alienate them. To make such compromises less painful to presenters, it is useful to remember that each intervention is but part of the overall movement toward safer sex and that successful performances, no matter how small, are another step in this direction.

THE COLLAPSIBLE-EXPANDABLE SCRIPT

For flexibility, scripts should always be collapsible and expandable so that the scenario fits the time available and immediate perceived needs of the audience. Sometimes a facilitator has hours, days, weeks, even months to work with participants, but at other times the job must be done in seconds. For example, a long workshop allows spiral learning or reiteration in ever deepening levels of experiential intensity; but in an outreach situation, a worker may have only time enough to give an outreach client condoms and a few words of advice before some prospective sexual partner or customer appears and the client is gone. Using our model in personal life, the expanded script might be one's overall, lifelong approach to a safer sex lifestyle while a collapsed script might be the structure and content of a particular sexual encounter.

In addition to flexibility, a collapsible-expandable script has other important advantages. Collapsing the script can help maintain a group's comfort or interest level and allow presenters to include important but touchy subjects such as genital piercing and urination ("water sports"), without overwhelming the audience. If during a performance it becomes apparent that an audience wants more information on prevention and a particular sexual variation, expanding the script can meet these special needs. If part of the presentation has stretched an audience's comfort level to the limit, expanding the script during subsequent options they are eager to hear about helps smooth over the sensitive topics.

THE ACTION

The action in formal safer sex productions consists of presentations by various experts and sexual community members, panel discussions, small group exercises, role plays, socio-dramas, explicit safer sex media, at home exercises and other dynamic techniques. The following examples and those in Appendix A provide a few illustrations. In outreach situations and actual sexual encounters, the action includes dramatic scriptings appropriate to the occasion. Extensive suggestions for both personal use and group processes can be found in "How To Create A Safe Sex Lifestyle" (McIlvenna 1987:105–187).

Non-Sexual Time

People can use non-sexual time, such as safer sex presentations, for learning about AIDS/STD prevention and planning what they would do in a sexual situation. This is a good time to study medical information and clarify safer sex guidelines.

In a workshop, it is important to emphasize the *range* of medical information and opinion: what is considered the most unsafe behavior, the possibly risky and the safest activities *under various conditions*. This impresses upon participants the situational risk or safety of any particular activity, and defuses potential resistance from the audience. We stress that transmission of AIDS/STDs is what is dangerous, not sex *per se*. We explain that if people knew for sure they were free of infection, safer sex would not be necessary; but that it is extremely difficult under most ordinary circumstances to assess accurately the complete situation. We stress that not all partners are knowledgeable or truthful about their HIV status,[17] that cofactors of HIV transmission such as other STDs can be silent infections (some hard to detect even with laboratory tests), and that there are serious, transmissible opportunistic infections which sometimes must be taken into consideration. Zero health risk in sex is impossible but evaluating each sexual encounter and taking extra precautions make the risks very manageable.

People often say they want simple answers, laundry lists of what to do and not to do. However, steps to insure sexual health are more complex than this. Furthermore, despite their demands, people often don't really *want* to be told what to do, or to be made to seem wrong. In fact, when presenters or members of an audience try to tell people what they ought to do or not to do, audiences often become hostile toward the presenters or get into arguments with each other. When this happens, the performance itself can be jeopardized and the basic concepts lost. To handle potential trouble of this sort, remind participants of the *range* of medical opinion and situational nature of risk, and stress the importance of sharing information rather than trying to reach a consensus or enforce conformity.

To avoid a strong sense of loss when discussing the perils of sex, it is helpful to provide a rich variety of safe activities and modifications of usual behavior (Table I). If time permits, participants can break into groups and discuss safer sex options and personal experiences. Results of small group processes can be shared with the larger group to increase impact.

Non-sexual time also can be used in personal life to shop for safer sex goods, think about appealing safer sex possibilities, plan dates, or talk with knowledgeable friends about their safer sex experiences. All these activities also can be incorporated into longer processes.

A particularly helpful activity during non-sexual time is the making of a "Yes, No, Maybe" list. The "Yes" part of the list consists of sexual activities a person knows s/he is comfortable with; the "No" part is activities the person is clear are definitely not an option; and the "Maybe" category contains sexual actions dependent upon other factors such as level of intimacy in the relationship, trust and knowledge of a partner's health status. This process of clarifying options in a non-sexual space creates confidence, enriches safer sex possibilities and helps making decisions under sexual conditions much easier.

Vague Stirring And Sexual Options

When people become aware of sexual feelings some react automatically and others think over their options. When typical reactions are brought to participants' awareness through various techniques, they become better able to use this part of the response cycle more constructively. If participants have a limited pattern of

TABLE I. A generic brand of prevention guidelines. These typical enriched safer sex guidelines were furnished by The Sexologists' Sexual Health Project.

A GENERIC BRAND OF PREVENTION GUIDELINES
- Risk increases with the number of partners in unprotected activities!
- Risk taking often increases when people are drunk or high on drugs!
- Risk factors change situationally!!

SAFE OR VERY LOW RISK
- SEXUAL FANTASIES of any kind
- PHONE SEX
- SEX TALK (romantic, simply informational or "talking dirty")
- FLIRTING
- SOCIAL (DRY) KISSING
- HUGGING
- BATHING TOGETHER (including erotic bathing)
- SENSUOUS FEEDING
- BODY MASSAGE (including erotic and non genital oral massage)
- BODY LICKING (on healthy, clean skin)
- SMELLING BODIES AND BODY FLUIDS
- TASTING OUR OWN BODY FLUIDS
- MUTUAL MASTURBATION—(hands and genitals in good condition)
- CONSENSUAL EXHIBITIONISM AND VOYEURISM—(showing off, watching)
- WATCHING SEX MOVIES AND VIDEOS
- READING EROTIC BOOKS AND MAGAZINES
- ENJOYING LIVE SEXUAL ENTERTAINMENT
- S & M GAMES (without bruising or bleeding)
- USING PERSONAL SEX TOYS

PROBABLY SAFE, POSSIBLY RISKY
- FRENCH KISSING
- FELLATIO WITH CONDOM (sucking penis using a rubber)
- FELLATIO/NO EJACULATE (sucking penis without taking sperm)
- PENO-VAGINAL INTERCOURSE WITH CONDOM (and spermicide)
- CUNNILINGUS—(oral-vaginal sex, safer with barrier and spermicide)
- ANAL SEX WITH CONDOM (safer to withdraw before ejaculation)
- ANALINGUS WITH LATEX (rimming through a rubber dam or condom)
- CONTACT WITH URINE (Water sports on unbroken skin)
- DIGITAL-ANAL SEX WITH GLOVE (assplay with latex or plastic glove)

UNSAFE
- VAGINAL OR ANAL INTERCOURSE WITHOUT A CONDOM
- UNPROTECTED ORAL-ANAL CONTACT (rimming)
- MANUAL-ANAL INTERCOURSE (anal fisting without a latex glove)
- MANUAL-VAGINAL INTERCOURSE (vaginal fisting without a latex glove)
- SWALLOWING OR ACCEPTING SEMEN VAGINALLY
- SHARING BLOOD (i.e. dirty needles for IV drugs or body piercing or careless menstrual blood play)

behavior, they can consider broadening the possibilities. If they have difficulty deciding what to do, people can work toward focusing their behavior.

This part of a process can be particularly helpful to those who equate sex with penetration and feel intercourse is the only correct way to deal with arousal. By opening up the possibility of entertaining other options, a person is helped to decrease frustration, expand sexual pleasure and increase the time available for better judgment. In safer sex terms, when a person has many ways to achieve total sexual satisfaction, modifying a favorite activity is not experienced as so much of a tremendous loss. In our experience, facilitators can serve an important function as role models by talking frankly and explicitly from time to time about their own choices or preferences and the options they know others use. This increases the ability of participants to discuss their own experience, problems, strengths and explore new safer sexual options. Discussing possible options flows directly into other stages of the socio-sexual response cycle plot line: safer sex fantasies, massage, dating, watching erotic videos, self exploration, sex with a partner, group sex and the rest of the socio-sexual response cycle.

Fantasy

Audiences must be reassured and encouraged to use fantasy in creating safer sex lifestyles. Many people forget that fantasy is not reality and feel guilty if their sexual fantasies are nontraditional, politically incorrect or otherwise "inappropriate." Nearly everyone fantasizes, but almost no one has the time, energy, ability or desire to act upon all that is fantasized. Most importantly, nobody will ever get AIDS or other STDs from a fantasy, *even if the activities in the fantasy are unsafe.*

Ordinary fantasy life can't force people to do things they don't want to do. But fantasies can be used to empower the decision to use safer sex. In educational settings participants can be encouraged to break into groups and create collective safer sex fantasies to share when the audience reconvenes. They can also be given safer sex fantasy homework to share anonymously the next day in class. Safe sex fantasy videos, books and short stories are particularly helpful. Of course, most of these options can be done in private life or can be suggested to clients.

The audience should be encouraged to include risk reduction negotiation, condoms, spermicides, dental dams, finger cots, latex gloves and other safer sex skills in their fantasies. To be most effective, participants should be instructed to let these elements of fantasy freely drift in and out of conscious. Hanging onto a theme can easily spoil the experience by turning fantasy play into work.

Masturbation

Although most people masturbate, they still must be reassured that it is a form of sex which is healthy.[18] Women's groups often like to call autoerotic practices "making love to (oneself, myself, yourself)." "Self-pleasuring" is another popular term. Masturbation is an ideal way to become familiar with our bodies, our sexual responses and a way to ease into or come out of a period of celibacy (non-partnered sexuality). Self pleasuring is an enjoyable way to show our partners the kind of stimulation we like and all the parts of our body that help to intensify pleasure. It is a safe and easy approach to exploring new ways of reaching sexual fulfillment, lengthening and intensifying orgasms, discovering new erotic potential and playing with multiple orgasmic potential. Masturbation is also an excellent time to begin experimenting with condoms; focusing on how they feel, what it takes to break them and how much lubricant to use inside to achieve the greatest sensation and yet keep condoms from slipping.

In a process, people can break up into dyads and discuss their masturbation patterns then discuss the experience with the whole group. This is particularly good for breaking down barriers and reluctance to learning enriched masturbation techniques. Passing around different types of vibrators, dildos, other sexual toys and catalogs advertising items for self pleasuring also helps. The use of latex masturbation videos such as *Robin Loves Rubbers* or "Cybil" in *The Complete Video Guide to Safe Sex* can be very helpful.[19] At home, enriched masturbation exercises accompanied by personal sharing about the experience with friends or a partner are also excellent learning techniques. Sharing helps people to develop comfort around condom communication and to find new ideas for condom exploration.

Safe Sex Dating

Some people are expert at dating, but many are not, especially people who have been used to meeting their sexual needs by having anonymous encounters. Good dating differs from "just getting together" in that the special time is planned. Like a gourmet meal, if the preparation was done well, the event flows with the kind of ease that adds to enjoyment and frees the participants to be more spontaneous during the event itself.

Handouts on dating, at home exercises, personal sharing between participants about exciting low risk dating experiences and ideas are all useful ways of helping a group enhance dating skills. Role plays and sociodramas are particularly useful in helping participants analyze personal dating problems and discover potential solutions. They also help people to learn safer sex negotiating skills and how to broach scary topics in effective ways.

It should be pointed out that dating provides more thorough time to make personal health disclosures, discuss topics such as AIDS concerns, prevention techniques, personal guidelines of what turns us on or off in sex, and reduces anxiety while increasing security and pleasure when sex actually occurs.

Touch And Physical Intimacy

Ordinarily, people live in a touch deprived society but in this age of AIDS, touch and physical intimacy are even more scarce. Just as sexual desire is a natural response of the body, so is the need to be touched, made to feel loved, valued, and protected and to provide these feelings to others.

There are many ways to approach touching in an educational setting. All hold certain basic elements in common:
   a. Creating a safe space for touching and intimacy,
   b. Empowering participants to say "yes" or "no,"
   c. Obtaining mutual consent and creating limits for specific forms of intimacy,
   d. Checking out health concerns before beginning,
   e. Staying within agreed upon limits during events,

f. Creating a rhythm of progressive intimacy and smooth re-entry into the ordinary world of non-touch, and

g. Providing time and space to debrief after the event is over.

Touching and intimacy exercises are sometimes called "sensate therapy" and require skill and sensitivity to conduct. They are infinitely valuable in terms of helping enrich and protect people's lives. When handled by experts, it is truly amazing how far people can stretch their limits and how long lasting and intense the experience can be.

Exercises include touch negotiation, "clothes on" techniques, clothes off experiences, sensuous bathing, feeding, hot tub floating and sometimes non-sexual practicing of barrier protection skills. The exercises can help diffuse sexuality and redefine both the nature of sex and the sexual response cycle from genital penetration and orgasm to a more total experience. As Loulan points out, diffuse touch helps people escape the tyranny of genital orgasm and redefines the sexual cycle as "a willingness to be sexual" (1984:71–76).

Touch and intimacy exercises must fit the time available, the comfort level of the participants, and the personal ability of the facilitator(s). But even in the most reserved audience, a little touch can make a safer sex presentation much more effective and can provide a safe place for people to clarify personal boundaries around touch and sex.

Sex Intimacy

This part of the plot is handled very differently according to the mixture of factors which affect the complete performance: audience composition and expectations, locale where the event takes place, expectations and limits of the sponsors, training of the staff, local laws, and so forth. Whatever the contour of the intervention, it is important to have as full a range of sexual orientations and repertoires represented as possible. Never assume even in an event advertised for a specific group that all present are *only* heterosexual, homosexual, bisexual, lesbian, or that nobody is into S&M, bondage, and other sexual options.

Common to all presentations at this part of the socio-sexual response cycle is learning proper use of barrier protection and helping the audience become desensitized to seeing and touching safer sex technology. This may be limited to a discussion or may be quite elaborate. In addition to demonstrations on penis models and use of instructional videos or handouts, various techniques can be employed to give the experience a more lifelike quality without being a sexual experience.

One very good exercise is "The Condom Relay" in which teams compete with one another to see which group can apply condoms to an artificial penis *correctly* in *several different ways* and the *fastest*. The altered state of consciousness, excitement and confusion induced by competative play are very similar to what many people experience using condoms in actual sexual situations. During condom relays people increase condom skills and recognize ways they need to improve. Many learn the value of going slowly when incorporating condoms into their sexuality and of making the experience a part of sensuality rather than something to be done quickly.

Another good technique is to distribute lubricants, condoms, rubber dams, and other latex products to participants and invite them to open the packages, taste, and play with the contents. To demonstrate how strong condoms are, and for fun, they can be put over hands and feet or be placed over the head and inflated. People can be shown how to turn condoms into erotic toys by blowing them up to the size of a penis or breast and tying a knot in the end. Anything that associates prevention with enjoyment is in order. A positive experience in a group environment is extremely effective at normalizing and eroticizing protection!

The "sex" part of the sexual response cycle provides a superb opportunity to use safer sex media. Many sexual communities are accustomed to accessing sexual information through visual and auditory stimulation. Of course, in a public context they still need to be prepared and desensitized since their private learning customs may not translate well into a public workshop environment otherwise. In addition to using one or two media selections, multimedia presentations are extremely helpful. Sexologists often show many safer sex images at the same time. The impact of 7 to 20 simultaneous explicit risk reduction videos, films, and slides on an audience is most impressive. Since there are too many images for people to concentrate on only one selection, their eyes wander, taking in a great number of activities. A well balanced mixture saturates an audience with an encyclopedic collage of safer sex options and a tremendous enthusiasm for prevention experimentation when a sexual situation comes along.

In presenting the sexual part of the socio-sexual response cycle people should be made aware that high plateaux of excitement involve a state of altered consciousness which makes it hard to concentrate on everything that is going on. This is when condoms may break but go unnoticed; fingers may go into one partner's body, become covered with potentially infected material and then be placed into the other partner without thinking; or other accidents may occur. Danger is greatly reduced by first practicing under conditions of low risk (such as intercourse between the legs), changing condoms before becoming sexually deeply involved and taking extra precautions such as withdrawing the condom-sheathed penis before ejaculation.

Repose

In the socio-sexual response cycle, after orgasms, ejaculation(s), or when sexual excitement begins to recede, there is a period of time when people re-enter the non-sexual world. They may reflect on or re-evaluate their experience(s), consider what to do next, or just relax. In a safer sex program, after the "climax" it is time to answer any remaining questions, pass out additional information, and help participants decide how to use the experience as they return to "life in the world out there." People often become deeply attached to one another in longer processes and it is important to help them prepare for separation and returning to their ordinary lives. Closing rituals are often useful.

CONCLUDING REMARKS, APPLAUSE AND A FEW TOMATOES

Performers and educators are always eager for applause, flowers, glowing press reviews, and congratulations for their performances. On occasion, of course, they also must be ready to duck tomatoes and learn from mistakes in order to continue growing. Now that the curtain is descending on this particular performance, let us reflect upon the safer sex movement, our treatment of safer sex interventions and how sex-positive approaches can grow.

The Applause

The general popularity and continuing growth of the safer sex movement is one source of applause. As we noted in the beginning, not only do sexually active people want sex-positive healthy lifestyles, they are contributing time, effort and money to promote them. The epidemiological indications that safer sex interventions are playing a successful part in stemming transmission among those groups most actively involved in the movement are another reason for tremendous ovation.

Although moralists and politicians sometimes bemoan the sexualization of modern society and conduct morality crusades against AIDS prevention materials, it is difficult to find propaganda created by the masses admonishing the public to stop having sex. On the other hand, as our abbreviated catalogue of safer sex intervention shows, popular culture abounds with examples of imaginative, erotic prevention strategies to make sex safer, healthier, and disease free.

We also have pointed out that elements of the safer sex movement have diffused to many countries throughout the world. For example, group sex, safer sex masturbation clubs and parties which originated in the United States have been adopted by France, Germany, Holland, Belgium and Australia. Other nations have contributed striking innovations to the movement as well. In Holland safer sex workshops and parties are advertised on public television and safer sex explicit media appealing to different orientations is shown monthly on late night television. Sweden and Denmark distribute condoms and HIV prevention materials both to citizens traveling abroad and to those entering their countries. In Great Britain, safer sex workshops are popular and safer sex artifacts abound (i.e., T-shirts with slogans such as "Don't be a meanie, protect your weanie," and stickers in public restrooms advising the public to use condoms when engaging in penetration sex).

THE REVIEWS

We stressed in our introduction that there is an interdependent relationship between formal safer sex educational interventions and strategies generated by grass-roots sexual subcultures. We also stressed that safer sex interventions take advantage of existing cultural forms and incorporate members of sexual worlds into building their own safer sex subcultures. We observed when anthropologists, sexologists and other professionals become participant observers in the sexual cultures served, they are able to incorporate community initiated safer sex interventions into their educational models as well.

We demonstrated that an enormous variety of safer sex interventions have developed over the last decade of the AIDS pandemic. And using a dramaturgical approach, we suggested that the myriad of strategies can be organized for analysis by looking at interventions as cognitively related performances or dramatic scriptings, much like a genre of plays.

To accommodate an immense variety of locales, contexts, and participants, we applied a dramaturgical concept, interactional theater, to these ever changing aspects of safer sex interventions. This allowed us to redraw or eliminate boundaries between life's theaters, stages, audiences and players as necessary to create an integrated account of safer sex strategies. As we allowed our audiences and players to interact, exchange roles, and become co-players in the dynamic processes of workshops and social life, our dramaturgical model acquired motion or action—dramatic scripting. And we stressed the importance of choosing forms of interactional theater which make best use of an audience's cultural background and style of accessing sexual information.

We gave the action in our model purposeful direction by creating a plot line based upon a sexological perspective of sexual encounters, the socio-sexual response cycle. We pointed out that this plot line provides a continuum which covers all phases of sexuality from non-sexual time to vague stirrings, arousal, choosing options, sexual expression, and repose to non-sexual time again. The rationale given for applying the socio-sexual response cycle to safer sex interventions was that individuals have different strengths and weaknesses along the cycle continuum which affect their ability to prevent HIV/STD infection or transmission. By addressing the entire continuum, we are able best to meet both the individual and group needs of an entire audience.

The plot line was illustrated with examples taken from formal interventions, outreach strategies, and actual safer sex encounters. We pointed out that in real life people move back and forth in the socio-sexual response cycle and have differing interests and safer sex needs. While some performances incorporate the entire cycle, shorter interventions focus upon those points along the continuum most essential to specific audiences. We stressed that all dramatic scriptings should begin where the audience has the most interest and highest comfort level and proceed to more challenging but necessary levels. To accommodate both people and programs it was suggested that performances use a collapsible-expandable script.

Throughout the article we stressed that the dramaturgical interactional model produced could be used to create novel interventions which meet the changing matrix of individual, social, and cultural variables found in everyday HIV prevention contexts. To employ the model, strategists were advised simply to exchange the variables of new situations for the examples given in the text and proceed systematically through the model by picking and choosing dramaturgical and gaming concepts which best fit the task at hand.

Ducking and Throwing Tomatoes

We direct our criticism to safer sex in general and to the social context in which it exists, and reserve the right to deal with any strong negative reactions to our model for a later time. Let us begin with seldom raised but particularly important problems concerning risk reduction guidelines.

From a technical point of view, we noted safer sex performances are epidemiologically only as effective as the basic guidelines are correct. Unfortunately there is not enough collaboration between medical experts and prevention specialists to ensure that the guidelines are as good as they should be. The guides have remained little changed since 1985 and are focused narrowly upon HIV from the perspective of preventing the healthy from becoming infected. They do not adequately address the prevention of STD cofactors which facilitate HIV transmission or sexual health maintenance for those with HIV disease.

Experts in safer sex intervention contribute to the problem by seldom teaching about the prevention of STD cofactors which are implicated in HIV transmission and which often-times hasten the progression of HIV disease (for example syphilis, herpes, chlamydia, gonorrhea, chancroid, hepatitis, papillomavirus (HPV), cytomegalovirus (CMV), et cetera).[20] Educators also seldom point out to audiences in need of such information that many of these diseases can become serious, even fatal opportunistic infections. Further, safer sex currently does not address teaching vulnerable populations how to prevent or identify *sexually transmissible* opportunistic infections such as tuberculosis and various skin disorders.

Safer sex educators need to become as comfortable with pathology as they are with sex to be most effective. Audiences need to know what STDs look like, where in/on the body they are located, when they are silent but contagious and how they can be prevented. As an example, herpes is a serious problem both for those infected with HIV and the general public, yet autoinnoculation and transmission through touching lesions or kissing are almost never addressed. Educators must redouble efforts to work productively with medical experts to perfect more thorough guidelines in order to carry the safer sex movement forward.

It also is urgent that epidemiologists become more informed about sexual behavior. They need to increase their comfort level and look intently at sexual patterns in both educational and commercial materials to learn what people actually do during sex and how this might affect transmission. Educators and the public urgently need the medical profession to overcome cognitive dissonance and role discrepancy in sexual matters and apply their knowledge of STD infection to the full range of actual sexual behavior. From our perspective, in the context of AIDS, avoiding explicit often stigmatized sexual behavior is not professional, admirable, moral, lofty, noble, or demure; however, it is common.

Just as safer sex is only as good as the accuracy of guidelines, so also it is limited by the quality of barrier protection available. Some attention is being paid to the strength of condoms but regulatory standards and manufacturers' practices limit condom width and length so much that they do not adequately fit millions of men. Further, the most readily available brands are still relics of the past; thick, smelly and horrible tasting—serious barriers to condom use. The entrance of Japanese prophylactics into the American market has forced manufacturers to focus more upon the sexual appeal of condoms; how they feel, smell, taste. But new, more "user friendly" barrier devices (such as the internal condom and products using materials with a more skin-like feel than latex) have lingered over 10 years in testing and production.

An area of much more serious neglect is the testing and development of chemical prophylaxis. While condoms and lubricants should be used together, millions of people use protective lubricants rather than condoms during sex. Lubricants are already commonly acceptable for most people because they decrease friction and can increase sexual pleasure, yet research on HIV/STD chemical prophylaxis during sex is almost nonexistent.

Medical researchers and epidemiologists have known since 1972 that in laboratory tests nonionic surfactants such as nonoxynol-9 kill common STD pathogens[21] and since 1985 have had evidence that these mild, detergent like substances kill HIV in the test tube.[22] However it is almost impossible to find *in vivo* studies which evaluate the safety and effectiveness of surfactants in *anal intercourse* or *oral sex* and very little has been published on nonoxynol-9 and HIV/STDs during actual vaginal intercourse. *In vivo* studies of nonoxynol-9 and vaginal intercourse are usually limited to retrospective analyses and anecdotal reports. We need sexologically sophisticated studies of chemical prophylaxis under the full range of actual sexual conditions.

The reasons for negligence in this area is extremely disquieting. An official very highly placed in the Center for Disease Control said privately to one of the authors (as the Second International Conference on AIDS in Paris 1986), that he thought it was wrong not to conduct research on chemical prophylaxis and that eroticizing sexual health was the greatest advance since contact tracing and the discovery of penicillin. Then he added, "The government isn't going to help people safely engage in behavior which is against the law in many states and which many people find obnoxious."

Manufacturers are also partly to blame for the lack HIV/STD chemical prophylaxis development. They often point out that most of the likely chemical candidates are so common and readily available there is almost no way to make money after proving their worth in HIV prevention. Manufacturers informally say that the cost of development, lack of potential monetary reward, and governmental obstacles to appropriate research have stymied their prevention research efforts for many years. In one example, a manufacturer concerned about the 1978 gonorrhea epidemic in the gay/bi community wished to test a nonoxynol-9 product's effectiveness during anal intercourse and submitted a protocol to the appropriate governmental agency. The agency forced the manufacturer to change the focus of investigation to gonorrhea and vaginal intercourse, a topic which had been studied for many years.

Nonoxynol-9 is far from the perfect solution to chemical prophylaxis. It can be irritating to some users (especially those who have many partners in quick succession or experience imbalance in the flora and acidity of the vagina). Further, in strong concentrations, nonoxynol-9 has sexually disagreeable qualities such as a very strong taste and numbing effect. Researchers, manufacturers and governmental agencies must apply themselves to finding new forms of chemical pro-phylaxis and the public must urge them in this endeavor.

Finally, both safer sex educators and medical specialists need to address the AIDS/STD risks of the general population more continuously and energetically. We must stop moving from one "high risk" group to another and lowering educational efforts when a group begins to make significant progress. As Cutler and Arnold (1988) point out, we must be consistent and coordinate medical, educational interventions to be successful. There is ample evidence that all sexually active people are at risk for STDs associated with HIV infection. Half-measures of education and prevention insure continuation of the problem.[23]

SEX-POSITIVE OR NEGATIVE—WHERE WILL HIV PREVENTION GO?

AIDS is the worst STD to attack humankind since the ages when syphilis was incurable. Safer sex does not exist alone but is embedded in a total cultural context; one which until very recently was extremely sex-negative. As the AIDS crisis deepens, there are pressures to meet the challenge with mandatory testing, laws against transmission, incarceration and quarantine.

In this new era, we must learn from mistakes that were made in campaigns against venereal diseases of the past. No society has ever been able to contain STDs by law, decrees, and draconian measures. The past ineffectiveness of STD quaran-tines, massive roundups, and the closing of sexual institutions in the United States are documented extensively by Brandt (1985) in *No Magic Bullet*. But a much more illustrative example of the futility and danger of such approaches is furnished by Nazi Germany.

In the early 1930s, brothels were closed and syphilitic populations were isolated and even destroyed to purify the race. Since Hitler's approach to syphilis has parallels to repressive AIDS agendas today, let us reflect upon a passage from *Mein Kampf* as we weigh prevention strategies:

Public life must be freed from the stifling perfume of our modern eroticism . . . The right of personal freedom recedes before the duty to preserve the race. . . . It is a half-measure to let incurably sick people steadily contaminate the remaining healthy ones. . . . if necessary, the incurably sick will be pitilessly segregated—a barbaric measure for the unfortunate who is struck by it, but a blessing for his fellow men and posterity. The passing pain of a century can and will redeem millenniums from sufferings.

The struggle against syphilis and the prostitution which prepares the way for it is one of the most gigantic tasks of humanity . . . because we are facing, not the solution of a single question, but the elimination of a large number of evils which bring about this plague . . . the sickening of the body is only the consequence of a sickening of the moral, social, and racial instincts. [Hitler 1943:255–256]

Far from stamping out syphilis through the elimination of infected citizens and sexual culture, Nazi tactics actually contributed to an increase in the size of the problem by driving the disease underground: in fact syphilis grew to such proportions that the Nazis were forced to reopen government regulated brothels to contend with the epidemic (Bleuel 1974:42, 303–309).

The safer sex movement creates a dramatic contrast to most approaches of the past and initial experience gives hope that sex-positive strategies will succeed where punitive measures have not. The direction we take in fighting AIDS will not impact society until a cure is found. The discovery of new STDs as well as the resurgence of old diseases in more pernicious forms make it evident that the world will never be free of sexually transmitted diseases. Further, it is obvious that most people will never stop having sex, be monogamous with only one lifetime partner, or suddenly become totally open and honest about sexual matters with partners.

As we look into the future, our best hope for containing STD epidemics appears to be social transformation through the creation of a new, health-supportive culture of sex. Working to prevent disease while preserving and enhancing sexuality offers not only a chance to protect millions of people but also an opportunity to improve the quality of life itself.

NOTES

1. Dramaturgical approaches are common in both the social sciences and helping professions. The methods used here are derived from interactionist theory, discussed further in the text. Erving Goffman provides a particularly helpful introduction both to interactionist theory and the use of theatrical models in the analysis of "everyday social life." Especially helpful are *Frame Analysis* Chapter 5, "The Theatrical Frame" (1974:124:155), *Encounters: Two Studies in the Sociology of Interaction* (1961), and *Relations in Public* (1971). Another important guide to the approach we use is *A Sociology of the Absurd* (Lyman and Scott 1970).

   Throughout the article we use the term "intervention" in a special way. Interventions are usually performed by specialists upon patients, clients, or treatment groups. We accept this definition but also use the term to include self help activities: prevention strategies ordinary people can perform upon themselves. An intervention can involve a solitary individual (as when a person practices condom use during masturbation), pairs, groups, or entire subcultures and societies. We also use "intervention" to refer to the purposeful diffusion and assimilation of safer sex practices (for example the spread of masturbation clubs throughout the Western world as a way to have group sex without transmitting HIV).

2. The authors work on an international level, giving presentations throughout the United States, and in Mexico, The Netherlands, Spain, France, Great Britain and Sweden. However, our work reflects some of the West Coast perspectives in which our initial research and the development of educational models took place. However, our experience in other geographical areas has taught us that the model we present is not limited to geography. It is simply necessary to modify elements to take into account regional and cultural variations.

   It is impossible to acknowledge and give recognition to every deserving person and group working in the safer sex movement or to utilize all their examples. This is not a review article and the movement is immense—international in scope. Likewise, we are unable to thank by name all with whom we have collaborated in AIDS prevention research and work over the last decade. However, we should like to give special acknowledgment to a few of the individuals and organizations contributing to the theory and information contained herein: Ralph Bolton and Joseph Carrier for their strong encouragement and contributions to the article; Maggi Rubenstein, Laird Sutton, Ted McIlvenna, Jerry Zientara, Carol Queen, Dan Ford, Janet Taylor, Michael Sanderson and Andres Gonzales of The Institute for Advanced Study of Human Sexuality; The AIDS Steering Committee and John DeCecco and John Elia of the Center for Research and Education in Sexuality of San Francisco State University; Buzz Bense and other members of the Coalition for Healthy Sex; Norma Wilcox, Myrna Alma, Cynthia Slater and Jim Garner of The Sexologists' Sexual Health Project; Paul Gibson, Lisa Stoller, Susan McCreedy and Jacque McCright of the San Francisco Centers for Disease Control Regional Sexually Transmitted Diseases/Training Center; Sam Puckett, Les Pappas, David May and Chuck Frutchi of The San Francisco AIDS Foundation; James D'Eramo and the staff of the

800 Men Study of New York's Gay Men's Health Crisis; Gerald Lander and Wesley Harris of the Santa Cruz AIDS Project; Daniel Bao of the Condom Resource Center; and Rhio Dante, Seth Munter and Gerard Koskovitch of The Stanford University AIDS Education Project.

We would also like to recognize the additional following groups: The Healing Order of K'thar Sissies, the Revolting Sexologists From Hell, the San Francisco Jacks, the Amsterdam Jacks, the Jack 'n Jills, Mother Goose Productions, the Haight Ashbury Clinic, and Larkin Street Youth Services.

Of course, while we deeply appreciate the help of others, we absolve them from responsibility for errors the article might contains.

3. When we refer to "the safer sex movement," we are using Roberta Ash's definition of social movements:

> A social movement is a set of attitudes and self-conscious action on the part of a group of people directed toward change in the social structure and/or ideology of a society and carried on outside of ideologically legitimated channels or which uses these channels in innovative ways. [Ash 1972:1]

Randy Shilts (1988) describes the evolution of the safer sex movement within the overall context of AIDS in *And The Band Played On*. Also see *The Complete Guide to Safe Sex* (McIlvenna 1987) for a thorough discussion of safer sex theory, its evolution and role in the AIDS pandemic. As background material, excellent treatment of the interrelationships between sexually transmitted diseases (STDs), social movements, and medicine are provided by Allan M. Brandt (1985, 1988), Cutler and Arnold (1988), and David Pivar (1973).

To clarify terminology, "AIDS" technically refers to the end stages of human immunodeficiency virus (HIV) infection, while "ARC" refers to early symptomatic stages of HIV infection. "HIV" or "HIV disease" is quickly replacing "AIDS" to refer to HIV infection in all its various stages and the hybrid AIDS/HIV is common. However, since "AIDS" is still the most general expression it often will be used here interchangeably with AIDS/HIV, HIV, HIV infection, ARC and HIV disease.

While "safer sex" is used throughout this article, the ambiguous terminology for the safer sex approach and supporting medical guidelines is constantly debated. "Safe Sex" and "Safe Sex Guidelines" are the original terms developed; "Safer Sex" often is used to point out that any sexual situation has its possible risks; and "Safe(r) Sex" is a compromise meaning that while activities such as solitary masturbation are totally safe in themselves, other activities have important elements of risk but can be made "safer" (i.e., unprotected oral sex can be made safer by using condoms) and some high risk activities (such as unprotected anal and peno-vaginal intercourse) can be made less dangerous or "safer" by *both* using condoms *and* withdrawing before ejaculation.

4. Of course, safer sex is not just limited to the groups who first developed the concept or to movements of sexual social reform. Now safer sex interventions are found in approaches quite independent from the movement's origins. For background on the sex field and sexual social movements see Haeberle (1978:460–487), Kirkendall and Whitehurst (1971), Bullough and Bullough (1977:213–228), Altman (1973) and Horowitz and Liebowitz (1968:280–296).

It can be argued that sex researchers like Alfred Kinsey started the modern sexual revolution by bringing sophisticated techniques to the study of sex and lifting the sex field out of an ethnocentric morass of traditional customs and folkways. It can also be argued that social movements of sexual change made it possible for sex researchers to rise above their conventional biases and for agents of social welfare (therapists, social workers, applied social scientists, etc.) to take a supportive rather than punitive approach to their work. Whatever the etiology, there is a substantial population of citizens and professionals from many fields who now hold a sex positive perspective and act upon their persuasion in the pursuit of sexual health and culture change.

5. In the parlance of the sociology of deviance, the "unsafe sex as illness" frame is a form of the "welfare" or "medical model" approach to social problems. Unfortunately, the biases we have pointed out are inherent in these models (Horowitz and Liebowitz 1968:280; Mercer 1973:77). Eliot Freidson discusses the general limitations in an article with the suggestive title "The Production of Deviant Populations" (1973:126).

We do not think it is the intent of researchers who study the relationship of health problems to unsafe sex to become agents of sexual social control. However their research bias sometimes fosters the impression that "normals" do not have problems with prevention guidelines while "deviates" are unable to comply.

Some medical approaches to AIDS prevention overlap and are extremely productive contributions to safer sex theory and techniques, i.e., the "Health Belief Model" (HBM), and other variations of health behavior modification theory. However, analyses of these models often recognize a limited ability to deal with socio-cultural variables and a need to grow in this area. For example, "The Health Belief Model in Understanding Compliance with Prevention Recommendations for AIDS: How Useful?" (Montgomery et al. 1989:303–323) and "Health Education Models in AIDS Prevention" (Chesney 1987).

There is a considerable literature on the effects of alcohol/drugs and HIV transmission. A good starter bibliography should include Ostrow et al. (1990:759–765), Stall and Ostrow (1989:57–73), Stall et al. (1986:359–371), Ostrow (1987:15–29) and MacGregor (1988:47–72). This research serves many excellent purposes. However, from the perspective we are presenting here, there is a curious and disquieting silence about the relationship of high risk behavior to unstigmatized conditions such as boredom, touch deprivation and the desire for unrestrained physical intimacy.

6. A Norwegian study of continued unsafe sex forcefully acknowledges and highlights the points made above (Prieur 1990). After noting that her respondents regarded unprotected intercourse and the exchange of bodily fluids as normal, cherished, traditional ways of expressing intimacy, trust, passion and love the author states:

Sex is more than actions and positions. Actions carry meanings. Accepting semen has been an important value in the gay culture, a way of showing devotion and belonging. Unsafe sex can be an expression of positive values and of good feelings. . . . this way of showing feeling [is] like a language where you cannot just invent new words and expect to be understood. Specific acts are linked to specific feelings, and it might be difficult to express these feelings in any other way.

When we started this research, some of us were surprised that gay men still had unsafe sex. Why can't they change their sex life, it must be more important to survive than to keep on having sex in the same way as before?. . . . We are used to thinking that every evil is caused by another evil. If this were true, continued practice of unsafe sex would be caused by a lack of self-control, by drinking, drugs, or just plain madness. This is a view that stems from a simple rational choice model . . . But the world is not that simple . . . a wider understanding of rationality is needed: one that includes longing and love as motives for action. [Prieur 1990:113–115]

Prieur further quotes an American anthropologist, Lee Kochems (1987), on this matter:

Informants have expressed to me that intercourse without a condom brings them 'closer', it's more 'intimate'. They often express a desire for a 'feeling of oneness' or 'sharing'. Expressions like 'I want you inside me' or 'I need you to come in me', or 'I want to cum in you, to be part of you', as phrases used in sexual encounters indicate a desire for a joining, a oneness or incorporation in one another's physical being.

Although Kochem's informants were also gay, in our experience their statements could just as well have been made by an enormous number of heterosexuals and bisexuals.

7. The definition of games used here is that of interaction theorists who:

treat social situations—in which two or more persons or groups are in communication with one another and are engaged in goal-directed action—in terms of a game theoretical framework, at least in its simple social-psychological form. [Lyman and Scott 1970:29]

8. A feature on Safe Sox explains:

The idea is to keep condoms readily at hand and to invite safe-sex conversation between potential partners. "And it's a good way to advertise," explains MAPP [Midwest AIDS Prevention Project] president Craig Covey, "especially in summer, when people are wearing shorts." [The Advocate 1991:81]

9. An audience can react very negatively when performers are unfamiliar with the sexual practices of a particular subculture, have prejudices against its cherished customs, or are insensitive to a group's values. For example those who disapprove of anal intercourse have difficulty making erotic suggestions about how to engage in ass play safely. Unsympathetic presenters sometimes betray themselves and alienate their audience by wincing or frowning when the subject of anal or vaginal fisting comes up.

At the other extreme, those who insist that everyone be comfortable with all sexual variations run the risk of alienating audiences so badly that people will not listen to important advise about the sexual practices they do feel comfortable about.

10. As Huizinga notes in his pioneering anthropological study of play:

> . . . play is not "ordinary" or "real" life. It is rather a stepping out of "real" life into a temporary sphere of activity with a disposition all its own. . . . What the "others" do "outside" is no concern of ours at the moment. Inside the circle of the game the laws and customs of ordinary life no longer count. We are different and do things differently. [1964:8–12]

> Also see Humphreys (1970:46) and Taylor (1986:117–136).

11. The most dramatic high profile intervention strategy we are aware of is as follows: On weekend nights, a Midwestern safer sex outreach worker drives a "condommobile" to lovers lanes and other sexually active locales, puts a revolving green light on top of the car to help people locate the dispensary and gives away prophylactics. About 200 contacts are made per weekend. Another dramatic outreach includes hanging bags of condoms and lubricants from tree branches where people congregate for sex. In Jalapa, Veracruz, and Guadalajara, Mexico, peer outreach workers distribute condoms and information in plazas, parks, and sexually active theater balconies. In Mexico City public baths, where dating couples and others often go to have sex in private rooms, some attendants have been recruited to distribute condoms and lubricants in addition to traditional powders, lotions and soft drinks.

12. As Goffman writes:

> . . . the very forms of behavior employed to celebrate and affirm relationships—rituals such as greetings, inquiries after health, and love-making—are very close in character to what would be a violation of preserves if performed between wrongly related individuals. . . . And it is hard to see how it could be otherwise. For if an individual is to join someone in some kind of social bond, surely he must be doing so by giving up some of the boundaries and barriers that ordinarily separate them. [1971:58–59]

13. Many people express to us that any type of sex other than peno-vaginal intercourse in the dark seems perverse to them. Some fear that if they come to like latex it will become a "fetish," and they will value having sex with condoms more than having sex with a particular partner. Such fears are reinforced by areas of academia which continue to promote ethnocentrism as science. For example, the American Psychological Association's official diagnostic manual, the DSM III, pp. 44–45, first labels heterosexual intercourse as the standard of sexual health, then clumsily excludes homosexuality from the list of sexual disorders, and subsequently lumps all other sexual variations together as pathology—sexual violence shares the same label with those playing S&M love games, the prowling peeper is not distinguished from the couple who like to look at each other's bodies, and so forth.

14. The points above deserve further discussion. Public educational institutions for children and adolescents are another arena where calls for chastity are often promoted as the only truly acceptable approach to prevention. A well studied example which advocates this perspective is the "Sex Respect Curriculum" or "Just Say No" approach. Wilson and Sanderson (1988:10–11) found the Sex Respect Curriculum teaches excellent assertiveness skills, but since "no" is the only acceptable answer to all sexuality, the program is counterproductive in helping young people to think independently, develop personal sexual identity, or know how to say "yes" to sexuality when that is the appropriate answer. Michelle Fine in an extensive analysis of sexual health education models, "Sexuality, Schooling, and Adolescent Females: The Missing Discourse of Desire" (1988:29–53), found that young women who tried to follow the "Just Say No" approach experienced more unwanted pregnancies and STD infections than those who acknowledged their enjoyment of sexuality and intention to continue being sexual. The latter were more likely to learn about barrier protection, obtain prophylactics and use them.

The Sex Information and Education Council of the U.S. has issued an excellent report on the controversy around youth and sexual health education (SIECUS 1988). An age graded protocol for pre-adolescent prevention is presented by Mary Valentich and James Gripton in "Teaching Children About AIDS" (1989).

15. Progressive desensitization is also effective in making audiences comfortable with graphic examples

of AIDS/STD infections. Such materials help audiences identify and avoid visible infections and can motivate participants to use safer sex.

16. We are thinking here of groups which are strongly dedicated to morality training, abstinence, and monogamy as the first and only line of acceptable AIDS prevention. Safer sex is not opposed to abstinence and monogamy, nor are interventions based upon traditional values always against incorporating a safer sex approach. In fact, many prevention programs include elements of each but with differing balance and emphasis.

An approach to better serving institutions with a narrow prevention focus is to give performances which fit within their ideological framework while on their turf (such as Catholic universities) but *also* give presentations at places frequented by the same clientele *not* defined as institutions of traditional values—bars, dance halls and other "off campus" establishments. This allows administrators to avoid criticism while helping those who seek more than moral armament to get the information they need. To borrow a phrase, it allows all concerned to "Praise the Lord and pass the ammunition."

17. Relying upon the honesty and devotion of others instead of using safer sex is extremely dangerous. It is very hard for many people to be honest about sexual matters. For example, Cochran and Mays in a study of 665 college students found that 20% of the men and 4% of the women reported they would lie about having a negative HIV-antibody test in order to have sex; and while 32% of the males and 23% of the females were dating more than one person at the same time, 68% of the men and 59% of the women kept the fact a secret from their partners (1990:774).

Another researcher using a statistical probability model to compare consistent condom use with careful selection of partners by heterosexuals otherwise not at risk for AIDS makes an extremely convincing argument for putting one's trust in the condom before putting it in others (Wittowski 1990:143–145). Wittowski's work was stimulated by another probability study which takes the point of view that since many find risk reduction guidelines hard to follow, and since the U.S. rate of infection among heterosexuals is relatively low, people should be advised to choose a low risk partner carefully and basically forget about condoms and other safer sex precautions (Hearst and Hulley 1988:2428–2432).

From working with many couples in monogamous or purportedly monogamous relationships, we have found that the more intensely the couple insists upon sexual faithfulness, the harder it becomes to be honest or cope with infidelity if and when outside sex occurs. We stress that couples should look at monogamy as a lifestyle rather than a physical health measure and use safer sex. If children are desired, couples should get tested for HIV, and other STDs before becoming pregnant.

18. Of course, the amount and acceptability of masturbation as a sexual option differs by ethnicity, race, social class, age, and individual sexual patterns (Kinsey et al. 1948, 1953 passim; DeMartino 1979; Cassidy and Porter 1988; Sorensen 1973:131–143).

19. These and many other safer sex videos are available from The Exodus Trust, 1523 Franklin St., San Francisco CA 94109.

20. A guide to HIV and STDs is to be found in the following sources: Pepin, et al. (1989); Mertens, Hayes, and Smith (1990); Cochran, Keidan and Kalechstein (1990); Nelson, Ghazal and Wiley (1990); Peterson (1988); and Byrne et al. (1989).

21. For example, see Food and Drug Administration: *Vaginal Contraceptive Drug Products for Over-the Counter Human Use*; Establishment of a Monograph; Proposed Rulemaking. (Federal Register, December 12, 1980; pp. 82014–82049). Also see Singh, Cutter, and Utidjian (1972), "Studies on the Development of a Vaginal Preparation Providing Both Prophylaxis Against Venereal Disease and Other Genital Infections And Contraception. II. Effect in vitro of Vaginal Contraceptive and Non-contraceptive preparations on Treponema pallidum and Neisseria gonorrhoeae:" British Journal of Venereal Disease 48:57–64.

22. "Birth-control Spermicide Eyed As AIDS Protection" San Francisco Chronicle, January 31, 1985. Anonymous;

Bruce Voeller, a researcher and president of the Mariposa Foundation, . . . announced yesterday that nonoxynol-9, the active ingredient in many spermicides, was found to kill the AIDS virus during laboratory tests conducted by the federal Centers for Disease Control last year. . . . Centers for Disease Control spokesman Don Berreth said the substance killed the AIDS virus—HTLV-III—

in the laboratory. But he said clinical trials on people are needed to determine if it can prevent them from contracting AIDS.

23. The following references make clear the real versus idealized nature of American sexuality. They also bring home the extreme danger AIDS and other STD's pose to *all* sexually active people regardless of orientation, age, race, religion, occupation, marital and socio-economic status: Darrow (1988); Brooks-Gunn and Furstenberg (1989); Cates (1986); Wilson and Sanderson (1988); Fine (1988); Talashek, Tichy and Epping (1990); Ostrow (1986); Dembert, Finney, and Berg (1990); and Kinsey et al. 1948, 1953. Problems illustrated with half measures are made clear by Stall et al. 1990.

REFERENCES CITED

Advocate
  1991   Sock It To Me. 574:81.
Altman, D.
  1973   Homosexual Oppression and Liberation. New York: Discus Books.
Ash, R.
  1972   Social Movements in America. Chicago, IL: Markham Publishing Co.
Becker, M., and J. Joseph
  1988   AIDS and Behavioral Change to Reduce Risk: A Review. American Journal of Public Health 78:394–411.
Beckstein, D. L.
  1990   AIDS Prevention in Public Sex Environments: Outreach and Training Manual. Santa Cruz, CA: Santa Cruz AIDS Project.
Bleuel, H. P.
  1974   Sex and Society in Nazi Germany. Translated by H. Fraenkel. Philadelphia, PA: J.P. Lippincott Co.
Brandt, A. M.
  1985   No Magic Bullet: A Social History of Venereal Disease in the United States Since 1980. Oxford: Oxford University Press.
  1988   AIDS in Historical Perspective: Four Lessons from the History of Sexually Transmitted Diseases. American Journal of Public Health 78(4):367–371.
Brooks-Gunn, J., and F. Furstenberg
  1989   Adolescent Sexual Behavior. American Psychologist 44(1):249–257.
Bullough, V., and B. Bullough
  1977   Sin, Sickness, and Sanity: A History of Sexual Attitudes. New York: The New American Library.
Byrne, M., J. Taylor-Robinson, P. Munday, et al.
  1989   The Common Occurrence of Human Pappillomavirus Infection and Intraepithelial Neoplasia in Women Infected by HIV. AIDS 3:379–382.
Cassiday, C. M., and R. Porter
  1988   Ethnographic Perspectives on Nonpenetrative Sexual Behavior. Washington, DC: AIDSCOM.
Cates, W.
  1986   Epidemiology and Control of Sexually Transmitted Diseases. In Sexually Transmitted Diseases. Y. M. Felman, ed., Pp. 1–23. New York: Churchill Livingston.
Chesney, M.
  1987   Health Education Models in AIDS Prevention. Paper Presented at the NIMH/NIDA Working Conference on Women and AIDS: Promoting Healthy Behaviors.
Cochran, S., J. Keidan, and A. Kalechstein
  1990   Sexually Transmitted Diseases and Acquired Immunodeficiency Syndrome (AIDS): Changes in Risk Reduction Behaviors Among Young Adults" Sexually Transmitted Diseases 17(2):80–86.
Cochran, S., and V. Mays
  1990   Sex, Lies, and HIV New England Journal of Medicine 322(11):774.

Cutler, J. C., and R. C. Arnold
   1988   Venereal Disease Control by Health Departments in the Past: Lessons for the Present. American Journal of Public Health 78(4):372–376.
Dale, E.
   1954   Audio Visual Methods in Teaching. New York: Dryden Press.
Darrow, W.
   1986   Sexual Behavior in America: Implications for the Control of Sexually Transmitted Diseases. In Sexually Transmitted Diseases. Y. M. Felman, ed. Pp. 261–280. New York: Churchill Livingston.
DeMartino, M.
   1979   Human Autoerotic Practices: Studies on Masturbation. New York: Human Sciences Press.
Dembert, M., L. Finney, and S. Berg
   1990   Epidemiology of Reported Syphilis Among U.S. Navy and Marine Corps Personnel, 1985–87. Sexually Transmitted Diseases 17(2):95–98.
Fine, M.
   1988   Sexuality, Schooling, and Adolescent Females: The Missing Discourse of Desire. Harvard Educational Review 58(1):29–53.
Food and Drug Administration
   1980   Vaginal Contraceptive Drug Products for Over-the Counter Human Use; Establishment of a Monograph; Proposed Rulemaking. Federal Register, December 12, pp. 82014–82049.
Friedson, E.
   1973   The Production of Deviant Populations In Deviance: The Interactionist Perspective. E. Rubington and M. S. Weinberg, eds. Pp. 125–127. New York: The Macmillan Company.
Goffman, E.
   1961   Encounters: Two Studies in the Sociology of Interaction. Indianapolis, IN: Bobbs-Merrill.
   1971   Relations in Public. New York: Harper Colophon.
   1974   Frame Analysis. New York: Harper Colophon.
Haeberle, E. J.
   1978   The Sex Atlas. New York: The Seabury Press.
Hearst, N., and C. B. Hulley
   1988   Preventing the Heterosexual Spread of AIDS: Are we Giving our Patients the Best Advice? Journal of the American Medical Association 259:2428–2432.
Hitler, A.
   1943   Mein Kampf. Translated by R. Manheim. Boston, MA: Houghton Mifflin.
Horowitz, I. L., and M. Liebowitz
   1968   Social Deviance and Political Marginality: Toward a Redefinition of the Relation between Sociology and Politics. Social Problems 15:280–296.
Huizinga, J.
   1964   Homo Ludens: A Study of the Play Element in Culture. Boston, MA: The Beacon Press.
Humphreys, L.
   1970   Tearoom Trade: Impersonal Sex in Public Places. Chicago, IL: Aldine.
Kinsey, A. C., W. Pomeroy, C. Martin, and P. Gebhard
   1948   Sexual Behavior in the Human Male. Philadelphia, PA: W.B. Saunders.
   1953   Sexual Behavior in the Human Female. Philadelphia, PA: W.B. Saunders.
Kirkendall, L., and E. Whitehurst, eds.
   1971   The New Sexual Revolution. Buffalo, NY: Prometheus Books.
Kochems, L. M.
   1987   Meanings and Health Implications: Gay Men's Sexuality. Paper presented at the Annual Meeting of the American Anthropological Association. (Quoted by Prieur 1990).
Loulan, J. A.
   1984   Lesbian Sex. San Francisco, CA: Spinsters Ink.
Lyman, S., and M. Scott
   1970   A Sociology of the Absurd. New York: Appelton-Century-Crofts.
MacGregor, R.
   1988   Alcohol and Drugs as Co-factors for AIDS" In AIDS and Substance Abuse. L. Siegel, ed. Pp. 47–72. New York: Haworth Press.

McIlvenna, T., ed.
   1987   The Complete Guide to Safe Sex. San Francisco, CA: Specific Press.
Mercer, J.
   1973   Labeling the Mentally Retarded. *In* Deviance: The Interactionist Perspective. E. Rubington and
         M. S. Weinberg, eds. Pp. 77–87. New York: The Macmillan Company.
Mertens, T. E., R. Hayes, and P. Smith
   1990   Epidemiological Methods to Study the Interaction Between HIV Infection and Other Sexually
         Transmitted Diseases. AIDS 4:57–65.
Montgomery, S., J. Joseph, M. Becker, D. Ostrow, et al.
   1989   The Health Belief Model in Understanding Compliance with Preventive Recommendations for
         AIDS: How Useful? AIDS Education and Prevention 1(4):303–323.
Nelson, J., P. Ghazal, and A. Wiley
   1990   Role of Opportunistic Viral Infections in AIDS. AIDS 4:1–10.
Ostrow, D. G.
   1986   Homosexuality and Sexually Transmitted Diseases. *In* Sexually Transmitted Diseases. Y. M.
         Felman, ed. Pp. 205–220. New York: Churchill Livingston Inc.
   1987   Barriers to the Recognition of Links Between Drug and Alcohol Abuse and AIDS. *In* Acquired
         Immune Deficiency Syndrome and Clinical Dependency. P. Petrakis, ed. U.S. Public Health
         Service Monograph ADM 87–1513 Pp. 15–29.
Ostrow, D., M. VanRaden, R. Fox, et al.
   1990   Recreational Drug Use and Sexual Behavior Change in a Cohort of Homosexual Men. AIDS
         4:759–765.
Pepin, J., F. A. Plummer, R. Brunham, et al.
   1989   The Interaction of HIV Infection and Other Sexually Transmitted Diseases: An Opportunity for
         Intervention. AIDS 3(1):3–9.
Pivar, D.
   1973   Purity Crusade: Sexual Morality and Social Control, 1868–1900. Westport, CT: Greenwood
         Press.
Prieur, A.
   1990   Norwegian Gay Men: Reasons for Continued Practice of Unsafe Sex. AIDS Education and
         Prevention 2(2):109–115.
SARguide
   1977   Sexual Attitude Restructuring for a Better Sex Life. San Francisco, CA: National Sex Fo-
         rum.
Shilts, R.
   1988   And The Band Played On. New York: Penguin Books.
SIECUS
   1988   SIECUS Report 17(1).
Singh, B., J. C. Cutter, and H. Utidjian
   1972   Studies on the Development of a Vaginal Preparation Providing Both Prophylaxis Against
         Venereal Disease and Other Genital Infections And Contraception. II. Effect in vitro of Vaginal
         Contraceptive and Non-contraceptive Preparations on Treponema pallidum and Neisseria
         gonorrhoeae. British Journal of Venereal Disease 48:57–64.
Sorensen, C.
   1973   Adolescent Sexuality in Contemporary America: Personal Values and Sexual Behavior Ages 13–
         19. New York: World Publishing.
Stall, R., T. J. Coates, and C. Hoff
   1988   Behavioral Risk Reduction for HIV infection Among Gay and Bisexual Men. A Review of
         Results from the United States. American Psychologist 43:878–885.
Stall, R., M. Ekstrand, L. Pollack, et al.
   1990   Relapse From Safer Sex: The Next Challenge for AIDS Prevention Efforts. Journal of Acquired
         Immune Deficiency Syndromes 3:1181–1187.
Stall, R, L. McCusick, J. Wiley, et al.
   1986   Alcohol and Drug Use During Sexual Activity and Compliance With Safe Sex Guidelines for
         AIDS. Health Education Quarterly 13:359–371.

Stall, R., and D. Ostrow
    1989   Intervenous Drug Use, the Combination of Drugs and Sexual Activity and HIV Infection
           Among Gay and Bisexual Men: The San Francisco Men's Health Study. Journal of Drug Issues
           19:57–73.
Stewart, D.
    1969   A Learning-Systems Concept as Applied to Courses in Education and Training. *In* Educational
           Media: Theory into Practice. R. V. Wilman and W. C. Mierhenry, eds. Pp. 134–171. Ohio:
           Charles Merrill.
Talashek, M., A. Tichy, and H. Epping
    1990   Sexually Transmitted Diseases in The Elderly: Issues and Recommendations. Journal of
           Gerontological Nursing 16(4):33–40.
Taylor, C.
    1986   Mexican Male Homosexual Interaction in Public Contexts. *In* Anthropology and Homosexual
           Behavior. E. Blackwood, ed. Pp. 117–136. New York: Haworth Press.
Valentich, M., and J. Gripton
    1989   Teaching Children About AIDS. Journal of Sex Education and Therapy 15(2):92–102.
Wilson, S. N., and C. A. Sanderson
    1988   The Sex Respect Curriculum: Is 'Just Say No' Effective? SIECUS Report (September/
           October):10–11.
Wittkowski, K.
    1989   Preventing the Heterosexual Spread of AIDS: What is the Best Advice if Compliance is Taken
           into Account? AIDS 3:143–145.

APPENDIX A
THE INSTITUTE FOR ADVANCED STUDY OF HUMAN SEXUALITY
SEXOLOGICAL INSTRUCTOR/ADVISOR OF AIDS/STD PREVENTION

Condensed Script

INTRODUCTION

The program has the following goals:
1.   To increase participants' overall comfort with sex, their own sexuality, and the sexuality of others.
2.   To provide participants with those basic theoretical concepts, assumptions and sex affirmative perspectives of sexology necessary to carry out AIDS/STD prevention and sexual health maintenance programs.
3.   To give participants experience with a wide range of sexological safe sex skills, helping them to master the ones which they feel will most help them in their present and future AIDS/STD work.
4.   To give participants exposure to a variety of AIDS/STD prevention and sexual health maintenance programs, and to help them formulate such programs within their own service system.
   The program is NOT a personal or group therapy workshop. However, because sex, AIDS, illness and death are such powerful subjects of study, many personal issues often arise. For this reason, each participant belongs to a small group designed to enhance personal sharing, assist in personal growth and help attend the various individual problems which arise due to the character of the subject matter.

If issues cannot be resolved adequately in the small group or through consultation with the small group facilitator, participants should seek help from one of the three program facilitators. Some time is reserved in the program for issues of concern to the participants as a whole, and the SHARP program is a *training* program. Issues beyond the scope of the task at hand need to be kept at a minimum and ought not to interrupt the group process.

SHARP is very intensive. Therefore, it is extremely important that we all be sensitive to one another's feelings and take responsibility for our own wellbeing; get as much rest as possible and *be on time*.

We each have issues which are difficult for us—such as sexual language, visual material, touch and nudity. No one is required to participate in any of the workshop exercises. However, attendance *is* required. If you must leave for any reason, participants are expected to notify a small group facilitator or the faculty. STAFF: David Lourea, Maggi Rubenstein, and Clark Taylor equally share responsibility for running the workshop. Each has different strengths and skills.
Small Group Facilitators are: Jerry Zientara, Janet Taylor, Mike Sanderson, Robyne Lewis, and Bernardo Useche

Saturday—November 3, Day 1

10:00–11:00	REGISTRATION. Plan to eat brunch before 11 as the lunch break will be very short today. Fill in sex history. *On your name card below your name, write something you like about yourself.*
10:45–11:00	Safe Sex slides shown in SAR room. *Laird.*
11:00–12:00	INTRODUCTION. *Maggi.*
12:00–12:15	RELAXATION EXERCISE. *David.*
12:15–12:30	BREAK.
12:30–12:45	BASIC ASSUMPTIONS. *Maggi, Laird.* Assumption Slides.
12:45–1:10	REVIEW MEDICAL ASPECTS OF TRANSMISSION. *Clark.*
1:10–2:15	GRIEVING PROCESS AND SAFE SEX. *David, Laird-tape.* Male Couples Facing AIDS.
2:15–3:00	Quick lunch break. Make new name card and *write one of your favorite forms of self pleasure* below your name. BE SURE TO WASH YOUR HANDS BEFORE RETURNING TO SAR ROOM.
3:00–3:45	INTRODUCTION TO SENSATE THERAPY. *Clark.*
3:45–5:00	SAFE SEX AND FANTASY LIFE. Fantasy media. *Laird, Maggi, Clark, Michael* and *Maggi.*
5:00–5:15	BREAK
5:15–6:30	SAFE SEX AND MASTURBATION. *Clark, Janet, David* and *Laird.*
6:30–6:40	HOMEWORK ASSIGNMENT—Spend at least 30 minutes exploring, pleasuring your body and/or masturbating in a new way. Also feel free to fantasize in a new way if this helps you explore your body. *Clark.*
6:40–7:30	SMALL GROUPS.
7:30–9:00	DINNER AND SOCIALIZING AT THE INSTITUTE. *Maggi, David* and *Clark.*
8:30–9:00	Small Group Facilitators meeting.

Sunday—November 4, Day 2

9:00–9:30	Coffee, tea and socializing. *Make a new name card and write down one of your personal favorite erotic zones* below your name.
9:30–10:15	CONDOMS & LUBRICANTS. *Laird, Clark.*
10:15–11:30	BEGINNING VERBAL AND SENSATE SKILLS. *Clark* and *Sheryl*
11:30–11:45	BREAK.
11:45–1:00	SAFE SEX AND THE SOCIO-SEXUAL RESPONSE CYCLE. *Maggi, Michael* and *David*
1:00–2:00	LUNCH BREAK. Make up a new name card and *write your current sexual orientation(s)* below your name before afternoon class begins.
2:00–2:15	THE RANGE OF SEXUAL BEHAVIOR. *David.*
2:15–4:15	BASIC GROUP SHARING OF SEXUAL ORIENTATIONS, LIFE-STYLES & AIDS. *Maggi, Laird.*
4:15–4:30	BREAK.
4:30–6:15	MULTI-MEDIA PROCESS. *Laird, Maggi, Clark, David.*
6:15–6:20	Homework Assignments. *Two parts.*

MAKE THREE LISTS.
1. What I feel sexually safe doing and want to do.
2. What I would feel sexually safe and be willing to do under certain circumstances (be clear about the circumstances).
3. What I do not feel safe doing and do not want to do under *any* circumstances.

WRITE A SAFE SEX FANTASY or write out why you don't want to do the exercise. After you have written the fantasy out once, go over it and figure out ways to make the activities in it safer and sexier. **BRING YOUR WRITTEN HOMEWORK TO CLASS WITH YOU TOMORROW!!** *Also, bring a towel and a pair of soft socks with you to class tomorrow for sensate focus work. David.*

6:20–6:30	BREAK.
6:30–7:30	SMALL GROUPS. Feedback, check-in, name tag feedback.
7:30–8:00	Small Group Facilitators.

EVENING FREE.

Monday—November 5, Day 3

9:00–9:30	Coffee, tea and socializing. Make a new name tag and *write one of your favorite sex words* below your name.
9:30–10:00	Feedback and HOMEWORK PROCESS. *David.*
10:00–11:00	COMMUNICATION EXERCISE. *David.*
11:00–11:15	BREAK
11:15–12:45	PANEL. THE RANGE OF HIV INFECTION. *Patti Britton, Michael Sanderson, David Lourea, Joan Baker.*
12:45–1:45	LUNCH BREAK. Make a new name tag and under your name write down one of your *favorite sex toys.*
1:45–3:15	ROLE PLAYS. *Maggi.*
3:15–3:30	BREAK.
3:30–5:30	SENSATE FOCUS. Boko-Maru ritual (foot bathing, massage, psychic detoxification by DR. WOOF! *Jerry Zientara.*

5:30–5:40   HOMEWORK ASSIGNMENT. **RUBBER EXPLORATION NIGHT**. (see *The Complete Guide To Safe Sex* for suggestions.) *Clark*.
5:50–6:50   SMALL GROUPS.
6:50–7:50   Small Group Facilitators meeting.
EVENING FREE.

Tuesday—November 6, Day 4
9:00–9:30   Coffee, tea and socializing. Make a new name tag and write below your name *something you like to do with a partner*.
9:30–10:00   Feedback on homework. *David*.
10:00–11:30   LATEX PANEL. *David, Janet, Carol* and *Robert*.
11:30–11:45   BREAK.
11:45–12:30   HOW TO TAKE A SEX HISTORY. *David*.
12:30–1:30   LUNCH BREAK. Make a new name card including *one of the parts of your body you like to have touched a lot*.
1:30–3:00   THERAPY ISSUES. *Maggi* and *David*.
3:00–3:15   BREAK.
3:15–4:00   DATING AND INTIMACY SKILLS IN A SAFE SEX LIFESTYLE. *Clark*.
4:00–6:15   ADVANCED SENSATE THERAPY SKILLS. *Clark, Robin, and Carol*.
6:15–6:30   BREAK.
6:30–7:30   Small Groups check-in.
7:30–8:30   Small Group facilitators.
OPTIONS NIGHT—OPEN.

Wednesday—November 7, Day 5
9:30–10:00   Check-in and feedback. *David*.
10:00–1:00   INTIMACY SKILLS. *Robin & Ray*.
1:00–1:30   Large or small group check-in (according to group decision).
AFTERNOON AND EVENING FREE—REST, RECUPERATION, FUN AND GAMES (list of options provided).

Thursday—November 8, Day 6
9:00–9:30   Coffee, tea and socializing. Make a new name tag including *one of your favoriate non-penetration things to do with condoms &/or lubricants*. Media in the SAR room.
9:30–10:00   Feedback. *Maggi*.
10:00–11:30   IV DRUG USERS, DOWNTOWN POPULATIONS, YOUTH AND INNOVATIVE SAFE SEX PROGRAMS. *Clark introduces panelists*.
11:30–11:45   BREAK.
11:45–1:15   CONDOMONIUM. *Clark, Sheryl, Jerry, Janet, Daniel* and *Robyne*.
1:15–2:30   Lunch break. *On your new name tag write one of your favorite safe sex activities*.
2:30–3:00   MEDIA. *Laird*.
3:00–4:15   BREAK.
4:30–5:45   ROLE PLAYS. *David*.
5:45–6:00   BREAK.

6:00–7:00   Small Groups.
7:00–7:30   Small Group Facilitators. Jerry Zientara talks with facilitators about Sensorium.
EVENING FREE.

Friday—November 9, Day 7
9:00–9:30   Coffee, tea and socializing. Make a new name tag indicating *a creative erotic safe sex experience you've had (or would like to have)*. Media in the SAR room.
9:30–10:45   GROUP SAFE SEX PROGRAM. *Laird, David*.
10:45–11:00   BREAK.
11:00–12:30   PLAYSHOP. *Clark*.
12:30–2:00   LUNCH BREAK. On your new name tag *add a safe sex activity you never told a partner you would like to do*.
2:00–3:00   TRUE CONFESSIONS OF SAFE SEX WORKERS. *David*.
3:00–3:30   FILMS, VIDEO. *Clark, Laird*.
3:30–3:45   BREAK.
3:45–5:15   WOMEN AND AIDS PANEL. *Maggi, Margo, Robin*.
5:15–7:30   Small groups plus dinner.
7:30–8:00   Costuming and preparation for eveing program at IASH.
8:00–10:30   SENSORIUM. A guided experience to facilitate deeper expansion of awareness. A celebration of our transformation into Sexological Instructor/Advisors of AIDS/STD Prevention.

Saturday—November 10, Day 8
9:00–9:30   Coffee, tea and socializing. Make a new name tag indicating *something you've never tried sexually but would like to*.
9:30–10:45   Watch video of Sensorium and debrief. *Maggi, Jerry, Laird and staff*.
10:45–11:00   BREAK.
11:00–12:30   S+M SAFE SEX PRESENTATION. *David facilitates*.
12:30–2:15   Small groups convene and go to lunch together for long lunch.
2:15–3:00   WORKING WITH MIDDLE AMERICA ON SAFE SEX. *Clark introduction. Patti Brinton, Daniel Bao* and *Michael Bouchard*.
3:00–3:30   BUILDING AIDS PROGRAMS WHILE LIVING DAY-TO-DAY IN THE MIDDLE OF THIS CATASTROPHE. *Andres Gonzales*.
3:30–4:15   SEX AND DISABILITY. *Carolyn Long* and *Burt Paris*.
4:15–4:30   BREAK.
4:15–5:15   CLOSURE and RITUAL. *Maggi, Jerry and staff*.
5:15–5:30   EVALUATION.
5:30–6:00   SMALL GROUP LEADERS CLOSURE.

Medical Anthropology, Vol. 14, pp. 285–306
Reprints available directly from the publisher
Photocopying permitted by license only

AIDS and the IV Drug User: The Local Context in Prevention Efforts

Merrill Singer, Zhongke Jia, Jean J. Schensul, Margaret Weeks, and J. Bryan Page

Key words: IV drug use, AIDS prevention, ethnography, medical anthropology

The AIDS epidemic has focused an unprecedented level of attention on the behavioral patterns of intravenous drug users (IVDUs), especially the manner and social setting in which they inject drugs into their bodies and the nature of their sexual practices. As IV drug users have emerged as a group significantly at risk for contracting and transmitting HIV infection (Des Jarlais, Friedman, and Stoneburner 1988; Des Jarlais and Friedman 1987; Haverkos 1988; Hahn et al. 1989), concern has been voiced about effective approaches for AIDS prevention for this population (Galea, Lewis, and Baker 1988; Hubbard et al. 1988; Conviser and Rutledge 1988; Friedman, Des Jarlais, and Sothern 1986; Newmeyer 1988; Valdiserri 1989). Unfortunately, there is a shared recognition among AIDS workers that "information [on IVDUs] is scanty in many relevant areas" (Turner, Miller, and Moses 1989:186).

Over the last several years, the National Institute on Drug Abuse (NIDA) has funded National AIDS Demonstration Research (NADR) projects designed to test AIDS prevention efforts for IVDUs in 25 cities around the country and in Puerto Rico. These projects are contributing to an emergent understanding of the extent of HIV infection, drug and needle use practices, sexual behaviors, and level of AIDS awareness in this population.

Participants in these projects are active IVDUs or the sexual partners of IVDUs (Young 1989; Weddington et al. 1990). As defined by NADR protocols, an IVDU is

MERRILL SINGER *is Deputy Director of the Hispanic Health Council, 98 Cedar Street, Hartford, CT 06106. He is Chairperson of the American Anthropological Association Task Force on AIDS and is the Principal Investigator on Project COPE, A National AIDS Demonstration Research Project (NADR) funded by the National Institute on Drug Abuse.*

ZHONGKE JIA *is a demographer and the Chief Data Analyst at the Hispanic Health Council.*

JEAN J. SCHENSUL *is the Executive Director of the Institute for Community Research in Hartford and Co-Principal Investigator on Project COPE. She has been engaged in community action research for 20 years.*

MARGARET WEEKS, *Project Director of Project COPE, is a cultural anthropologist who specializes in women's issues.*

J. BRYAN PAGE *is Professor of Psychiatry at the University of Miami and has been involved in ethnographic research on drug use for 18 years. He is Project Ethnographer on the Community and Behavioral Strategies for HIV Reduction Project, the Miami NADR study.*

an individual who has used drugs intravenously (or otherwise injected drugs) during the last six months. The NADR projects specifically attempt to include street IVDUs who are not currently (nor for the last 30 days have been) in drug treatment. Recruiting this "hard core" IV drug using population into a research demonstration project requires diligent, committed street outreach by indigenous outreach workers who know and can operate comfortably in local neighborhoods where potential project participants can be contacted.

Preliminary data from the national dataset produced by these projects (Sowder 1989; Brown 1990) cast doubt on the accuracy of the public image of the IVDU as "a criminal, a willful degenerate, a hedonistic thrill-seeker in need of imprisonment and stiff punishment" (Goode 1984:218). Moreover, these studies provide a means of challenging the reified and overly homogeneous portrayal of IVDUs commonly found in media accounts of the AIDS crisis. Because they are simultaneously carried out in a number of cities using standardized instrumentation, these studies offer the opportunity for the comparative examination of the relationship between IVDUs and their local social context and the use of this information in designing locally grounded and situationally appropriate prevention efforts. As Page et al. (1990:69) emphasize, "Generic approaches to preventing HIV contagion developed in New York or Miami may not succeed in Minneapolis or Oakland." Prevention of AIDS in a highly at-risk group like IVDUs, it is argued here, must be sensitive to local differences in the target population, their ideational and behavioral patterns, and their configuration of risk behaviors. Consequently, effective prevention must be grounded in an awareness of the local setting in which IVDUs reside (Siegal 1990).

In this paper, following a review of the concept of "local context" in the urban anthropology literature, we compare findings from the Hartford AIDS demonstration research project (Project COPE) with data from the Miami Community Outreach Project. (C. McCoy et al. 1990; H. McCoy, Dodds, and Noland 1990). The purpose of this comparison is to demonstrate variation among IVDUs residing in two contrasting cities located in very different regions of the country and to indicate the importance of this variation in AIDS prevention efforts.

TWO LOCAL CONTEXTS: MIAMI AND HARTFORD

As Hastrup and Elsass (1990) recently have affirmed, a distinctive feature of anthropology is its concern with the social context in which thought and action unfolds. Anthropologists concerned with life in the city have variously construed the nature of the social context under study. Eames and Goode note,

One vital distinction [is] between those to whom urban means the *locus or setting within which the study is pursued* (anthropology in the city), and those to whom the *urban itself is the prime focus on study* (anthropology of the city). [Eames and Goode 1977:30–31, emphasis in the original]

In anthropology *in* the city studies, the city is conceived of as the location in which the activity or group of interest can be found, but the city itself is not an object under examination. By contrast, anthropology *of* the city research "emphasizes the urban context as a major variable influencing life" (Eames and Goode 1977:33). However, even among those who work within the anthropology of the city tradition, alternative approaches to context can be found. For some, the concern is with contrasts between the urban and other types of social environments (e.g., villages). This approach focuses on identifying the defining characteristics of urban living. Other researchers question the utility of attempting to understand the city as an abstract universal and instead are concerned with contrasting cities drawn from disparate culture areas of the world.

In the mid-1970s, an extension of the latter approach emerged with the recognition that there are significant dissimilarities between cities located in the same culture area or nation-state. As Press (1975:29) noted at the time, "only recently has there developed a real momentum toward recognizing important differences between urban milieus." Within the resulting *city-as-local-context perspective*, attention has been directed to the nature of particular cities as products of interactions between their constituent components or between the latter and external forces. Thus, Leeds (1968) demonstrated the ways contrasting economic and administrative structures in the Brazilian cities of Rio de Janeiro and Sao Paulo contribute to the formation of notably different working classes and local neighborhoods in the two cities. Similarly, Rollwagon (1972) and Price (1973) contrasted several Mexican cities in terms of demographic variables, regional location, history, and political economy and used these comparisons to explain differences in local lifeways. Within the U.S., several studies have used the local context perspective to explain variation in social life within two or more urban centers (Fox 1972; Smith 1975; Singer 1978; Backstrand and Schensul 1982). Fox (1972), for example, compared Newport, Rhode Island and Charleston, South Carolina in an effort to relate the growth of distinct forms of local governance and class formation in these cities to their contrasting histories and urban adaptive patterns. Focusing on the "same" subgroup in two different urban settings, Singer (1978) explained variation in community outreach efforts of the Lubavitcher Hassidim in Pittsburgh and Los Angeles in terms of the historical/compositional differences in the Jewish communities in the two cities. Finally, Backstrand and Schensul (1982) accounted for differences in the Puerto Rican communities of New York and Hartford, including the health behavior and health status of individuals within these communities, in terms of contrasting features of the two urban environments.

Within the AIDS field, there is growing awareness that the "relationship of IV drug use to HIV infection varies by gender, race, and ethnicity, *as well as by geographic location and culture*" (C. McCoy and Khoury 1990:419, emphasis added). In their study of IVDUs in treatment, Lange et al. (1988) found that geographic region was the strongest predictor of seropositivity. Local context factors, such as physical location, sociodemographic composition, density and size of the IVDU population, availability and desirability of particular drugs or combinations of drugs, level of police pressure on IVDUs, availability of syringes generally and sterile syringes in particular, established social traditions and locations for drug injection, local awareness and popular understanding of HIV infection, and needle use frequencies, may play a significant role in the level of AIDS risk for IVDUs in any setting. For example, Mascola et al. (1989) explain low rates of HIV infection among IVDUs in Los Angeles in terms of the rarity of large shooting galleries in the city, while Chaisson et al. (1987) note that as contrasted with New York and New Jersey, heterosexual IVDUs in San Francisco do not commonly share needles with gay IVDUs, a pattern known to play an important role in the rapid transmission of the virus in a previously low prevalence city (Battjes and Pickens 1989).

Local influence on IVDU behavior is especially significant because of the socially insulated nature of this activity. It is well known that it is through established social networks that IVDUs

obtain daily information on the availability, cost, and quality of drugs. And it is through "associates" that financial resources are often pooled to buy [drugs] and it is with "walking partners" that users often hustle money, cop, and shoot their drugs. [Beschner and Bovelle 1985:99]

Consequently,

most IV drug users do not appear to travel extensively. In addition to limited economic resources, the need for a constant supply of drugs reduces their mobility, although they appear to travel some, especially to locations where friends can help them obtain drugs. [Turner, Miller, and Moses 1989:235–236, emphasis added]

Moreover, there is a demonstrated ability of HIV infection to be transmitted rapidly within local areas. Increases in seropositivity rates among IVDUs of 10–50% in a 3–4 year period have been observed in New York, Edinburgh, Scotland, and Milan, Italy (Novick et al. 1986; Novick, Truman, and Lehman 1988; Robertson, Bucknall, and Welsby 1986; Angarano et al. 1985; Moss 1987). As Des Jarlais, Friedman, and Stoneburner (1988:152) question:

Are periods of rapid spread inevitable among IV drug users, or are there local conditions that can prevent rapid spread? Answering this question will require additional risk-factor research in a variety of locations and some coordination of the studies so that the findings can be readily compared across geographic areas.

The importance of local context factors in IV drug use and HIV infection is underscored by briefly comparing features of the two cities of concern to this paper.

Miami is a Sunbelt multicultural tourist and migration center in which ethnic groups from the Bahamas, the West Indies, and Central and South America converge in large numbers. Hispanics, particularly Cubans, form a plurality in the city (approximately 35% of the total population) (Page et al. 1985). Miami is also characterized by its high number of AIDS cases. Only six cities in the U.S. report a higher cumulative case total. Further, only New York has a higher number of pediatric AIDS cases than Miami. Between June 1988 and May 1989, the incidence of AIDS per 100,000 population was 47.5 in Miami, a rate that was surpassed only by Jersey City, New York, Newark, and San Francisco (Centers for Disease Control 1989).

Research on drug use in Miami has a long history and was already well established before the initiation of the NADR study in 1987 (Wiedman and Page 1982; McCoy et al. 1990). Prior research had revealed that: 1) African American IVDUs tend to be concentrated in identifiable neighborhoods; 2) white IVDUs are scattered throughout Dade County; and 3) IV drug use among Hispanics, especially Cubans, is comparatively limited (McBride et al. 1986).

Initial outreach in Miami to locate and recruit IVDUs for the NADR study focused on several African American neighborhoods, with the intention of building network connections with white drug users through contacts in the African American community. While contacts with white IVDUs were established in this way, the sparse networks they had with other white drug users limited the sample size of this subgroup (Page et al. 1990). Consequently, among the first 560 participants in the Miami sample who agreed to a blood test for HIV infection, 74% were African American, 17.6% were white, and 7.4% were Hispanics (see Table I). Many of the participants in the Miami study were recruited from "neighborhoods where unemployment is high, as is violent crime, crime against property, and drug use" (Page et al. 1990:63). However, these neighborhoods

are not grim in the same way that other cities' slums are grim. They have ample open spaces, and the buildings are not tall enough to block out the constant sunlight. The air is very clean for a big city. Still these places can be oppressive. Heat and humidity are almost as constant as the greenness, lasting eight to ten months a year. By July and August, people who have been living in the squalor of publicly subsidized housing in crowded conditions can become surly and unpredictable. . . The drugs make living in . . . slum neighborhoods more bearable. . . [Page and Smith 1990:304]

Raising money for the purchase of drugs is an important component of "taking

TABLE I. Demographic characteristics and seropositivity of street IV drug users: A comparison between Miami and Hartford.

	Percent of Tested		Percent of Positive	
Category	Miami	Hartford	Miami	Hartford
All subjects	560	166	26.2	45.2
Gender				
Male	81.0	83.7	23.7	45.3
Female	19.0	16.3	36.8	44.4
Race				
White	17.6	6.6	14.3	27.3
African American	74.1	43.4	28.6	50.0
Hispanic	7.4	49.4	29.3	43.9
Other	0.9	0.6	—	—
Age				
18–25	7.0	12.3	10.3	24.0
26–35	47.4	50.5	25.8	35.9
36–45	35.5	30.4	29.3	41.9
46–62	10.2	5.9	28.6	66.7
Duration of Drug Injection				
0–5 years	15.6	17.5	15.1	28.6
6–10 years	21.5	20.0	21.8	28.1
11–15 years	17.4	17.5	29.2	57.1
16–20 years	25.5	17.5	33.3	50.0
21–25 years	14.1	7.5	23.1	66.7
26 or more years	6.0	2.5	39.4	75.0

*The Miami data are taken from Clyde B. McCoy and Elizabeth Khoury, 1990 "Drug Use and the Risk of AIDS." *American Behavioral Scientist* 33(4):422.

care of business" among IVDUs. Field studies in Miami found that IVDUs raise money through a wide variety of strategies, including panhandling near public transit stations or hospitals. In addition, ethnographic interviews with Miami IVDUs revealed that many "had, at one time or another in their lives, traded sex for money or drugs" (Page et al. 1990:63). Drug injection was found to take place in various locations, including shooting galleries or "get-off houses" as they are known in Miami.

> The most common variety of get-off is the small apartment in which the client pays an entry fee at the door and may pay for additional services, such as rental or purchase of syringes and a "doctor's" or a "hit-man's" assistance in the injection process. . . . Customers . . . often arrive with their own cocaine and/or heroin and syringes bought elsewhere. Bags of drugs bought and delivered by runners serving the get-offs are stapled at the top, so that the dealers' reputation for selling units of reliable quantity and the runners' integrity will not be questioned. [Page et al. 1990:64]

Field observation suggests that "IVDUs in Miami do not usually share syringes and needles, yet they engage in several other behaviors during the course of getting off that place them at risk of infection" (Page et al. 1990:68), including renting unclean needles at get-off houses.

As contrasted with Miami, Hartford is a comparatively small city. However, unlike its popular images as a New England Yankee settlement or a bastion of insurance industry wealth, Hartford is the fourth poorest city in the country, with an ethnic composition that is roughly 45% African American, 30% Hispanic, and 25% white. Over 25% of households in the city have incomes below the poverty level and over 30% are on welfare (Backstrand and Schensul 1982; Singer and Borerro 1984).

Also unlike Miami, there is no long tradition of IV drug use research in Hartford, and consequently far less is known about behavioral and other patterns in the local IVDU subculture. The Connecticut Alcohol and Drug Abuse Commission (CADAC) estimates that 1.9% of the statewide population in Connecticut 12 years of age and older use narcotics and cocaine intravenously. In urban areas such as Hartford, CADAC data suggest that IV drug use is greater than the state as a whole, and involves 2.5–3% of the adolescent and adult population. Based on this information, it is estimated that there are about 3500 IVDUs in Hartford (Pereira and Henrickson 1988). Experience of the Hartford Dispensary, a methadone drug treatment center, suggests considerably higher figures, perhaps as many as 12,000 IVDUs in a city with a total population just over 130,000. Combining these two "informed guesstimates" (Butynski et al. 1987), the Hartford Health Department estimates approximately 8,000 IVDUs in the city. Based on the sociodemographic characteristics of IVDUs seeking HIV antibody testing and the reported cases of AIDS in the local IVDU population, it is believed that approximately 80% of IVDUs in Hartford are male and 20% female. Using data on persons in drug treatment, police arrest records for drug-related crimes, and diagnosed cases of AIDS, it is estimated that the racial composition of Hartford's IVDU population is 16% white, 44% African American, and 40% Hispanic (Pereira and Henrickson 1988). The majority of Hispanics in Hartford and the vast majority of the Hispanic IVDUs are Puerto Rican. Reports of drug treatment agencies, police records, and the experience of Health Department HIV antibody testing sites indicate several identifiable areas of the city are characterized by especially high rates of IV drug use. These include three housing projects, a southend Puerto Rican neighborhood, and a northend African American neighborhood. Hartford Dispensary AIDS outreach prevention workers have also identified a number of bars in white neighborhoods in which white IVDUs congregate.

Focus group research and informant interviews with IVDUs conducted as part of the Hartford NADR project suggest that while shooting galleries exist in Hartford, their density, even in high drug use areas, is comparatively low. As one IVDU interviewed in Project COPE by the lead author explained with reference to common places used to inject drugs:

Most of the time we'd find a patch of woods and just walk into it. It's kind of hard in the city, but there are enough spots you can go to. There's plenty of alleys you know, back parking lots, little stretches of woods. A lot of times I'd come back to the YMCA and get off, but after a while they picked up on that pattern, they're not stupid. There were a couple of dope fiends living there at the time. We'd get off outside, we'd get off in the car, or sometimes in garage bathrooms, you get off in restaurant bathrooms. Any place where there was water and you had a little degree of privacy you'd shoot up, you didn't care who saw you as long as it wasn't the police.

Focus group interviews also revealed that many Hartford IVDUs drive to New York to purchase drugs. Commonly these individuals rent or borrow needles from IVDUs in New York prior to their trip back to Hartford (Singer et al. 1990).

Possession of needles without a prescription is illegal in Connecticut.[1] Consequently, IVDUs are cautious about carrying "works" (drug injection equipment) with them for fear of being arrested. The effect is seen in the lead author's field notes from a IVDU focus group interview:

Several participants said that diabetics are a common source of needles, they regularly sell them to addicts. One participant talked about a women who regularly does this because she needs the money, but she feels bad about it and tries to tell her customers to use bleach. In fact, this participant indicated that he had tried to help her get bleach out to IV users, but had not had much success. But access to needles does appear to be a problem, needles are used and reused often. New needles are in demand, not because they are HIV-free, but because they are not clogged up or broken. Participants described how needles get used and passed around for so long that the needle is bent, the rubber gasket is missing, and wax or petroleum jelly is used to keep it somewhat closed. When someone shows up on the street or in a gallery with a new needle, everyone wants to use it. [Singer, field notes]

In Hartford, IV drug use is the primary source of new AIDS cases (Connecticut Department of Health Services 1989). As of March 30, 1990, 54% of diagnosed adolescent and adult AIDS cases in the city were among heterosexual IVDUs and another 10% were among gay/bisexual IVDUs (Connecticut Department of Health Services 1990). Palm notes:

The AIDS "profile" in Hartford is distinctive. In contrast to the rest of the country, AIDS here is found more often among IV drug users than among homosexuals. And, proportionately, more women here are infected than is true on a national level. . . . [The Department of Health] estimates conservatively that more than 6,000 Hartford residents are currently infected with the virus and perhaps 20,000 more are at risk for infection because of causative drug and sexual behaviors. That means that Hartford, although it is only the 112th largest city in the country, ranks 50th in the number of AIDS cases per capita. [Palm 1989:37]

NADR FINDINGS ON IV DRUG USERS: A TWO CITY COMPARISON

Reported data on demographic characteristics of research participants, sero-positivity rates, AIDS risk associated with needle use practices and sexual behavior, injection location, sources of injection equipment, and drug use frequency from the Miami NADR study are available for comparison with findings in Hartford (McCoy and Khoury 1990; Page 1990). Data were limited to 560 IVDUs from Miami and 347 from Hartford. Statistical analyses utilized frequency distributions, crosstabulations, analysis of variance, and chi-square tests. Four demographic variables (gender, ethnicity, age, and duration of drug injection) were examined for each city. Three categories of needle using behavior (needle-related AIDS risk, injection setting, and sources of needle supply) were constructed as variables to examine inter-city differences. Drug use variables were used to analyze similarities in injection and noninjection use patterns. Finally an index of sexual risk behavior was used to classify participants in terms of number of IVDU sex partners, nature of sexual practices, and condom use.[2]

Socio-Demographic Characteristics and HIV Infection

The sociodemographic characteristics and HIV infection rates of IVDU NADR participants in Miami and Hartford are reported in Table I. Rates of seropositivity are notably higher in Hartford generally as well as across gender, ethnic, age, and duration of drug injection categories. Differences in seropositivity are especially evident among males, African Americans compared to Hispanics, older addicts, and individuals with longer histories of intravenous drug use in the two cities. While female IVDUs have a noticeably higher rate of seropositivity than males in Miami, in Hartford gender is not significantly associated with infection. In fact, the rate of infection among males in the Hartford sample is 48% higher than the rate among males in the Miami sample, but among females the Hartford rate is only 17% higher. Conversely, unlike Miami, age is significantly related to serostatus in Hartford (P = .03), with IVDUs in the older age sets having notably higher rates of infection. Moreover, while rates of infection are at similar levels for African Americans and Hispanics in Miami, in Hartford seropositivity is higher among African Americans (50%) than among Hispanics (43.9%). Greater similarity is seen when comparing IVDUs in the two cities in terms of age and length of involvement in the IV drug subculture. For Miami, the median age of participants is 35 years and the median duration of drug injection is 14 years, compared to 34 and 15 years respectively for Hartford.

Miami researchers also report that 52% of the IVDUs in their study have at least a high school diploma, while 37% have not graduated from high school. Thirty-nine percent are unemployed, 30% report occasional work, and 27% have either full- or part-time employment. In addition, 29% report that their major source of income is obtained illegally, 24% have traded sex for money, 21% have traded sex for drugs, and 43% have been in jail (McCoy and Khoury 1990). Finally, 22% of the Miami sample lack permanent housing and are living in either a shelter, a welfare boarding home, or on the streets.

IVDU participants in the Hartford study report less formal education, with only 27% being high school graduates. Hispanics report the least amount of formal education, with only 19% reporting completion of high school. While 5% of African Americans in the Hartford sample report 8 years or less of education, for Hispanics this figure is 22%. White participants report the highest level of education among the three ethnic groups in the sample. Similar to Miami's rate, 30.8% of the individuals in the Hartford IVDU sample report that illegal activities provide their major source of income. However, only 11.5% have traded sex for money and 7.8% have traded sex for drugs, noticeably lower proportions than in the Miami sample. Again, while homeless rates among participants are similar in the two cities (20.4% for Hartford), a far higher percentage of Hartford respondents (83%) report having been in jail. A check of Connecticut Department of Correction records for 244 Hartford participants that failed to return for their 6 month follow-up interview revealed that 133 (55%) have been arrested since the beginning of Project COPE, 11% for drug-related charges. Seropositivity was significantly related to having been in jail or prison among Hartford respondents (P = .005).

These data reveal *four dimensions of contrast* (seropositivity patterns and rates, educational backgrounds, involvement in sex trade, and arrest histories) among IVDUs in Hartford and Miami. To some degree these contrasts reflect differences in the ethnic composition of the two samples (e.g., a larger percentage of Hispanics in the Hartford sample). However, arrest rates and involvement in sex trade would appear to reflect differences in local social environments, while positivity patterns may be tied to both drug use patterns and geographic proximity to New York, an epicenter of HIV infection.

Drug Use and Drug-related AIDS Risk

Comparisons between Hartford and Miami in AIDS risk among IVDUs associated with needle sharing and the use of unclean needles is reported in Table II. In both cities, only a small percentage of participants report consistently safe needle use behavior during the previous six months (i.e., avoiding of needle sharing, borrowing, and renting, or using only new or cleaned needles), however safe needle practices are somewhat more frequent among both male and female IVDUs in Miami. More marked contrasts are seen when comparing the percentage of participants who engage in the most risky set of needle use practices. While 9.7% of males and 7.7% of females in Hartford report the riskiest injection patterns (i.e., sharing with two or more persons, renting or borrowing needles, and not always using clean needles), in Miami these frequencies are 34.3% and 25.9% respectively.

Comparing the percentages reported in Table II in terms of sharing avoidance, sharing with one person, and sharing with two or more persons, it is clear that needle sharing is much more common among Miami IVDUs than it is among

TABLE II. Needle risk behavior of street IV drug users during the past six months.

Risk Behavior Category	Miami		Hartford	
	Male (%) N = 447	Female (%) N = 108	Male (%) N = 282	Female (%) N = 65
1. Doesn't share, doesn't rent/borrow always uses new/clean needles	11.8	15.7	9.6	11.5
2. Doesn't share, but does always use clean/new needles	1.3	0.0	9.3	9.1
3. Doesn't share, but doesn't always use clean/new needles	7.0	2.8	4.4	4.9
4. Doesn't share, but does rent/borrow, doesn't always use new/clean needles	3.4	3.7	9.6	7.7
5. Share with one person	3.8	6.5	3.4	5.6
6. Share with one person and rents/borrows needles	0.7	0.0	9.4	9.4
7. Share with one person and doesn't always use new/clean needles	5.9	9.3	5.5	6.6
8. Share with one person, rents/borrows needles, doesn't always use clean needles	11.4	16.7	9.6	8.0
9. Share with two or more persons	8.6	7.4	9.8	10.5
10. Share with two or more persons and rents/borrows needles	2.9	4.6	9.6	9.1
11. Share with two or more persons and doesn't always use new/clean needles	9.1	7.4	9.9	10.1
12. Share with two or more persons, rents/borrows needles, doesn't always use clean needles	34.3	25.9	9.7	7.7

*The Miami data are taken from Clyde B. McCoy and Elizabeth Khoury, 1990 "Drug Use and the Risk of AIDS." *American Behavioral Scientist* 33(4):424.

Hartford IVDUs. More Hartford IVDUs avoid needle sharing altogether than their Miami counterparts, and among those who do share, Hartford IVDUs are more likely than their Miami counterparts to share with only one person. These patterns are consistent for both males and females in the two samples. On the other hand, Hartford IVDUs are more likely to report renting or borrowing needles than Miami IVDUs. Again, this pattern exists for both male and female IVDUs. Table III indicates that the key variable here is borrowing of needles. While about 52% of Miami respondents report never borrowing needles, this figure is only 44% in Hartford, and Hartford IVDUs are also more likely to borrow needles more than half the time than those in Miami. Also, it is clear from Table III that IVDUs in Miami are much more likely to report that they obtain their needles legally, obtain new needles before "shooting up," and use needles only once. Less access to new needles in Hartford would appear to contribute to a greater tendency to borrow needles. These contrasts suggest local context variables that have influenced the development of critical differences in the configuration of *drug use rituals* (Agar 1977) among Hartford and Miami IVDUs.

These differences also are seen in Table IV, a comparison of places where IVDUs inject drugs. Hartford IVDUs are less likely than Miami participants to report that they "shoot up" at social gatherings (where sharing is more expected). Also, confirming focus group interviews, only 7% of Hartford IVDUs report using shooting galleries more than half the time, compared to 12% in the Miami sample. Instead, abandoned buildings, on the street, at home, and "other places" (perhaps the wooded areas referred to in the focus group interviews) are more common sites for injecting drugs in Hartford. Importantly, shooting galleries in Hartford appear to be riskier places for contracting HIV infection than those in Miami. While 29% of respondents who shoot up in galleries less than half the time and 52% who always shoot up in galleries all of the time were HIV positive in Miami, for Hartford these infection rates were 49% and 100% respectively. Given the higher level of sero-positivity among IVDUs in Hartford, and greater likelihood that participants know someone who has become sick with or died of AIDS, Hartford IVDUs may be attempting to restrict their involvement in the riskiest needle use patterns.

Inter-city differences also obtain with reference to drug use frequencies (Table V). While most participants in both cities report having injected cocaine in the past 6 months (93% in Miami, 97% in Hartford), Hartford IVDUs are much more likely to report injection of heroin and speedball (a combination of heroin and cocaine). Moreover, Hartford IVDUs are considerably more likely to report shooting these drugs every day, especially heroin. While only 33% of Miami IVDUs report intravenous drug use once or more a day, 76% of Hartford respondents report this level of intravenous drug use. And more frequent injection of cocaine in Hartford is significantly related to seropositivity ($P = .01$). By contrast, Hartford IVDUs are much less likely to report use of noninjection drugs like alcohol, marijuana and crack, and are notably less likely to report daily use of these drugs. Much larger percentages of Miami IVDUs report not having used cocaine and heroin in a noninjected form (e.g., smoking, snorting) while Hartford IVDUs are much more likely to report daily smoking or snorting of heroin than Miami IVDUs. Overall, these drug use patterns suggest that Miami IVDUs have broader, less frequent

TABLE III. Settings for drug injection among street IV drug users.

Setting	Miami (%) N = 720	Hartford(%) N = 318
Own place		
Never	27.3	29.6
Half the time or less	37.6	28.6
More than half the time	35.1	41.8
Friend's place		
Never	29.9	33.1
Half the time or less	49.1	45.5
More than half the time	18.2	21.3
Social gathering		
Never	78.2	85.0
Half the time or less	18.9	13.4
More than half the time	2.9	1.6
Dealer's place		
Never	73.6	78.7
Half the time or less	21.2	19.0
More than half the time	5.2	2.2
Shooting gallery		
Never	57.5	58.3
Half the time or less	30.3	34.7
More than half the time	12.1	7.0
Abandoned building		
Never	58.1	51.0
Half the time or less	33.0	41.1
More than half the time	8.9	8.0
On the street		
Never	69.2	58.4
Half the time or less	25.0	36.5
More than half the time	5.8	5.1
Other place		
Never	87.9	76.5
Half the time or less	10.0	22.2
More than half the time	2.1	1.3

*The Miami data are taken from J. Bryan Page, 1990 "Shooting Scenarios and Risk of HIV-1 Infection." American Behavioral Scientist 33(4):485.

polydrug use repertoires, while Hartford IVDUs tend to be more focused on frequent injection of cocaine or heroin alone or in combination or the smoking/snorting of these drugs. Lower levels of crack use in the Hartford sample may help explain lower rates of exchanging sex for drugs/money in the city. Smoking of crack has been tied to high-risk sexual activity, including prostitution, among women (Friedman et al. 1988; Rolfs, Goldberg, and Sharrar 1990).

In sum, a comparison of NADR findings for Hartford and Miami suggests noteworthy differences in both needle use practices and drug use patterns, differences that may be important in implementing prevention programs that are in tune with the constellation of risk behaviors present in each locale.

TABLE IV. Sources for syringes and needles among street IV drug users.

Sources	Miami (%) N = 720	Hartford(%) N = 318
Rented used works		
Never	61.5	65.0
Half the time or less	34.1	29.7
More than half the time	4.4	5.4
Borrowed used works		
Never	51.8	44.3
Half the time or less	40.4	43.7
More than half the time	7.8	12.0
Procured needles legally		
Never	82.5	96.2
Half the time or less	7.4	1.6
More than half the time	10.1	2.2
Used new needles only once		
Never	45.6	56.0
Half the time or less	31.1	38.2
More than half the time	23.3	15.8
Obtained needle in a sterile wrapper		
Never	11.3	17.0
Half the time or less	27.2	30.3
More than half the time	61.5	52.7

*The Miami data are taken from J. Bryan Page, 1990 "Shooting Scenarios and Risk of HIV-1 Infection." American Behavioral Scientist 33(4):486.

Sexual Risk Patterns

Beyond their risk for HIV infection through the use of contaminated drug injection equipment, IVDUs are also at risk for the contraction or transmission of the human immunodeficiency virus through sexual contact (Lewis et al. 1990; Nemoto et al. 1990; Robert et al. 1990). As H. McCloy et al. (1990:432) note, "Sexual behaviors which have been shown to contribute to the risk of HIV infection include multiple sex partners, number of sexual exposures, condom usage, and type of sexual activity during intercourse." Comparisons for sexual risk behaviors are reported in Table VI. In this index, risk scores are recorded for three types of sexual practices relative to the use or nonuse of condoms and whether or not sex partners are also IVDUs. Sexually active individuals with the least risk on the index are those who report that they have no IVDU sex partners and engage in only vaginal sex with a condom, while those at greatest risk have two or more sexual partners who are IVDUs and engage in anal intercourse without a condom.

Overall, Hartford respondents tend to be concentrated at the lower risk end of the sexual risk index, while Miami respondents are more likely to show up at the higher risk end. Hartford IVDUs, especially males, are much more likely to report that their sexual partners are not IVDUs. And among those with IVDU sex partners, Hartford respondents are less likely to have more than one partner who injects drugs intravenously. There are ethnic differences in these sexual patterns however. While most Hispanic IVDUs in the Hartford sample report no IVDU sex

TABLE V. Frequency of drug usage by street IV drug users during the past six months.

Category	Miami				Hartford			
	Never Use (%)	Once a week (%)	2 to 6 times a week (%)	Once a day (%)	Never Use (%)	Once a week (%)	2 to 6 times a week (%)	Once a day (%)
Noninjected Drugs								
Alcohol	9.9	24.2	18.5	47.3	19.3	37.7	13.8	29.1
Marijuana	21.1	41.1	13.3	24.1	32.3	39.3	13.9	14.5
Crack	19.5	23.4	15.1	39.6	25.9	44.4	8.6	21.0
Cocaine	33.5	28.1	13.5	21.6	20.7	47.1	13.0	19.2
Heroin	68.5	9.2	4.1	4.6	41.6	31.7	5.0	21.7
Injected Drugs								
Cocaine	6.0	35.4	24.3	33.8	2.5	22.7	15.6	59.2
Heroin	35.1	27.4	14.2	19.5	4.7	16.9	9.1	69.3
Speedball	38.0	23.4	12.8	22.2	4.3	25.3	7.9	62.5
Methadone	75.6	0.4	0.8	0.2	50.0	40.0	—	10.0
Other Opiates	74.5	8.4	1.6	1.2	48.9	31.9	4.3	14.9
Barbiturates	78.1	1.8	1.4	0.2	78.6	14.3	—	7.1
Tranquilizers	76.5	2.0	0.6	0.0	75.0	12.5	12.5	—
Amphetamines	75.4	6.1	1.4	1.6	75.0	20.8	—	4.2
PCP	76.2	0.8	0.6	0.2	—	—	—	—

*The Miami data are taken from Clyde B. McCoy and Elizabeth Khoury, 1990 "Drug Use and the Risk of AIDS." American Behavioral Scientist 33(4):425

TABLE VI. Sexual risk of street IV drug users .

Risk Behavior Category	Miami		Hartford	
	Male (%) N = 388[a]	Female (%) N = 96[b]	Male (%) N = 265[c]	Female (%) N = 62[d]
No sex partners	5.0	12.5	21.8	12.9
No IVDU sex partners, vaginal sex with condom	2.2	3.4	14.9	8.8
No IVDU sex partners, vaginal and oral sex with condom	2.4	2.2	0.6	0.0
No IVDU sex partners, vaginal sex without condom	9.8	10.1	39.1	17.6
No IVDU sex partners, vaginal and oral sex without condom	13.9	10.1	3.7	0.0
No IVDU sex partners, anal sex with condom	0.5	0.0	1.2	0.0
No IVDU sex partners, anal sex without condom	1.9	0.0	7.4	2.9
One IVDU sex partners, vaginal sex with condom	1.9	1.1	3.7	20.6
One IVDU sex partners, vaginal and oral sex with condom	1.1	3.4	0.0	0.0
One IVDU sex partners, vaginal sex without condom	5.2	18.0	19.3	38.2
One IVDU sex partners, vaginal and oral sex without condom	9.5	22.5	1.2	5.9
One IVDU sex partners, anal sex with condom	0.3	3.4	0.6	0.0
One IVDU sex partners, anal sex without condom	5.2	0.0	3.7	8.8
Two or more IVDU sex partners, vaginal sex with condom	0.8	0.0	1.2	0.0
Two or more IVDU sex partners, vaginal and oral sex with condom	0.8	0.0	0.0	0.0
Two or more IVDU sex partners, vaginal sex without condom	6.8	7.9	1.2	0.0
Two or more IVDU sex partners, vaginal and oral sex without condom	25.8	18.0	0.0	0.0
Two or more IVDU sex partners, anal sex with condom	0.5	0.0	1.2	0.0
Two or more IVDU sex partners, anal sex without condom	11.4	0.0	0.6	0.0

*The Miami data are taken from Clyde B. McCoy and Elizabeth Khoury, 1990 "Drug Use and the Risk of AIDS." *American Behavioral Scientist* 33(4):428.
a: Of the 447 men surveyed, 59 were unknown on at least one risk factor and were not included.
b: Of the 108 women surveyed, 7 were unknown on at least one risk factor and were not included.
c: Of the 265 men who are IV drug users during the past six months, 58 did not have sex with others.
d: Of the 62 women surveyed, 8 did not have sex with others in the past six months.

partners, African American participants are about equally likely to report either no IVDU or one IVDU sex partner. Both Hartford and Miami IVDUs with no IVDU sex partners or one IVDU sex partner tend not to use condoms, thereby increasing their sex risk level.

Also, Hartford IVDUs are much less likely to report multiple sex partners during the last six months than Miami IVDUs (42% vs. 77%), and among individuals who report multiple partners, Hartford respondents report fewer partners. Fifty-nine percent of Miami respondents with multiple partners report having between 2–6 partners and 41% report more than 6 partners; these figures compare with 77% and 24% respectively for Hartford. This pattern suggests that Hartford IVDUs are less sexually active than those in Miami, which may be related to their more frequent IV injection patterns (Wieland and Yunger 1979; Mirin et al. 1980; Mendelson and Mello 1982). This interpretation is supported by the data on the percentage of respondents who report having had no sex partners at all during the last six months. In Miami, 6.6% of the IVDUs in the sample report sexual abstinence during this period, while in Hartford the rate is 20%. Among females in these two samples, the same level of abstinence (12.5% in Miami vs. 12.9% in Hartford) is found, rates are notably different among men (5% in Miami vs. 21.8% in Hartford) however. This greater interest in IV drug injection rather than sex was graphically expressed by a respondent from the Hartford sample who commented, "I'd jump over 20 naked women for a bag of cocaine."

This interpretation also is consistent with findings showing that compared to the Miami respondents, individuals in the Hartford sample report a lower incidence of sexually transmitted diseases. In the Miami sample, almost half (49%) indicate a history of gonorrhea (compared to 13% for Hartford), 20% have had a history of syphilis (compared to 22% for Hartford), and 13% have had genital sores (compared to 5% for Hartford).

These comparisons further underscore the importance of examining local context factors. Not only are drug use patterns different in Hartford and Miami, sexual risk among IVDUs also differs in these two settings. And, as suggested above, it is likely that these two characteristics are related, creating differing risk profiles among IVDUs in the two cities.

DISCUSSION

IVDUs are highly at risk for HIV infection because of the use of needles and other injection equipment contaminated with the virus, the frequency with which they have one or more sexual partners who are also intravenous drug users, and their involvement with unsafe sexual practices. Enrollment of IVDUs in drug treatment is a critical step in limiting risk for HIV infection. Currently, it is estimated that there are as many as 1.2 million IVDUs in the U.S. and that only about 148,000 of them are in treatment at any point in time (Boffey 1988). Consequently, expansion of drug treatment, easy and rapid intake to treatment upon request, the implementation of indigenous case finders and culturally appropriate treatment modalities, and treatment-based AIDS education/counseling are all vital components of AIDS prevention for IVDUs. However, these are not sufficient conditions for eliminating the spread of HIV infection in the IVDU population and from IVDUs to their sexual partners and children. As Valdiserri notes,

Although to many, terminating drug use would seem to be the ideal solution to AIDS prevention among [IVDUs], it is, like so many of our responses to AIDS, neither easily implemented nor universally acceptable to all the individuals at risk. Merely making treatment opportunities available will not ensure that all addicts will enter treatment. [Valdiserri 1989:177]

As researchers in the Heroin Lifestyle Study of 124 male out-of-treatment IVDUs found, "80 percent . . . held treatment in disrepute and of these, 75 percent expressed particular concerns about methadone maintenance" (Beschner and Bovelle 1985:160). Also, expansion of treatment does not ensure that clients will remain in treatment or that they will not return to drug use some time afterward. In their drug treatment follow-up study for a number of different treatment modalities, Hubbard et al. (1984) found that only about one-third of clients report not returning to their pretreatment drug of choice during the follow-up period. Contrary to folk beliefs, however, the best retention rates were found among methadone maintenance clients. Finally, AIDS risk among IVDUs is not limited to their drug use behaviors. IVDUs also face substantial risk from unsafe sexual contact.

Alternative AIDS prevention efforts for IVDUs beyond drug treatment clearly are needed. Various types of prevention have been attempted, including street outreach education, bleach distribution, educational media and poster campaigns, IVDU community group promotion efforts, and sterile needle exchange programs (Wiebel 1988; Newmeyer et al. 1989; Singer, Irizzary and Schensul 1991; Liebman et al. 1990). In Hartford, Project COPE has implemented and is testing the efficacy of community-based, culturally sensitive intervention for African American and Puerto Rican IVDUs (Singer, Owens, and Reyes 1991; Weeks, Grier, and Dyton 1990). Other NADR projects are testing several alternative AIDS prevention approaches and evaluating their effectiveness using follow-up post-intervention data collection on changes in AIDS risk. The ultimate goal of the NADR initiative is the dissemination nationally of project models that demonstrate superior effectiveness in reducing risk behaviors. In the implementation of AIDS prevention programs, however, the comparisons reported here point to the importance of grounding prevention in a clear-sighted and ethnographically holistic awareness of the local context and its impact on the configuration of IVDU behaviors and beliefs. As Bateson and Goldsby (1988:69) cogently note:

There is an old story about a group of blind men and an elephant in which each man, because he tactilely explores a different part of the animal, comes away with a different conception of the whole. And so it is with AIDS.

ACKNOWLEDGMENTS

The authors would like to thank Lani Davison for her helpful comments on an earlier version of this paper. The Hartford study reported here was supported by grant R18 DA05750 from the National Institute on Drug Abuse.

NOTES

1. Recently the Connecticut State Legislature passed a bill that authorizes the implementation of a needle exchange program in New Haven. Possession of specially marked needles distributed by this program will not be illegal in New Haven. Possession of needles and syringes without a prescription remains illegal in Hartford.
2. Construction of these variables follows the Miami presentation of the data in McCoy and Khoury (1990) and Page (1990).

REFERENCES CITED

Agar, M.
   1977   Into that Whole Ritual Thing: Ritualistic Drug Use among Urban American Heroin Addicts. *In* Drugs, Rituals and Altered States of Consciousness. B. Du Toit, ed. Pp. 137–148. Rotterdam: A. A. Balkema.
Angarano, G., G. Pastore, L. Monno, F. Santantion, N. Luchena, and O. Schiraldi
   1985   Rapid Spread of HTLV-III Infection Among Drug Addicts in Italy. Lancet 2:1302.
Backstrand, J., and S. Schensul
   1982   Co-evolution in Outlying Ethnic Communities: The Puerto Ricans of Hartford, CT. Urban Anthropology 11:9–38.
Bateson, C., and R. Goldsby
   1988   Thinking AIDS. Reading, MA: Addison-Wesley.
Battjes, R., and R. Pickens
   1989   Introduction of HIV Infection Among Intravenous Drug Abusers in Low Prevalence Areas. Journal of Acquired Immune Deficiency Syndromes 2:533–539.
Beschner, G., and E. Bovelle
   1985   Life with Heroin: Voices of Experience. *In* Life with Heroin. B. Hanson, G. Beschner, J. Walters and E. Bovelle, eds. Pp. 75–107. Lexington, MA: Lexington Books.
Boffey, P.
   1988   AIDS Panel Backs Wide Drive in U.S. New York Times, 3 March: B5,B7.
Brown, B.
   1990   Preliminary Findings from the National AIDS Demonstration Research Projects. Paper presented at the National Association of State Alcohol and Drug Abuse Directors Conference. New Orleans, LA.
Butynski, W., N. Record, P. Bruhn, and D. Canova
   1987   State Resources and Services Related to Alcohol and Drug Problems, Fiscal Year 1986. Washington, DC: National Association of State Alcohol and Drug Abuse Directors.
Centers for Disease Control
   1989   HIV/AIDS Suveillance Report, June:1–16.
Chaisson, R., A. Moss, R. Onishi, D. Osmond, and J. Carlson
   1987   Human Immunodeficiency Virus Infection in Heterosexual Intravenous Drug Users in San Francisco. American Journal of Public Health 77(2):169–172.
Connecticut Department of Health Services
   1989   Acquired Immunodeficiency Syndrome in Connecticut: Annual Surveillance Report. Hartford, CT: State of Connecticut, Department of Health Services.
   1990   Acquired Immunodeficiency Syndrome (AIDS): Surveillance Report for March 30, 1990. Hartford: State of Connecticut, Department of Health Services.
Conviser, R., and J. Rutledge
   1988   The Need for Innovation to Halt AIDS Among Intravenous Drug Users and Their Sexual Partners. AIDS and Public Policy 3(1):43–50.
Des Jarlais, D., and S. Friedman
   1987   HIV Infection among Intravenous Drug Users: Epidemiology and Risk Reduction. AIDS 1: 67–76.

Des Jarlais, D., S. Friedman, and R. Stoneburner
 1988   HIV Infection and Intravenous Drug Use: Critical Issues in Transmission Dynamics, Infection
         Outcomes, and Prevention. Reviews of Infectious Disease 10(1):151–158.
Eames, E., and J. Goode
 1977   Anthropology of the City. Englewood Cliffs, NJ: Prentice-Hall.
Fox, R.
 1972   Rationale and Romance in Urban Anthropology. Urban Anthropology 1:205–233.
Friedman, S., D. Des Jarlais, and J. Sothern
 1986   AIDS Health Education for Intravenous Drug Users. Health Education Quarterly 13(4):383–393.
Friedman, S., C. Dozier, C. Sterk, T. Williams, Jo Sothern, D. Des Jarlais, et al.
 1988   Crack Use Puts Women at Risk for Heterosexual Transmission of HIV from Intravenous Drug
         Users. Paper presented at the Fourth International AIDS Conference, Stockholm.
Galea, R., B. Lewis and L. Baker
 1988   A Model for Implementing AIDS Education in a Drug Abuse Treatment Setting. Hospital and
         Community Psychiatry 39(8):886–888.
Goode, E.
 1984   Drugs in American Society. New York: Alfred A. Knopf.
Hahn, R., I. Onorato, T. Jones, and J. Dougherty
 1989   Prevalence of HIV Infection among Intravenous Drug Users in the United States. Journal of the
         American Medical Association 261:2677–2684.
Hastrup, K., and P. Elsass
 1990   Anthropological Advocacy: A Contradiction in Terms? Current Anthropology 31(3):301–312.
Haverkos, H.
 1988   Overview: HIV Infection Among Intravenous Drug Abusers in the United States and Europe.
         In Needle Sharing Among Intravenous Drug Abusers: National and International Perspectives.
         R. Battjes and R. Pickens, eds. Pp.7–17. NIDA Research Monograph 80. Washington, DC: U.S.
         Department of Health and Human Services.
Hubbard, R., J. Rachal, S. Craddock, and E. Cavanaugh
 1984   Treatment Outcome Prospective Study (TOPS): Client Characteristics and Behavior Before,
         During and After Treatment. *In* Drug Abuse Treatment Evaluation. F. Tims and J. Ludford, eds.
         NIDA Research Monograph 51. Washington, DC: Department of Health and Human Services.
Hubbard, R., M. E. Marsden, E. Cavanugh, J. Rachal, and H. Ginzburg
 1988   Role of Drug-Abuse Treatment in Limiting the Spread of AIDS. Reviews of Infectious Diseases
         10(2):377–384.
Lange, R., F. Snyder, D. Lozovsky, V. Kaistha, M. Kaczaniuk, J. Jaffe and the ARC Epidemiology
Collaborating Group
 1988   Geographic Distribution of Human Immunodeficiency Virus Markers in Parenteral Drug
         Abusers. American Journal of Public Health 78(4):443–4446.
Leeds, A.
 1968   The Anthropology of Cities. *In* Urban Anthropology. E. Eddy, ed. Pp. 31–47. New York:
         Praeger.
Lewis, D., J. Watters, and P. Case
 1990   The Prevalence of High-Risk Sexual Behavior in Male Intravenous Drug Users with Steady
         Female Partners. American Journal of Public Health 80(4):465–466.
Liebman, J., D. McIlvaine, L. Kotranski, and R. Lewis
 1990   AIDS Prevention for IV Drug Users and Their Sexual Partners in Philadelphia. American
         Journal of Public Health 80(5):615–616.
Mascola, L., L. Lieb, K. Iwakoshi, D. McAllister, T. Siminowski, M. Giles, G. Run, S. Fannin, and I.
Strantz
 1989   HIV Seroprevalence in Intravenous Drug Users: Los Angeles, California, 1986. American
         Journal of Public Health 79(1):81–82.
McBride, D., et. al.
 1986   Drugs and Homicide. Bulletin of the New York Academy of Medicine 62(5):497–508.
McCoy, C., D. Chitwood, E. Khoury, and C. Miles
 1990   The Implementation of an Experimenal Research Design in the Evaluation of an Intervention to
         Prevent AIDS among IV Drug Users. Journal of Drug Issues 20(2):215–223.

McCoy, C., and E. Khoury
    1990   Drug Use and the Risk of AIDS. American Behavioral Scientist 33(4):419–431.
McCoy, H. V., S. Dodds, and C. Nolan
    1990   AIDS Intervention Design for Program Evaluation: The Miami Community Outreach Project. Journal of Drug Issues 20(2):223–243.
McCoy, H. V., C. McKay, L. Hermanns, and S. Lai
    1990   Sexual Behavior and the Risk of HIV Infection. American Behavioral Scientist 33(4):432–450.
Mendelson, J., and N. Mello
    1982   Hormones and Psycho-sexual Development in Young Men Following Chronic Heroin Use. Neurobehavioral Toxicology and Teratology 4(4):441–445.
Mirin, S., R. Myer, J. Mendelson, and J. Ellingboe
    1980   Opiate Use and Sexual Function. International Journal of the Addictions 4:1–24.
Moss, A.
    1987   AIDS and Intravenous Drug Use: The Real Heterosexual Epidemic. British Medical Journal 294:389–390.
Nemoto, T., L. Brown, K. Foster and A. Chu
    1990   Behavioral Risk Factors of Human Immunodeficiency Virus Infection Among Intravenous Drug Users and Implications for Preventive Interventions. AIDS Education and Prevention 2(2):116–126.
Newmeyer, J.
    1988   Why Bleach? Development of a Strategy to Combat HIV Contagion among San Francisco Intravenous Drug Users. In Needle Sharing among Intravenous Drug Users: National and International Perspectives. R. Battjes and R. Pickens, eds. Pp. 151–159. NIDA Research Monograph 80. Washington, DC: U.S. Department of Health and Human Services.
Newmeyer, J., H. Feldman, P. Biernacki, and J. Watters
    1989   Preventing AIDs Contagion Among Intravenous Drug Users. Medical Anthropology 10(2–3):167–176.
Novick, D., M. Kreek, D. Des Jarlais, T. Spira, E. Khuri, J. Ragunath, V. Kalyanaraman, A. Gibl, and A. Miescher
    1986   LAV among Parenteral Drug Users. In Problems of Drug Dependence 1985: Proceedings of the 47th Annual Scientific Meeting, L. Harris, ed. NIDA Research Monograph 67. Washington, DC: U.S. Department of Health and Human Services.
Novick, L., B. Truman, and J. Lehman
    1988   The Epidemiology of HIV in New York State. New York State Journal of Medicine 88:242–246.
Page, J. B.
    1990   Shooting Scenarios and Risk of HIV-1 Infection. American Behavioral Scientist 33(4):478–490.
Page, J. B., D. Chitwood, P. Smith, N. Kane, and D. McBride
    1990   Intravenous Drug Use and HIV Infection in Miami. Medical Anthropology Quarterly 4(1):56–71.
Page, J. B., L. Rio, J. Sweeney, and C. McKay
    1985   Alcohol and Adaptation to Exile in Miami's Cuban Population. In The American Experience with Alcohol. L. Bennett and G. Ames, eds. Pp. 315–332. New York: Plenum.
Page, J. B., and P. Smith
    1990   Venous Envy: The Importance of Having Functional Veins. The Journal of Drug Issues 20(2):291–308.
Palm, C.
    1989   The Persistence of AIDS: A Cautionary Tale. Hartford Monthly, May:37–39, 64.
Pereira, L., and M. Henrickson
    1988   Demographic Estimates of Intravenous Drug Use in Hartford. Hartford, CT: Hartford Health Department AIDS Prevention Program.
Press, I.
    1975   The City as Context: Cultural, Historical and Bureaucratic Determinants of Behavior in Seville. Urban Anthropology 4(1):27–35.
Price, J.
    1973   Tijuana: Urbanization in a Border Culture. South Bend, IN: University of Notre Dame Press.

Robert, C.-F., J.-J. Déglon, J. Wintsch, J.-L. Martin, L. Perrin, M. Bourquin, V. Gabriel, and B. Hirschel
    1990   Behavioural Changes in Intravenous Drug Users in Geneva: Rise and Fall of HIV Infection, 1980–1989. AIDS 4:657–660.
Robertson, J., A. Bucknall, and P. Welsby
    1986   Epidemic of AIDS Related Virus (HTLV-III/LAV) Infection among IV Drug Abusers. British Medical Journal 292:527–529.
Rolfs, R., M. Goldberg, and R. Sharrar
    1990   Risk Factors for Syphilis: Cocaine Use and Prostitution. American Journal of Public Health 80(7):853–857.
Rollwagon, J.
    1972   A Comparative Framework for the Investigation of the City-as-Context: A Discussion of the Mexican Case. Urban Anthropology 1:68–86.
Siegal, H.
    1990   Intravenous Drug Abuse and the HIV Epidemic in Two Midwestern Cities: A Preliminary Report. Journal of Drug Issues 20(2):281–290.
Singer, M.
    1978   Chassidic Recruitment and the Local Context. Urban Anthropology 7(4):373–383.
Singer, M., and M. Borrero
    1984   Indigenous Treatment for Alcoholism: The Evidence for Puerto Rican Spiritism. Medical Anthropology 8(4):246–273.
Singer, M., C. Flores, L. Davison, G. Burke, Z. Castillo, K. Scalon, and M. Rivera
    1990   SIDA: The Economic, Social, and Cultural Context of AIDS among Latinos. Medical Anthropology Quarterly 4:73–117.
Singer, M., R. Irizarry, and J. J. Schensul
    1991   Needle Access as an AIDS Prevention Strategy for IV Drug Users: A Research Perspective. Human Organization 50(2):142–153.
Singer, M., P. Owns, and L. Reyes
    1991   Culturally Appropriate AIDS Prevention for IV Drug Users and their Sexual Partners. In Community-Based AIDS Prevention. Pp. 234–239. Washington, DC: U.S. Department of Health and Human Services (DHHS Publication No. [ADM] 91–1752.
Smith, M. E.
    1975   A Tale of Two Cities: The Reality of Historical Differences. Urban Anthropology 4:61–72.
Sowder, B.
    1989   A Preliminary Look at National AFA-Reported Behavior Change. Paper presented at the First Annual NADR National Meeting. Washington, DC:
Spencer, B.
    1989   On the Accuracy of Current Estimates of the Numbers of Intravenous Drug Users. In AIDS: Sexual Behavior and Intravenous Drug Use. C. Turner, H. Miller, and L. Moses, eds. Pp. 429–446. Washington, DC: National Academy Press.
Sufian, M., S. Friedman, A. Neaigus, B. Stepherson, J. Rivera-Beckman, and D. Des Jarlais
    1990   Impact of AIDS on Puerto Rican Intravenous Drug Users. Hispanic Journal of Behavioral Sciences 12(2):122–134.
Turner, C., H. Miller, and L. Moses, eds.
    1989   AIDS: Sexual Behavior and Intravenous Drug Use. Washington, DC: National Research Council.
Valdiserri, R.
    1989   Preventing AIDS: The Design of Effective Programs. New Brunswick, NJ: Rutgers University Press.
Weddington, W. et al.
    1990   Risk Behaviors for HIV Transmission among Intravenous-Drug Users Not in Treatment— United States, 1987–1989. Morbidity and Mortality Weekly Review 39(16):273–276.
Weeks, M., M. Grier, and R. Dyton
    1990   Comparisons of Culturally Oriented Community-Based AIDS Intervention Programs for IV-Drug Users and their Sexual Partners. Paper presented at the annual meeting of the Northeastern Anthropological Association, Burlington, VT.

Weibel, W.
   1988   Combining Ethnographic and Epidemiologic Methods in Targeted AIDS Interventions: The Chicago Model. *In* Needle Sharing among Intravenous Drug Users: National and International Perspectives. R. Battjes and R. Pickens, eds. Pp.137–150. NIDA Research Monograph 80. Washington, DC: U.S. Department of Health and Human Services.

Wiedman, D., and J. B. Page
   1982   Drug Use on the Street and on the Beach: Cubans and Anglos in Miami, Florida. Urban Anthropology 11(2):212–226.

Wieland, W., and M. Younger
   1979   Sexual Effects and Side Effects of Heroin and Methadone. *In* Proceedings of the Third Conference on Methadone Treatment. Pp. 50–53. Washington, DC: National Institute on Mental Health.

Young, P.
   1989   NIDA's NADR Project. Network 1(1):1–2.

Medical Anthropology, Vol. 14, pp. 307–322
Reprints available directly from the publisher
Photocopying permitted by license only

Sex, Drugs and Videotape: The Prevention of AIDS in a New York City Shelter for Homeless Men

Ida Susser and M. Alfredo González

This paper documents a process of social change through participant observation. During the course of research a group response was facilitated by a team of residents, staff and researchers. The social context, a shelter for homeless men in New York City, will be presented first, emphasizing those aspects of resident living that are germane to HIV transmission. Next, we describe the group response, the creation of a video. This activity gave numerous insights to the investigators into how the men perceived the homeless state and something of their relationships to others within and outside the institutions. In particular, their views on women and sex were expressed in the video. The insights gained by the men and the investigators are analyzed in terms of a self-help strategy which was effective in conveying information about HIV transmission and prevention.

Key words: AIDS prevention, homeless men, drug use, New York City

INTRODUCTION

The goal of the project described in this paper was to explore the possibility of promoting social changes relevant to the prevention of HIV transmission. Politicians and scientists now give ample lip service to education as a primary tool needed for the control of the HIV epidemic (Baltimore and Wolff 1986) but grassroots experience with preventive approaches shows that the need is for strategies far more fundamental than has ever been implied by "education" (Stall 1988; Stall et al. 1990; Matiella 1988; Martin and Stroud 1988; Christiano and Susser 1989; Singer 1990; Fullilove et al. 1990). Thus preventing HIV infection demands of both individuals and groups that they modify many intimate, historically-rooted, habitual social relations. People can hope to set the needed behavior changes in motion, in a community or social group, only if first they achieve some understanding of the

IDA SUSSER *is a member of the faculty in the doctoral program in Anthropology at the Graduate School and University Center of the City University of New York, 33 West 42nd Street, New York, NY 10036 and is Professor of Community Health at the School of Health Sciences, Hunter College, City University of New York. Dr. Susser is the author of* Norman Street: Poverty and Politics in an Urban Neighborhood *and has conducted extensive research on poverty and health in the United States and Puerto Rico. Her research interests include gender, social movements and politics.*

M. ALFREDO GONZÁLEZ *is an AIDS activist and a Ph.D. candidate in the Anthropology program of the Graduate School and University Center of the City University of New York, 33 West 42nd Street, New York, NY 10036. His main research interests are AIDS, poverty and politics. He is currently involved in a project evaluating efforts to maintain mentally ill men out of city shelters.*

social organization within the group, and second, if they discover ways to facilitate social movements of the required kind.

This paper documents a process of social change through participant observation.[1] During the course of research, a group response was facilitated by a team of residents, staff and researchers. The social context, a shelter for homeless men in New York City, will be presented first, emphasizing those aspects of resident living that are germane to HIV transmission. Next, we describe the group response, the creation of a video. This activity gave numerous insights to the investigators into how the men perceived the homeless state and something of their relationships to others within and outside the institutions. In particular, their views on women and sex were expressed in the video. These insights, learned by the men as well as by the investigators, are analysed in terms of a self-help stratagem which seemed to be effective in HIV transmission and prevention.

THE SOCIAL CONTEXT

Community, Location and Shelter: Risks and Resources

The shelter for homeless men, our focus of study, is located in a community which is at high risk for HIV infection. The seropositivity rate for men in a neighboring hospital is about 18 per cent (St. Louis et al. 1990). The risks for HIV infection among homeless men are in part a function of the rates in this community with which they interact and within which they find sexual partners or share needles (Murphy 1988).

The higher the rate of HIV infection in any community, the greater the risk for "risky" behaviors. It would therefore not be surprising if the shelter in question has one of the highest prevalence rates of seropositivity among non-institutionalized populations in the U.S., because even compared to other residents in the community, risks can be expected to be higher in shelters. The very state of homelessness implies alienation from a fixed abode and family, which in turn encourages sexual encounters of a casual nature (many partner changes, ignorance of the partner's risks). Transmission of the infection will also be more frequent if men lack responsibility for passing on infection to partners as both casual sex and drug use reduce responsibility for self and partner. This is also a high risk population in that an appreciable proportion of residents have past or present experience with parenteral drug use. Survey data confirm our own fieldwork that 38% of men who stay at the shelter are or have been involved with drugs in some way (E. Susser, Struening, and Conoven 1989). Our research suggests that the most common substance used by men in 1988–89 was cocaine, administered intravenously. Thus a significant source of HIV infection is likely to be needle sharing.

A sexually active population with a high prevalence of drug use faces multiple risks in the spread of HIV. Therefore, the implementation of educational programs focused on needle cleaning and condom use would be two areas around which men at the shelter could organize for HIV prevention. Such efforts would involve behavior change among shelter residents in their contacts with the wider community. In this sense, interventions at the shelter would serve as important conduits for information and practice throughout the network of city-wide interactions in which the men who stayed at the shelter participated.

Just as people with AIDS from poorer minority communities have not been diagnosed as readily, so they have had greater difficulty in developing organizations to combat AIDS than people from more prosperous groups (Singer et al. 1990). The combination of high risk with lack of resources in poor communities makes the analysis of instances of self-expression and mobilization crucial for understanding how such communities can work to prevent the spread of AIDS and, as we learned from the gay community, how they can learn to initiate health care practices in which patients have greater control (Feldman 1986; Stall 1988; Susser and Jagemann 1989).

Life in the Shelter

In describing life in the shelter and its significance for the HIV epidemic, we refer briefly to the physical environment and the staff. Next we discuss how shelter residents make a living, first in terms of formal employment and secondly in the informal or illicit economy. This is an essential backdrop to the marketing of illicit drugs and to sexual encounters mentioned above. We also consider the institutional responses to AIDS. Lastly, we look in more depth at contacts between the men resident in the shelter and the wider community.

The Armoury Shelter (a pseudonym, as are all proper nouns in this paper) stands on the corner of two streets on the crest of a hill overlooking a rundown neighborhood. Seen from the bus-stop at the bottom of the hill, it is an impressive red brick structure, outlined against the sky. Four sets of stairs lead up to the level where the shelter is located. Residents of the shelter "hang out" across the street from the main entrance. Opposite is a vacant lot that in summertime is full of vegetation. At the back is an abandoned building behind which is a "shooting gallery," (a place where drug users can go to borrow needles and inject drugs).

Clients must enter the shelter through a metal detector. Employees are not checked for weapons and use a different doorway. At the entrance is a security point where people sign in and state their destination. A long staircase leads upstairs to the second floor where 300 men sleep in a large dormitory. The floor of the dormitory is divided into three unequal sections: one for the handicapped, another for men with psychological problems, and a third large section for everyone else. On the same floor are tables where men sit to have their meals and two television sets around which they gather.

Some men stay in the shelter for a single night while others remain for several months or even years. At entry every man is assigned a locker. The locker is reserved for three days after the last night that a man spent at the shelter; following that, the contents are thrown away and the locker is assigned to the next entrant. This practice illustrates the tenuous ties between the men and the shelter.

Over 150 people staff the shelter, in addition to 12 security guards. Shelter staff, depending on their office, interact with residents in different ways. Maintenance and custodial staff make up the largest proportion. They frequently employ residents to perform tasks, acting more as supervisors than as workers. Social workers and caseworkers help residents apply for public assistance, look for housing, and finance medical care. Community workers provide special services for mentally ill and disabled homeless, and a doctor holds a clinic on the premises.

Making a Living

Shelter residents vary widely in their need for wealth and in their success in acquiring it. We categorized the strategies they use broadly as "formal" and "on the streets." Formal sources of income include "regular work," the shelter work program, and public assistance. "On the streets" was sub-classified as legal, questionable, and illegal.

Formal Employment.   Securing "regular" work from a homeless shelter is not easy. An example that demonstrates the difficulties were the experiences of Angel, a young man regarded by shelter employees as a model resident. Thus Angel often talked about returning to school and regarded life in the shelter as a temporary expediency. Like many in the shelter, he referred to others as having problems and in conversation distanced himself from "homeless men" in general.

Angel wanted to apply for a job as a sidewalk guard, watching over goods laid on tables in front of a store. He had first to prepare a resumé. In order to type the resumé, he used his institutional contacts (at the shelter) to gain access to a university computer. Only an exceptional homeless person would have first the presence to walk into a university computer room and then the technological facility to prepare the resumé. Next, he had the common problem of providing an address. Homeless men do not like to use the shelter as an address since they say that it causes employers to prejudge them negatively. Angel used a friend's address. He also had to give names of references, which can be difficult for a man without connections among stable households. Angel provided names of shelter workers, without identifying them as such.

Having surmounted the hurdles of resumé, address and references, Angel was scheduled for a job interview. In order to appear for the interview, he borrowed clothes from shelter residents. However, he needed to iron a shirt. One resident of the shelter owned an iron. When Angel approached this man who controlled a variety of important resources in the shelter, he was told he could borrow the iron in exchange for sexual favors. Angel claimed, in recounting the incident to the fieldworker, that he preferred to go for his interview in a wrinkled shirt.

These were some of the obstacles involved in one man's search for a regular job. Still, some shelter residents did find jobs in fast-food restaurants and other low-paying work. One resident was employed as a nurse's aide in a hospital where he had been working for years. Since he had been hired before he became homeless, he had not been forced to confront the barriers faced by Angel. Although he had been homeless for two years he maintained his employment throughout. He was reluctant to participate in the video because it might disclose his homelessness to viewers who knew him from work.

Participation in the Shelter Work Program was required of all men, although enforcement was lax. The men were supposed to work for 20 hours to earn food tickets and to stay in the shelter for more than three weeks. They cleaned the floors and carried out kitchen and other unskilled tasks under the supervision of regular shelter employees. These jobs, seen as demeaning by shelter residents and paying only $12.50 a week, did not contribute significantly to making a living. Moreover, the requirement of shelter work allowed shelter employees to act more as work bosses than as staff, setting up negative hierarchical work relations between some employees and residents (see also Gounis and Susser 1990).

Financial assistance was available to some shelter residents in the form of Social Security Income (SSI) because they had been classified as disabled in some way, perhaps due to a history of mental disorder. Others, not officially disabled hence not qualifying for SSI, received public assistance. Social workers helped clients to complete forms to receive shelter services.

Work on the streets: legal, questionable and illegal.   Legal sources of work on the streets were two: can collecting and junk collecting. Both required an extensive amount of labor for low returns. Cans at five cents each are returnable at stores, machines in stores, and at a center set up by the homeless. Frequently store workers do not welcome wandering men and claim that they do not have time to take cans. Machines are often broken. Nevertheless, this remains a common source of income for men in the shelter. Others are junk collectors who follow a routine schedule of sifting through garbage early in the morning, filling shopping carts, and lugging their findings to sites where they can exchange them for money.

One questionable source of income involves the begging economy. Men frequently clean car windows at intersections and earn change, occasionally amounting to more than a dollar. Others ask shelter workers or acquaintances for subway tokens to go somewhere, then walk instead and save the token, as did one man when accompanied by our assistant.

Another questionable source of income is an informal shelter market. Residents sometimes appear at the shelter with new packaged goods, often with brand names visible, for sale. One man earlier institutionalized for mental disorder functioned well in this underground economy. He arrived one day with a pile of shirts to sell, then sold bottles of cologne, and another day fashionable handbags. The source of the goods was not disclosed to us. The shelter served as a marketplace for a variety of goods and at least one discharged resident later returned to the shelter to sell his wares. Hence, the shelter provided a familiar environment for trade and social interchange, one that was also profitably exploited in the drug trade, a topic to which we now turn.

An outright illegal source of funds was the drug trade, central to the spread of HIV. Although discussed here as providing income, the use and exchange of drugs in the life of shelter residents relates also to entertainment, sex, and social interaction with staff, police, and community.

In light of the legal and semi-legal alternatives outlined above, the sale of drugs was a lucrative business. However, in our interviews and fieldwork, although we found many drug users, primarily users of intravenous cocaine, only two residents were reported to sell drugs. Both these were regarded as petty traders—they were not the big-time dealers but were connected to larger dealers outside the shelter. In this sense, shelter residents served as reserve labor supply and market for the drug industry, rather than as managers and owners. One man who apparently some-times sold cocaine at the shelter was the brother of a reputedly larger dealer who lived outside the shelter.

The second so-called "part-time" dealer provides an example of how the meager resources available to homeless men elevate those with even a slight advantage in access to positions of power in the social networks. Joe was white, American-born, and receiving social security income on the basis of mental disability. He was able to accumulate prescription drugs through Medicaid. He sold these medications in order to buy cocaine for his own intravenous use. At the same time, he diligently put in his hours working for the shelter and actively participated in shelter activities, such as the theater and video project we shall describe. Joe knew numerous shelter residents and employees and served as a link between them. Joe had money to spend, and as a consequence of his multiple social connections and his available cash he had considerable influence among the residents. He could recruit people to work on various projects and he used his extra resources to build wider networks. Thus, as in the case of the resident who owned the iron, control of few resources can be manipulated into considerable influence in the almost cashless barter economy of the shelter. In light of widespread drug use, those who do sell drugs accumulate power quickly and effectively although they themselves may be only petty dealers from the point of view of the city drug market. As we discuss later, residents claimed that shelter workers were often suppliers of drugs (see also Gounis and Susser 1990).

In terms of intravenous drug use, obviously central to the spread of HIV infection, residents and guards said that residents use the bathrooms to inject cocaine and are likely to share "works" (drug equipment). Residents mentioned that the vacant lot opposite the shelter (where several bushes screened people from view) served both as a "shooting gallery" and a place to find women willing to have sex for money or drugs. "Works" could be rented for a few dollars and were reused constantly. Scenes of intravenous drug use and the exchange of sex for drugs featured prominently in the plans for the video created by shelter residents. Residents seemed aware of the importance of cleaning "works" and needles with bleach, but claimed that this was not commonly done around the shelter.

Sex in the shelter economy.   Within the shelter, sexual favors between men seemed to be bartered more than sold for money or exchanged for drugs, although we cannot document the extent of such practices. One man told us that he had worked as a transvestite prostitute outside the shelter. The sale of sex was certainly an available source of cash for some men in the shelter, whether or not they saw themselves as gay or bisexual. Thus in planning for the video, residents chose to portray a man, who was not self-identified as gay, exchanging sex with men because he badly needed cash. There were also women who spent time at the door of the shelter and in the vacant lot opposite who apparently exchanged sex with shelter residents and with other men for money or crack (smokable cocaine). While the men in the shelter claimed to inject cocaine, they described the women as using crack. As will be noted below, each of these issues was discussed among shelter residents and worked through in video scenes.

Topics such as the sale of drugs and sex are difficult to assess or discuss openly. For these reasons the video project became an important channel for residents, shelter workers and researchers to address such issues, while not attributing the behavior in question to any particular resident. In analyzing the video project below, we attempt to sort out further some of the perspectives on sex and drugs which emerged among shelter residents and workers.

Institutional Responses to AIDS

Lacking clear directives, the institutional responses to the AIDS epidemic found the staff at a loss, bewildered and inconsistent. At the time our fieldworkers entered the shelter in August 1988, no AIDS education had taken place in the shelter and no funding was available for it. This was in spite of the fact that by December 1987 both residents and staff knew that at least three residents had recently died of AIDS (Brown and Valencia 1987) and shelter staff had asked for a health educator to be appointed to the shelter.

Members of the shelter staff whom we interviewed at this time were under the impression that persons who were diagnosed as having AIDS were not permitted to remain at the shelter. For this reason shelter staff were uneasy about identifying AIDS cases. In fact, we were told by staff members that it was possible that doctors at the nearby hospitals might be purposely delaying diagnosis in order to avoid precipitating the eviction of PWA's (persons with AIDS) from the shelter system and into the streets. Nobody wanted the responsibility of finding housing for those evicted, since a PWA could not be re-admitted to the shelter. Hospital staff argued that their social workers were already too busy. Residents and staff themselves also were receiving ambiguous and inaccurate information about AIDS. When the shelter doctor was asked whether every client should be tested for AIDS, the minutes of the meeting note: "Dr. Paz replied that the clinic is not set up to test everyone for AIDS, also that the test is very costly and will only be done at a hospital upon request by the client." The Centers for Disease Control and public health officials in general were at this time recommending that people who thought themselves at risk should be tested. Considering the high incidence of drug use known to occur among the shelter population, the doctor's answer seems to undermine effective action. Since the test for HIV infection is free and available at a number of sites in New York City, such a statement was not only wrong but ran counter to the preventive health initiatives current then (and now).

The life of one security guard whom we interviewed gives an indication of the similarity of experiences between homeless men and staff employees and also demonstrates the significance of such relationships for AIDS education. James was an African American, born in New York City. He had a wife and two children and had held a variety of jobs. He used to shoot heroin with his younger brother. This brother with whom he had shared needles, had died of AIDS three years previously. James claimed that he had stopped using heroin over five years ago. After his brother died he had requested the HIV test and fortunately tested negative. When we started working in the shelter James became active in the video project and shared the loss of his brother to AIDS and his feelings about it with shelter residents. While remaining a security guard, he became one of a group of men in the shelter committed to educating others about the impact of AIDS.

Community Contacts

Although the shelter and its personnel formed an overarching institution with which homeless men had to interact, their social worlds were not defined by the shelter alone. In terms of work, amusement, sexual encounters, contact with the drug culture, shelter men moved in and out of the wider community. Many men did not even stay in the shelter on weekends. Some visited relatives or wives and children while others stayed with friends. One man with whom we spoke had been evicted by his mother because of mental problems. He fought with his brother and threatened to kill his sister. However, he returned to his mother's house daily for meals. Those who had goods to sell ranged throughout the city. Men with regular outside work appeared at the shelter only early in the morning and late at night. In fact, one of the grievances voiced by the Clients' Council concerned the 10 PM curfew. Men would prefer to return to the shelter later than 10 PM but were told the curfew could not be changed because of the need for a bed count after the curfew. This was a problem if a resident found a night job or any other employment that would not allow him to be back by 10 PM.

Thus the shelter was in no way a confined institution within New York City. It served as one gathering place among many for people trying to survive with few resources in an expensive urban environment where the majority of living spaces, eating places and stores are oriented toward the wealthier sector of the population. The immediate vicinity of this particular shelter was a poor run-down neighborhood where stores welcomed the daily business brought by 150 shelter employees. In contrast to residents and storeowners in other parts of the city, many local residents viewed the shelter as an extra resource rather than a threat to the area. As a consequence, should a shelter resident be infected and share needles or have sexual situations with people in his wider network, the lack of barriers in the community meant that HIV infection could spread through the neighborhood. However, on the positive side, the shelter could also serve as a resource to disseminate AIDS education.

SOCIAL RESPONSE TO AIDS

Knowledge, Attitude, Perceptions

Most residents had heard about AIDS. When questioned systematically, we found there were many misunderstandings about the disease. Some people were eager to have questions answered. Some men denied that they had any risk of being infected. Many of the men claimed they could tell whether someone was infected or not by the level of cleanliness of the person. In other words, men associated AIDS with other stigmatizing characteristics such as poor hygiene and disheveled appearance.

The shelter seemed to be divided into three groups with different attitudes: the drug users who argued that they were not at risk because they were not gay; the gay men who thought that the drug users were at most risk; and the few remaining men who thought they were safe because they were neither gay nor drug users.

Very few men envisioned the risk of heterosexual transmission of HIV. Although in general, men told us that they did not think they were at risk, they were, at the same time, aware of the categories of risky behaviors and appeared to be denying what they knew rather than truly ignorant of the risks.

Community workers suggested that there had been enough education about AIDS and that the next task was to try to change behavior. Both condoms and needle-cleaning kits which contained bleach were available for free in the office of the community mental health workers. They were laid out on a table next to information about HIV infection. People seemed reluctant to take them when someone was looking. When we did see people take supplies from the table they always made a joke. Interestingly, people were much less embarrassed to take condoms than needle-cleaning kits. In one case a man whom we had observed frequenting the "shooting gallery" across the street dropped a few kits which he was smuggling out of the office in a rolled magazine. Although there were no rules about how many kits could be taken he obviously felt that he did not want to be seen with them.

Condoms and cleaning kits were being used, and needed to be replenished periodically. Community workers were not sure whether they were being used appropriately by residents or whether they were simply sold for extra cash. Even if they were being sold, the fact that there was a market for such goods implies that some people were implementing preventive strategies against AIDS. However, these small beginnings were very far from being a social movement.

THE VIDEO PROJECT: THE MAKING OF A VOICE

The video project was suggested to our researchers by the community mental health director who had already worked with residents in a theater group, developing plays around the issues of housing and employment. Nevertheless, it would be misleading to describe the project as one that was initiated with clearly defined goals. Rather, the idea of making a video that would address HIV infection among the shelter residents emerged somewhat gradually from discussions between two of our researchers, one community worker, and a few residents. The decision to give the video a fictional rather than a documentary format was made early on and maintained quite firmly by the resident members. They argued that a documentary was too "clinical" and would fail to attract the attention of the shelter population. The initial purpose was clearly to develop a health education strategy. Later, as we show, other purposes were served by the activity that had not been anticipated at the onset.

In the next few weeks, a community worker, three researchers and a changing group of about four to six men from the shelter began work on an AIDS video. This work was to continue for the next six months although many of the men who attended early meetings dropped out while others joined the process. There were always enough men from the shelter interested in working on the video to continue the project, and overall about thirty men participated at one time or another. Initially, the group spent time viewing the results of previous attempts at video making at the shelter. In these videos, the camera was static and the effect was similar to filmed theater. The work was structured around a conversation of homeless men who shared their frustrating experiences when looking for work or housing. The actors cited their untidy appearance and lack of a home address as the major problems in finding a job. In these scenes, potential employers and landlords were portrayed as obtuse and unsympathetic. Thus, the video representations, although fictionalized, were not far from the realities people experienced in shelter life and they seemed at the same time to validate the homeless man's sense of himself in the face of adversity.

It turned out that the creation of the script for the AIDS video was also a way for residents to portray their lives and the conflicts in them. The collective nature of the work and the fact that no ideas were ever rejected, made the script long and complex. There were various written outlines of it but none of them encompassed all the scenes that different people thought were in it. The only basis on which a proposed "vignette" was rejected was "incorrectness" as evaluated by the team. This gave the video validity and meaning to the residents. The team was also very careful not to offend anyone and to project an image of homelessness with which they could identify.

We shall discuss here three of the unedited scenes and examine the statements about behavior, homelessness and AIDS contained within them. The first scene dramatizes attitudes about homosexuality, the second about women and the third illuminates, among other issues, the relationship in these representations between drama and reality.

In a scene suggested by shelter residents, a man from the shelter who is supposedly "straight" is picked up by a man in a car. The man was identified as a "bisexual building contractor." The relation between the two was monetary and the scene attempted to portray the risks for homeless men when trying to earn some money by selling sex. In this scene, the fact that an occupation had been ascribed to the man who was the source of HIV infection was a way to collapse the danger and stigma of HIV with the antagonistic position of those in the housing business. The man portrayed as the "enemy" had four counts against him from the point of view of shelter residents. He was an employer, and probably would not hire a shelter resident for legitimate work; he was in housing but had not provided housing for the homeless; he was bisexual and forced a heterosexual homeless man to sell sex in order to earn money; and, fourthly, he was supposed to infect that man with HIV. The shelter resident is portrayed as becoming infected with AIDS through his unfortunate shortage of cash.

The video scene described above incorporates a variety of negative stereotypes in the "enemy" and renders the behavior of the homeless man excusable through necessity. The scene was later dropped from the script when one of the staff members suggested that it made a negative statement about homosexuality. Thus, the process of inventing the script gives an indication of attitudes about employers, the housing business, and homosexuality. The fact that the scene was eventually dropped suggests that attitudes toward homosexuality may have changed through the discussion of the dramatization.

A second series of scenes dealt with the same hapless shelter resident and his girlfriend. There were many variants of this popular theme and we provide only one. In this dramatization the girlfriend, who is addicted to crack, solicits the shelter resident for sex in exchange for money to buy crack or other drugs. In the face of warnings from his friends about the danger of HIV infection and the farflung sexual connections of the woman, the resident leaves with the woman. As they leave, another shelter resident hands his friend a condom which our hero dramatically discards in the gutter. The girlfriend actively suggests that she wants only 'him' (no condom) and reinforces the discarding of the prophylactic. Once again, although this time the shelter resident is portrayed as interested in legitimate heterosexual sex, we see the intimate connections perceived between sex, drugs and the need for money in shelter life. This time the woman, as villain and temptress, addicted to drugs, lures the shelter resident towards sex and HIV infection.[2] We also see the representation of the "macho" man who fails to heed warnings and refuses to use a condom.

The third scene is slightly different from the first two. In this section, the security guard mentioned above whose brother had in reality died of AIDS, plays a security guard and evicts a man who is injecting heroin from the shelter bathroom. Next, the security guard, James, says, "Now, I'm not acting anymore, this is a true story" and proceeds to read an extremely moving poem which he wrote about his brother's death. The closeness of the video to real shelter life is reflected through this scene as the security guard acts the security guard and performs a task which he frequently is required to do in his daily routine. Then, he says he is no longer acting and becomes a human being grieving over a real loss.

Throughout the video, shelter residents play the roles of shelter residents involved in situations which our fieldwork and their comments suggest that they confront daily. Researchers, significantly, were cast in the roles of women, employers, and other outsiders frequently responsible in the drama for the spread of HIV infection. Thus, in fictional representation, shelter residents are able to replay issues which they must routinely face. In the collective process of creating the script and acting the parts, the groups developed a sophisticated knowledge of strategies for AIDS prevention. In portraying the obvious pitfalls threatening the beleaguered shelter resident they also were able to build their own confidence in adopting alternative ways of relating to New York City realities. They could discuss and reconsider issues of group stereotyping and dramatize the denial prevalent in the shelter.

Some problems which were never adequately overcome in the video project demonstrate the degree of exclusion of homeless men from the working population of New York City. People who stayed with the project had either just become homeless or were able to make a living in the ways described above, outside the formal economy. No men in steady jobs outside the shelter participated in the project. As one man explained to the researchers "In my job they don't know I live here, I can't take the risk that someone sees me in the video." Such men were enthusiastic about the project but formed the most inconsistent group in keeping appointments and remaining in the project. In their attempts to return to "mainstream" work, many had job interviews or had to apply for social benefits. Appointments conflicted with project meetings. After participating in the project for a while, several such men suddenly became aware of the stigma of homelessness as they saw their images in the context of the men' s shelter. They withdrew from the project altogether.

Those men with seemingly little intention of rejoining the "mainstream" had worked out their existence in terms of income, recreation and other issues which the men trying to establish themselves in more respectable walks of life had not solved. The men in the former group were more reliable, more easily located, and more self-reliant. They saw in the video a vehicle for militancy. They were happy to see their ideas about the "system" portrayed in a video. Eventually, this was the group that remained consistently in the project. Thus, while the video helped people to counteract negative views of the homeless man, only those men who had given up the possibility of participating in formal employment would take charge and reinvent their own images without fear.

As people participated in the video project they became much better informed about AIDS. They also confronted stereotypes of homosexuality and drug use through discussion of dramatic representations rather than live individuals. Thus, the process of developing the video led to a re-examination of a variety of topics including, but not restricted to, HIV infection.

CONCLUSION

Homelessness is an unanticipated consequence of rising property values, occurring simultaneously with job shortages, unemployment and poverty (Hopper, Susser, and Conover 1987). The drug-culture is part cause, part effect of similar factors. Homelessness, drug use and poverty in turn affect the nature of sexual encounters, and all conspire to favor the spread of HIV infection. The shelter is not an isolated phenomenon, but a microcosm reflecting the interplay of these forces in the larger society.

Life in a men's shelter in New York City involves a variety of strategies for survival. People participate in both the formal and informal economy, and drugs and sex are part of this economy. In New York City, where HIV infection is a major risk and the primary cause of death for men between the ages of 25 and 45, the population which circulates among the shelters and streets is particularly important to mobilize. It represents people who may be at high risk of receiving and transmitting the infection but who are difficult to reach. Our research suggests that institutional responses to the problem up to now have been ambiguous, ambivalent and ineffective. Because of the lack of institutional commitment and the many problems homeless men face, they may find it harder to implement preventive strategies and be in greater need of mobilization than other sectors of the society. Since this is a changing population with strong community links, effective prevention strategies implemented by men in the shelters could also have reverberating effects throughout a wider population of urban poor.

The video project, as one instance of collective action among men in a shelter, gives us some insight into both possibilities and problems in the development of effective community organizations to deal with AIDS. The video representations reflect the tensions surrounding views of homelessness, unemployment, social services, homosexuality and drugs. While homeless men are portrayed by society as villains or victims, the video embodies the militant, self-conscious efforts of men to assert their humanity and their rights in the face of continuous social barriers and insult. In the collective process of creating the video, the men rebuilt and re-analyzed their sense of themselves. However, while the video itself represents an attempt to control the environment and develop an effective voice, the portrayal of homeless men as hapless victims rather than self-conscious critical actors suggests that residents are not yet fully aware of their own political situation or their potential for collective organization. The video reflects views of the poor as passive victims at the same time as dispelling views of the homeless man as villain. Thus, it reflects only a partial recreation of the homeless man. In a reversal of current hegemony, the villains in these videos are to be found among the owners of bureaucratic representatives of the state but the residents do not paint themselves as potential self-conscious actors or heros.

A second important characteristic of the videos is the perspective on women which emerges. While the homeless man is portrayed as passive victim, poor, hustling women are portrayed as classic "EVE-il" lurers. Clearly, in the process of developing effective community-wide organizations such perspectives on women will have to give way to an understanding of the needs of poor women and their own potential for collective organization. HIV prevention depends on effective implementation of safe sex methods between men and women. Such preventive strategies will be hindered by unequal and hostile gender relations. Unless such issues are confronted in a variety of ways, as they may be in the process of collective organization, it is unlikely that effective preventive and community-wide strategies will emerge. However, since women are not allowed in the shelter (only select women shelter employees are even allowed to walk across the hall where the men stay), there were few women involved in the collective effort. If poor women had been included in the project, they could have negotiated, or perhaps the more appropriate word might be struggled for, a more realistic and politically conscious representation of women in the final drama.

At this point, we might compare the prevailing attitudes towards men and to HIV infection discovered among pregnant women living in a women's shelter in New York. For these women, as for the men, the shelter represented not a total institution, but a temporary, necessary but disliked form of life, interrupting rather than reinforcing whatever stability they had achieved in their relations with the men in their lives (Christiano and Susser 1989). In practice, the policy of gender-segregation imposed on the shelters could be encouraging high-risk sexual behavior.

Role-playing is here recognized as revealing the perceptions and motivations of the players. There are many comparable examples: thus the women residents of the Bedford Correctional facility have organized themselves as a self-help community to inform residents about HIV infection, to instruct, equip and empower women about the risks of heterosexual transmission, and to inform them also *not* to fear causal contacts with those known to be HIV positive. Much of this educational "curriculum" was developed in the form of short fictional vignettes, dramatized by the women. Here, too, role playing—for example, about how a man might react when the woman proposes that he use a condom—is a vital part of the experience, for players and audience. Similarly, in a New York mental ward, patients played out the roles of both doctors and clients, revealing *pari passu* the limited function they saw for the doctor in supporting clients resolve to prevent infection (Enfield and Cournos 1990).

It seems plausible to compare the role of the homosexuals in the team making the video with that which poor women could have had if they had been in it. Not all gay men working on the video were open about their sexuality, but a few were. Their presence provided the monitoring for "correctness" of the images used in the script and they also contributed insights into the gay life and homosexual activities of the shelter. As work progressed on the video project no abuse was directed against those identified openly as gay. We believe that the physical environment in which our work took place, the CSS office, helped to create harmonious work relationships by providing a stage where the informal rules and laws of the shelter floor did not apply. Instead, the possibility of a new space for hetero- and homosexuals was provided where each might negotiate new ways of regarding the other.

In summary, we suggest that in this particular setting, among men in a New York City shelter, effective HIV prevention involves a process of re-evaluation and re-creation of a sense of identity through collective action. Homeless men must face the difficulties of life in the streets, and the neglect or actual obstructionist policies of service institutions in addition to the negative stereotypes of poverty, unemployment, and homelessness. These views were partially overcome in this case through a collective attempt to create a dramatic representation by shelter residents for shelter residents. The video project represented a step taken by shelter residents themselves in reshaping their conscious views of themselves and their potential to confront hazards such as HIV infection along with the numerous other issues with which they are forced to battle. In this sense, the action research triggered a response of group self-help. Nevertheless, issues which emerged in this process were not in any way fully resolved, and continuous staff-client interaction will be essential to maintain and reinforce this nascent social movement.

ACKNOWLEDGMENTS

We would like to acknowledge the help received from the Robert F. Wagner, Sr. Institute of Urban Public Policy, City University of New York, U.S. Department of Education, Grant No. 4-2-000701-0 and also the encouragement and assistance of Dr. Anke Ehrhardt, Director, and Dr. Zena Stein, Co-Director, of the HIV Center for Clinical and Behavioral Studies, Columbia University, New York, N.Y. Grant No. MH 43520 NIMH/NIDA.

NOTES

1. The findings reported here are based on participant observation combined with more formal interviews conducted intensively for one year, 1988–89. Three fieldworkers including one of the authors (Alfredo González, a Spanish-speaking graduate student in Anthropology; Tamara Apollon, a Haitian graduate student in Anthropology; and Sheryl Heron, an African-American graduate student in Community Health Education) worked for three months under the training and coordination of Ida Susser. Alfredo González continued participant observation at the shelter and worked on the video for the following year.
2. For a discussion of the woman portrayed as the bringer of disease in history, see Teichler (1990).

REFERENCES CITED

Baltimore, D., and S. Wolff
  1986 Confronting AIDS: Directions for Public Health, Health Care and Research. Washington, DC: National Academy Press.
Brown, D. B., and E. Valencia
  1987 Community Support Systems Program at the Franklin Avenue Men's Shelter. Funding Request for Additional Needs, 1988–1989.
Christiano, A., and I. Susser
  1989 Knowledge and Perceptions of HIV Infection among Homeless Pregnant Women. Journal of Nurse Midwifery 34:318–322.
Feldman, D.
  1986 AIDS, Health Promotion and Clinically Applied Anthropology. *In* The Social Dimensions of AIDS: Method and Theory. D. Feldman and T. Johnson, eds. Pp. 145–159. New York: Praeger.
Fullilove, M. T., R. E. Fullilove, K. Haynes, and S. Gross
  1990 Black Women and AIDS Prevention: A View Towards Understanding the Gender Rules. Journal of Sex Research 27:47–64.
Gounis, K., and E. Susser
  1990 Shelterization and its Implications for Mental Health Services. *In* N. Cohen, ed. Psychiatry Takes to the Streets. New York: Guilford.
Hopper, K., E. Susser, and S. Conover
  1987 Economics of Makeshift: Deindustrialization and Homelessness in New York City. Urban Anthropology 14:183–236.
Martin, R., and F. Stroud
  1988 Delivering Difficult Messages: AIDS Prevention and Black Youth. *In* The AIDS Challenge. M. Quackenbush and M. Nelson, eds. Pp. 345–362. Santa Cruz, CA: Network Publications.
Matiella, A.
  1988 Developing Innovative AIDS Prevention Program for Youth. *In* The AIDS Challenge. M. Quackenbush and M. Nelson, eds. Pp. 333–344. Santa Cruz, CA: Network Publications.
Murphy, D.
  1988 Heterosexual Contact of Intravenous Drug Abusers: Implication for the Next Spread of the AIDS Epidemic. *In* AIDS and Substance Abuse. L. Seigel, ed. Pp. 89–97. New York: Harrington Park Press.
New York Times
  1987 New York City Lacks Space for Increase of the Homeless. 28 May:89–98.
St. Louis, M. E., R. J. Rauch, L. R. Petersen, J. E. Anderson, A. Schablec, and T. J. Dondero
  1990 Seroprevalence Rates of Human Immunodeficiency Virus Infection at Sentinel Hospitals in the United States. New England Journal of Medicine 323:213–218.
Shilts, R.
  1986 And the Band Played On. New York: St. Martin Press.
Singer, M., C. Flores, L. Davison, G. Burke, Z. Castillo, K. Scanlon, M. Rivera
  1990 SIDA: The Economic, Social, and Culture Context of AIDS Among Latinos. Medical Anthropology Quarterly 4(10):72–114.
Stall, R.
  1988 The Prevention of HIV Infection Associated with Drugs and Alcohol Abuse During Sexual Activity. *In* L. Seigel, ed. AIDS and Substance Abuse. Pp. 73–88. New York: Harrington Park Press.
Stall, R., S. Heurtin-Roberts, L. McKusick, C. Hoff, S. Wanner-Lang
  1990 Sexual Risk for HIV Transmission Among Singles-Bar Patrons in San Francisco. Medical Anthropology Quarterly 4(1):115–128.
Susser, E., E. L. Struening, and S. Conover
  1989 Psychiatric Problems in Homeless Men. Archives of General Psychiatry 46:845–850.
Susser, I.
  1982 Norman Street: Poverty and Politics in an Urban Neighborhood. New York: Oxford University Press.

1989   The Structuring of Families in Homelessness. Paper presented in the Symposium on Homelessness at the Annual Meeting of the American Anthropological Association, Washington,
DC, November.

Susser, I., and C. Jageman
1989   Comparative Perspectives on AIDS. Proceedings of a Conference. New York: Hunter College.

Susser, I., and J. Kreniske
1987   The Welfare Trap: A Public Policy for Deprivation. *In* Cities of the United States. L. Mullings,
ed. New York: Columbia University Press.

Susser, M., W. Watson, and K. Hopper
1985   Sociology and Medicine. New York: Oxford University Press.

Teichler, P.
1988   AIDS, Gender and Biomedical Discourse: Current Contests for Meaning. *In* AIDS, the Burdens
of History. E. Fee and D. M. Fox, eds. Pp. 172–189. Berkeley, CA: University of California Press.

Medical Anthropology, Vol. 14, pp. 323–363
Reprints available directly from the publisher
Photocopying permitted by license only

Alcohol and Risky Sex: In Search of an Elusive Connection

Ralph Bolton, John Vincke, Rudolf Mak, and Ellen Dennehy

Since the publication of the 1986 article by Stall, McKusick, Wiley, Coates and Ostrow, the conclusion that drinking alcohol prior to or during erotic encounters increases the probability of engaging in high-risk sexual behavior has been widely accepted, despite some contradictory findings from research on this hypothesis. This paper presents the results of tests of the alcohol/risky-sex hypothesis in a cohort of gay men in Flanders, Belgium. Failing to find evidence to support the hypothesis of a general effect of alcohol on sexual risk taking, we argue that previous conclusions on this matter must be viewed with extreme caution, especially in light of the implications that this failure to replicate has for AIDS prevention programs. Cultural, social, and methodological factors that could account for this failure to replicate are discussed in the context of a review of the literature on this hypothesis.

Key words: AIDS, alcohol, sex, culture, gay men, Belgium

INTRODUCTION

At the beginning of the second decade of the AIDS pandemic certain propositions about the transmission of HIV, the etiologic agent, appear to be well established. The first is that the dominant mode of transmission in most countries to date is sexual, with both heterosexual and homosexual encounters serving as venues of transmission (Miller, Turner, and Moses 1990; Turner, Miller, and Moses 1989). The second is that not all forms of sexual behavior are equally effective in transmitting the virus and that in homosexual encounters unprotected anal intercourse is overwhelmingly implicated in transmission with efficiency of transmission higher for transmission from the insertive partner to the receptive partner than vice versa, and that in heterosexual intercourse, vaginal sex is the primary behavior involved in transmission with efficiency greater from the male partner to the female partner than vice versa (Darrow, Jaffe, and Curran 1988; Detels et al. 1989; Van der Graaf and Diepersloot 1989; Winkelstein et al. 1987; cf. McCoy et al. 1990). The third proposition is that knowledge about how HIV is transmitted may be necessary but

RALPH BOLTON *is Professor of Anthropology at Pomona College, Claremont, CA 91711. As a medical anthropologist, he has done research in Peru on susto, high-altitude sex ratios, and the behavioral effects of hypoglycemia. His current work focuses on AIDS prevention and gay male sexual behavior in Europe and the United States.*
JOHN VINCKE *is a sociologist whose research deals with AIDS prevention, gay culture, and phenomenological theories of the body.*
RUDOLF MAK *is a physician specializing in sexually transmitted diseases. He has done extensive work on AIDS prevention among female sex workers in Belgium. Both Vincke and Mak are affiliated with the State University of Ghent in Belgium.*
ELLEN DENNEHY *is a recent graduate of Scripps College.*

324/[186]   R. Bolton et al.

it is not sufficient to induce people to eliminate risky sexual practices from their sexual repertoires (Brendstrup and Schmidt 1990; McCusker et al. 1989b; O'Reilly 1988; Valdiserri et al. 1988; cf. Pleak and Meyer-Bahlburg 1990). The fourth is that rapid behavioral change is possible, and in many communities in which such high-risk practices were once quite prevalent, sexual risk-taking has declined remarkably (Coates et al. 1988; Kelly and St. Lawrence 1990; Kelly et al. 1989; Stall, Coates, and Hoff 1988; Martin 1986; Ekstrand and Coates 1990; Siegel et al. 1988). The fifth point is that despite information on transmission and despite changes in community sexual norms, some people continue to engage in high-risk practices (Hays, Kegeles, and Coates 1990; Kelly et al. 1990; Linn et al. 1989; Martin 1986; Valdiserri 1988).

In view of the failure of risk-reduction models which emphasize rational decision-making to account for the behavior of those who continue to take risks in the face of sufficient knowledge about the consequences of high-risk activities, many researchers have turned to the problem of trying to understand why high-risk behaviors continue to be practiced. The search for factors which influence individuals has concentrated on two types of variables: 1) psychological factors and the personality traits of risk-takers (e.g., fear, denial, perceptions of risk and efficacy, and self-esteem), and 2) social and situational determinants (e.g., community norms and social support) (Fisher and Misovich 1990; Miller, Turner, and Moses 1990; Valdiserri 1989; Kelly et al. 1990; Vincke et al. 1991). But probably the most widely cited behavioral co-factor for sexual risk-taking has been alcohol usage.

A considerable body of literature now exists on the supposed influence of alcohol on sexual risk-taking. Although the mechanisms whereby alcohol increases the likelihood of risky sex are not well understood, several studies have reported evidence for a relationship. Moreover, the proposition that alcohol increases risk-taking has been sufficiently accepted, perhaps as much because of American folk models of the effects of alcohol on responsible behavior as because of the evidence generated by AIDS researchers, that most AIDS prevention programs tend to place some emphasis on the role of drinking, and urge people to eliminate the consumption of alcohol in the context of sexual activity (e.g., Kus 1987; Ocamb 1989; Rolf et al. 1990–91; Stall 1988).

However, not all studies on this issue have provided confirmation of the hypothesis, or they have yielded support for a rather weak effect. Indeed, a recent overview of this research contained in a program announcement of the National Institute on Alcohol Abuse and Alcoholism (1991:3) referred to the association between alcohol use and sexual risk taking as "unstable" and indicated that the research on this issue among gay and bisexual men "does not show a consistent association between alcohol use and high-risk sex (or HIV infection)." In addition, the studies have come from only a few research centers with study cohorts drawn from a narrow range of populations. In this paper our goal is to test the hypothesis that alcohol consumption increases risk-taking in a different population in order to clarify some of the problems apparent in previous research conclusions.

The focus of attention in this paper is the hypothesized effects of alcohol on sexual risk-taking among gay men. The importance of understanding the relationship between drinking and risky sex cannot be overstated given the historical centrality of bars in the institutional structure of gay cultures in Western countries (Bell and Weinberg 1978; Jackman 1978; Judell 1978; Kelsey 1978; Newman 1978; Read 1980; Taub 1982; Witomski 1986). As Weinberg and Williams noted:

In all major cities in the United States the gay bar is the cornerstone of the gay community. Because there are few public locations where homosexuals are able to present their sexual orientations and preferences, the bar emerges as probably the single place that provides the terms and conditions necessary and sufficient for large numbers of homosexuals to congregate in public, engage in leisure-time socializing, and pursue sexual relationships.

Thus, homosexual males frequent gay bars for the consumption of alcohol, for meeting new friends and old, for entertaining and being entertained, for sitting, dancing, and getting drunk, for something to do, and, especially, for meeting sexual partners. [Weinberg and Williams 1974:45]

Although the institutional complexity of gay society has increased considerably since the time when Weinberg and Williams did their research, bars, and hence alcohol, continue to be intimately associated with the sexual lives of gay men.

One of the questions we are interested in is, To what extent is the cultural context a significant factor in determining the effect of alcohol on sexual behavior? Anthropologists have long discussed the variations in patterns of human behavior associated with alcohol consumption, stressing the significance of cultural interpretations of drunken comportment (MacAndrew and Edgerton 1969; Marshall 1979; Pittman and Snyder 1962). Clearly, knowledge about the influence of social and cultural contexts will be helpful in clarifying the mechanisms whereby alcohol influences sexual risk taking, if it in fact does so.

REVIEW OF THE LITERATURE ON HIGH-RISK SEX AND ALCOHOL

The seminal article on this hypothesis is one by Stall et al. (1986) who tested it in the context of an examination of a postulated general relationship between substance abuse and high-risk sex. Their data were gathered in 1985 from a sample of gay men in San Francisco, approximately half of whom were recruited from bars and bathhouses. They eliminated men in monogamous gay relationships. In this study a significant relationship was reported between a sexual risk score and how often during the preceding month the respondents had been drinking while having sex. Although the statistical significance reported was high, the authors did not present any measure of the degree of association between their variables. Instead, they indicated the percentages of respondents who fell into high, medium, and low risk categories for AIDS risk with respect to each level of drinking involvement.

Another finding from the above study was that changes in risk levels during the preceding year were associated with the consumption of alcohol during sex; those who remained at high risk were "2.3 times more likely to use alcohol during sexual activity" (Stall et al. 1986:364). Despite the associations found in the study, the authors state that the findings do not prove conclusively that alcohol causes/drives high-risk behaviors, but they go on to discuss the mechanisms which might, in fact, explain a relationship between these two phenomena.

A later study by Paul, Stall, and Davis (1989), however, which used a different sample (gay and bisexual men entering a substance abuse treatment program) and a different risk scale, found that high-risk sex was not associated with alcohol use. It also reported that unsafe sex while inebriated was more likely to be associated with drugs other than alcohol. They concluded that "unsafe sex while 'high' on drugs/alcohol is a more complex matter than 'disinhibition' or drugs impairing judgment."

McCusker et al. (1990) carried out a study of gay male clients of a health center in Boston. They found that maintenance of high-risk sexual activities was more frequent among men who continued to drink than among those who reduced their drinking. They note that respondents who drink and who report impaired judgment in connection with drinking were more likely to be at high risk than those who drink but do not think their judgment was impaired by alcohol.

Molgaard et al. (1988) discuss the relationship between alcohol and sexual practices, but they base their discussion on an unpublished study which found that individuals who decreased or eliminated alcohol use also decreased or eliminated the practice of anal sex and the number of their sexual partners. They provide no other evidence.

Plant's (1990a) review article only discusses the work by Stall and co-workers for gay men plus some questionably relevant studies on heterosexual samples in which there have been mixed results. For example, Bagnall (1989, personal communication to Plant) reported a significant association between alcohol consumption and high-risk sex for females, but not for males.

The MACS investigators, Ostrow et al. (1990:762), using still another high-risk-sex scale, found that there was no association between "any alcohol use or frequency of use and sexual risk, once we controlled for use of other drugs." They explained their inability to find evidence for a connection between alcohol and high-risk sex as follows: [it] "may be the result of the near universal use of alcohol in these cohorts and our lack of specific measures of alcohol use with sexual partners" (1990:764).

In another study, Stall et al. (1990b) again found a relationship among bar patrons in San Francisco between high-risk sex and alcohol and drug use. But in this study, alcohol use is not analyzed separately from drug use. Moreover, what these authors conclude is a relatively strong relationship between drugs/alcohol and risky sex is a correlation of .22, which suggests to us that even when combined with drug use, alcohol would contribute less than 5% of the variance in sexual risk-taking behavior among gay men.

Penkower et al. (1991), using MACS data again, reported that men who engaged in high-risk sex and who were heavy drinkers were more likely to seroconvert than were moderate or light drinkers and they were less likely to report using condoms during sex. The former finding, of course, relates not to the increased likelihood of engaging in high-risk behavior but of seroconverting if they do engage in such behavior, which is, of course, another issue entirely. In contrast, Gómez et al. (1990) report on a study of serostatus and alcohol consumption patterns among gay men in Columbia; they found no relationship.

Siegel et al. (1989) attempted to distinguish gay men who practice safe sex from those who practice risky sex in a New York City sample. Alcohol consumption (average number of alcoholic drinks per month during the past 6 months) was one of the variables that they entered into their discriminant analysis. This variable did not correlate with risky sex at a statistically-significant level.

Valdiserri et al. (1988), in contrast, did find a relationship between being "high" while having sex and failure to use condoms. Unfortunately, again, in their analysis these authors combined alcohol use with the use of other drugs, which in light of the findings of Ostrow et al. (1990), may be misleading.

Leigh (1990b), in yet another study of San Francisco gay men, found no relationship between alcohol consumption and risky sex, though she did find it for heterosexual men and women. Indeed, for the high-risk men, a lower proportionate amount of sex occurred in conjunction with drinking than for the men with lower risk levels. She concluded that when one controls for the amount of sex the individual has, the relationship between alcohol and high risk evaporates.

Martin and Hasin's (1991) research on gay men in New York City indicated the possibility of a relationship between oral sex and drinking behavior, although the evidence did not consistently support the hypothesis. What was consistent in their analysis was the conspicuous absence of any relationship between unprotected anal sex (insertive or receptive) and alcohol consumption or alcoholism.

For a largely heterosexual sample, Bagnall, Plant, and Warwick (1990) found no association between general alcohol consumption levels and condom use in vaginal sex, but they did find that when sex was combined with alcohol, there was a significant reduction in condom use. They emphasize, however, that most of their respondents were monogamous during the preceding year.

Table I provides an overview of the major features and findings of the studies discussed above (plus several others using samples of heterosexual adolescents or sex workers) which have tested the alcohol/risky sex hypothesis. Clearcut support for the hypothesis is found in only three of the 16 studies reviewed. Partial or ambiguous support is found in another six studies. Seven studies failed to find evidence to support the hypothesis. It is important to note that two of the three supportive studies were done in heterosexual adolescent (Hingson et al. 1990; Kraft, Rise, and Traen 1990). For the gay/bisexual samples, we find that only the original study by Stall et al. (1986) is fully supportive of the hypothesis; negative results are provided by six studies (Leigh 1990b; McCusker et al. 1989a; Paul, Stall, and Davis 1989; Siegel et al. 1989; Ostrow et al. 1990; Martin and Hasin 1991). Partial or ambiguous support could be argued for three studies (Valdiserri et al. 1988; McCusker et al. 1990; Stall et al. 1990), but in all three of these studies alcohol and other drugs are confounded, thereby making it impossible to determine whether drugs or alcohol or both are responsible for the relationships detected.

In this review of the literature, we have excluded some studies which purport to test the hypothesis of a relationship between drinking and risky sex because the indicators of risky sex were indirect and therefore not pertinent. For example, McKirnan and Peterson (1989a, 1989d) used as their measure of "AIDS-risk behavior" the number of sexual partners of their subjects (for a critique of "promiscuity" as a high-risk factor see Bolton 1992a, this issue). Bagnall, Plant, and Warwick (1990) cite several of these studies. In one such study Temple and Leigh (1990) failed to confirm a relationship between risky sex and drinking even though alcohol tended to be associated with encounters with new partners. Another study

TABLE I. Empirical studies on the relationship between alcohol consumption and high-risk sexual behavior.

Study	Study site	Sample size	Sample	Sex variables
Stall et al. (1986)	San Francisco	463	Gay men, recruited from bars, baths, ads, couples groups (excludes men in a monogamous relationship)	Risk scale based on riskiness of specific behaviors multiplied by frequency during previous month; subjects placed in three groups based on total risk
Valdiserri et al. (1988)	Pittsburgh	955	Gay/bisexual men who engage in anal intercourse; prospective AIDS cohort (MACS study)	Condom use; subjects asked if they always, most times, sometimes, hardly ever, or never used condoms when having sex
McCusker et al. (1989a)	Boston	278	Homosexually active men; clients of a community health center	Risk categories: 'safer' and 'unsafe' (receptive or insertive unprotected anal intercourse)
Paul, Stall, and Davis (1989)	San Francisco	115	Gay/bisexual men, participants in a substance abuse program	Risk scale based on riskiness of specific behaviors, from low (celibate) to high (unprotected anal sex outside a monogamous relationship)
Siegel et al. (1989)	New York City	100	Homosexual males, recruited by ads, fliers given out near gay establishments, physician referrals	Two risk groups: risky, engaging in any one of a set of ten items; safe, all other subjects; based on sexual behavior during previous month
Gomez et al. (1990)	Antioguia, Colombia	432	Clients of public clinic (bisexual men, 37%, homosexual men, 28%, heterosexual men, 22%, women, 13%)	Serostatus rather than sexual behavior
Hingson et al. (1990	Massachusetts	1050	Male and female adolescents, recruited by random digit dial telephone survey	Use of condoms: subjects divided into those who never use and those who always use condoms

(continued)

TABLE I. (*continued*).

Study	Study site	Sample size	Sample	Sex variables
Kraft, Rise, and Traeen (1990)	Norway	1827	Male and female adolescents, 17–19 years old; population-based random sample	Subjects asked if they used condoms during first experience of sexual intercourse
Leigh (1990b)	San Francisco	424	Men and women, all sexual orientations (includes only persons who are single or who have multiple partners)	Risk scores based on frequency of various sexual behaviors in previous 30 days; frequencies multiplied by risk weight; subjects grouped as low, medium or high risk
McCusker et al. (1990)	Boston	322	Homosexually active men; clients of a community health center	Risk categories based on sex practices previous six months; high/multiple, high/single, low (no anogenital or orogenital contact with exposure to ejaculate)
Ostrow et al. (1990)	Pittsburgh, Baltimore, Washington, DC, Chicago, Los Angeles	3916	Homosexually active men; MACS prospective AIDS cohort	Risk scale based on sexual behavior during previous six months; grouped into no risk, low risk, modified high risk, and high risk categories
Plant, Plant, and Morgan Thomas (1990)	Edinburgh, Scotland	205	Sex workers, 102 males and 103 females	Level of condom use (not specified further)
Stall et al. (1990b)	San Francisco	1344	Male and female patrons of gay and heterosexual bars	Risk scale with four levels based on sex during last 30 days: no risk, low risk, modified high risk, and high risk
Morgan Thomas, Plant, and Plant (1990)	Edinburgh, Scotland	209	Clients of male and female sex workers (3 female clients, 206 male clients)	Level of condom use (not specified further)
Martin and Hasin (1991)	New York City	604	Cohort of gay men	Risk scores based on annual frequency of oral sex and unprotected anal intercourse
Bagnall, Plant, and Warwick (1990)	Lothian region of Scotland	778	Nonrandom sample of men (350) and women (428), 75% heterosexual, 6% sexually inactive, 18% unknown sexual orientation, <2%	Trichotomized indicator of condom use for vaginal intercourse (always, sometimes, seldom)

TABLE I. (*continued*).

Study	Drinking variables	Support for hypothesis	Basic findings and comments
Stall et al. (1986)	Subjects asked if they drank often, sometimes, rarely or never while having sex during the past month	Yes	Statistically significant relationship found between drinking while having sex and sexual risk taking. Inspection of data suggest that only those who never drink while having sex account for the finding; no significant differences exist between other groups.
Valdiserri et al. (1988)	Subjects asked about number of partners with whom they were 'high' (drugs or alcohol) during sex: none, half or less, or more than half	Ambiguous	The study showed a statistically significant relationship between being "high" on alcohol and/or drugs and whether or not one uses condoms always vs never. Combining alcohol and drugs makes it impossible to determine the independent effect of alcohol; most studies show stronger drug/risky sex relationship.
McCusker et al. (1989a)	Subjects asked frequency of use of alcohol	No	Higher level of alcohol use was significantly related to subsequent adoption of safer sex practices. Alcohol was not associated in bivariate analysis with insertive anogenital intercourse.
Paul, Stall, and Davis (1989)	Subjects asked about episodes of alcohol consumption and being inebriated during sex	No	Risky sexual practices were found not be be associated with alcohol use. Drug use accounted for 75% of reported unsafe sex while inebriated.
Siegel et al. (1989)	Subjects asked to state average number of alcoholic drinks per month during previous six months	No	Statistically significant relationship between alcohol use and risky sex was not found ("approached" significance); drug use was potent predictor. Authors raise possibility that failure to support hypothesis was due to not asking specifically about use of alcohol during sex.
Gómez et al. (1990)	Use of alcohol (measures not specified)	No	This study found no relationship between serostatus and patterns of alcohol use. Serostatus in some research is used as a surrogate marker for risky sex.

(continued)

TABLE I. (*continued*).

Study	Drinking variables	Support for hypothesis	Basic findings and comments
Hingson et al. (1990)	Subjects asked to indicate the number of drinks per day in past month and if they had sex and used condoms when drinking (always, sometimes, never)	Yes	Heavy drinkers (five or more drinks per day) used condoms "always" less than did abstainers (29% v. 35%). Sixteen percent of subjects indicated they are less likely to use condoms after drinking than when having sex without drinking. But note, 8% said they were more likely to use condoms when drinking. Hence, 92% do not reduce condom use when drinking. Relationships in this study appear to be produced by small number of very heavy drinkers.
Kraft, Rise, and Traeen (1990)	Subjects asked if they had consumed alcohol immediately prior to first intercourse	Yes	Non-use of condoms was found to be statistically significantly associated with alcohol use prior to having sex for the first time. Exclusive focus on "first-time sex" (an event that is often highly charged emotionally) limits the conclusions to be drawn.
Leigh (1990b)	Subjects asked how often they had been drinking during sexual encounters (never, rarely, sometimes or often)	Partial, not for gay men nor for women	Study found statistically significant relationship between risk scores and having sex while under the influence of alcohol, but relationship disappeared when amount of sexual activity was controlled. For gay men there was a nonsignificant contrary trend: a lower proportionate amount of sex under the influence of alcohol for high-risk subjects. Statistically significant relationships existed for heterosexual men between frequency of sex while drinking and risk level and between risk level and partner drinking.

(*continued*)

Table I. (*continued*).

Study	Drinking variables	Support for hypothesis	Basic findings and comments
McCusker et al. (1990	Frequency of alcohol use and of alcohol use during sexual activity; perception of impaired judgment due to alcohol ingestion	Partial	Found that men who reduced alcohol intake were more likely to reduce high-risk sex practices, but at last visit, no statistically significant difference between men who continued to use drugs or alcohol during sexual activity and those who discontinued such use. Inspection of data suggests to us no difference between those who do not drink during sex and those who view themselves as not "impaired," and at best a weak relationship when one compares the abstainers with those who view themselves as "impaired" while having sex. Drugs appear to be responsible for the relationship, not alcohol.
Ostrow et al. (1990)	Frequency of alcohol use and of alcohol use during sex in past six months	No	The study found no association between any use or frequency of use of alcohol and sexual risk when controlling for other drugs.
Plant, Plant, and Morgan Thomas (1990)	Respondents asked to estimate proportion of clients under the influence of alcohol and to report own frequency of drinking during past week, amount last time, and during the previous seven days as well as extent of drinking while working	No	Levels of condom use not associated with alcohol consumption variables, nor with the proportion of clients estimated to be under the influence of alcohol when having sex.
Stall et al. (1990b)	Proportion of all sexual occasions in which the respondent used drugs or alcohol	Yes, with important qualifications	High risk subjects were reported to be more likely to be 'high' while having sex than were other subjects. Note, however, that the cause of the 'high' was "drugs and/or alcohol" combined. Thus, it is impossible to determine an independent effect for alcohol. Respondent-identified reasons for not using condoms included "alcohol or drugs with sex", but this was one of the least frequently cited reasons.

(continued)

TABLE I. (*continued*).

Study	Drinking variables	Support for hypothesis	Basic findings and comments
Morgan Thomas, Plant, and Plant (1990)	Respondents asked to estimate proportion of sex workers under the influence of alcohol and to report their own alcohol use during previous week, amount consumed last time and during previous week, and whether they drank during sexual contacts with sex workers	Yes, but weak	No significant association was found between estimate of alcohol use by sex workers and level of condom use, nor between respondents' alcohol consumption and anal or vaginal intercourse with female sex workers. A significant association was found between respondent's alcohol consumption during the preceding week (but not when having sex) and level of condom use (inverse relationship) by male clients of male sex workers during anal intercourse. Finding only one relationship among numerous tests suggests that this one may be due to chance, especially since a similar relationship did not occur with the more proximal indicator (sex while under the influence of alcohol).
Martin and Hasin (1991)	Alcohol consumption score based on frequency of drinking in a typical week during the preceding year times the usual number of drinks per drinking episode; recent alcohol abuse determined by NIMH Diagnostic Interview Schedule	No	For two of the three time periods, oral sex was associated with drinking, but unprotected anal intercourse, insertive or receptive, was unrelated to alcohol consumption; no differences between alcoholic and non-alcoholic groups in frequency of unprotected anal intercourse, and for only one time period a positive association between receptive oral sex and drinking.
Bagnall, Plant, and Warwick (1990)	Dichotomized indicator of amount of alcohol consumed on last drinking occasion; frequency of drinking before sex	Partial	Alcohol consumption levels not associated with condom use, but both men and women who combined alcohol and sex were significantly less likely to use condoms for vaginal intercourse; the authors note that 64% of the males and 81% of the females "at risk" had had sex with only one partner during the past year.

by Leigh (1990a) did not find a relationship between drinking and unsafe sex among gay men but did find a weak association between safe sex and alcohol use among heterosexual males and females in a diary sample, and in a survey sample an association between unsafe sex and heavy drinking was found among heterosexual women. Ekstrand and Coates (1990) found a relationship between unprotected anal sex in their 1985 data but not in their 1988 data, and Doll (1989) and Zielinski and Beeker (1989) found "a stronger association between high-risk sex and alcohol when it is used in combination with other drugs than when used alone" (National Institute on Alcohol Abuse and Alcoholism 1991).

Overall the pattern of findings suggests that the hypothesis of an association between risky sex and alcohol is not supported among gay men, or at a minimum, if an association exists a) it is weak at best, b) it is severely affected by the sociocultural setting, i.e. San Francisco in the mid-1980s, or c) it applies only to a small set of problem drinkers. Support for the hypothesis has depended heavily on a single study. Among heterosexuals, both adults and adolescents, the evidence for a link between condom use and alcohol combined with sex seems somewhat stronger, but even in studies on these populations the results must be considered inconclusive. Possible explanations for the rapid and widespread acceptance of the hypothesis as fact despite the weakness of the evidence will be considered in the discussion section below.

METHODS

Participants

The present study is part of a wide-ranging investigation of gay life in Flanders, Belgium, entitled the Gay Service Research Project (GSRP), which was begun in 1989 (Vincke, Mak, and Bolton 1990). Participants for the study were recruited in the Spring of 1989 throughout the Flemish region of the country. In order to constitute a cohort of gay and bisexual men that is as representative as possible of the population of Flemish men who have sex with men, a novel approach to recruitment was employed. Initial publicity for the project was generated in both the print and broadcast media. Interviews with R. Mak and J. Vincke were printed in Flemish newspapers with a general audience as well as in publications of the gay community, and other interviews were aired on television and on the radio. Following this publicity campaign, project personnel arranged to meet with the members of gay organizations throughout Flanders to explain the project and to enlist the assistance of key persons.

The key persons served as the recruiters for the project. Each key person was asked to sign up individuals in their social network for the GSRP. Key persons were instructed to make every effort to achieve diversity in signing up participants. Specifically, they were asked to recruit individuals of different ages and lifestyles, e.g., closeted versus non-closeted, partnered versus single, organizational members as well as non-members, and participants as well as non-participants in the public gay "scene" (e.g., bars and baths). While some individuals entered the cohort through the general publicity on their own or from having seen announcements posted in bars and bathhouses, most of the final cohort (379 men) were recruited by the key persons. While it cannot be demonstrated that this cohort is fully representative of all Flemish men who have sex with men, we believe that the recruitment techniques used reduced some of the biases that have been inherent in other studies on gay and bisexual men which have been based on individual volunteering, or on limited segments of the community (e.g., bar or bathhouse clients or members of gay social groups).

In order to reduce another common bias in AIDS research, namely the tendency to recruit individuals who are especially concerned about AIDS and health issues, the health components of the present study were placed in the context of a more comprehensive study of the gay subculture in Belgium. This was particularly important inasmuch as resistance to the AIDS issue is markedly strong in some gay communities in Europe, and many of the participants would have refused to participate if the study had been presented as one focussing on AIDS.

Participants were guaranteed confidentiality of data, and for those recruited by key persons, anonymity was also guaranteed since only the key persons knew the identities of the men they recruited. Data sets were identified by numbers which were supplied to participants for use in any future re-study using this cohort; key persons would contact them again to participate in follow-up research which is planned if funding is available.

No one was paid to participate in this project, but all participants were reimbursed for their travel expenses. Data collection took place in a central location in the country (Ghent), and participants came to the research site mostly by automobile or train.

Demographic characteristics of the cohort can be seen in Table II. The ages of the men ranged from 17 to 78 years, with just over 80% aged 21–40 (mean age = 33.8 years, standard deviation = 9.9). Teenagers as well as men over 50 are undoubtedly somewhat underrepresented in this cohort, in the case of the former because they may still be in the process of "coming out" to themselves as well as to others and in the case of the latter because they may be less active in gay social circles, hence less likely to have been tapped by a key person. As in most research on gay men, the cohort is more highly educated than the general population, with over 50% having some education beyond secondary school (university or non-university professional training). While 85.1% of these men are single, 14.9% are either currently married or were previously married. The sexual orientation and identity of the men in the cohort is shown in Table III.

The Interview Process

Interviewing in this study was done by computer. An interactive program was designed for use on personal computers. The research setting was a large classroom with 18 personal computers arranged on desks in rows. Each respondent was able to work at his own pace through the questionnaire which presented one question at a time to the participant. All questions were closed-ended, and a participant could not review and change answers once entered. Participants were given a brief introduction to using the computer; experience with computers was not necessary. The design mirrored the use of ATMs with which all informants were familiar.

TABLE II. Demographic characteristics of GSRP* cohort.

	n	%
Age (years)		
<21	7	1.8
21–30	151	39.9
31–40	159	42.0
41–50	35	9.2
51–60	17	4.5
>60	10	2.6
Education		
Legal minimum (to age 15)	14	3.7
No. of years above legal minimum:		
1–3	43	11.3
4–6	99	26.1
7–9	128	33.8
>9	95	25.1
Marital status		
Single	322	85.1
Married	20	5.2
Married, but separated	5	1.3
Divorced	27	7.1
Widowed	5	1.3
Religion		
Catholic	134	35.4
Protestant	3	0.8
Jewish	2	0.5
Humanist	74	19.4
Atheist	87	23.1
Other	31	8.1
Non-religious	48	12.6

*GSRP = Gay Service Research Project

TABLE III. Respondents' self-identification of their sexual orientation.

Sexual orientation	n	%
Exclusively homosexual	251	66.2
Predominantly homosexual, slightly heterosexual	96	25.3
Predominantly homosexual, some heterosexual	21	5.5
Equally homosexual and heterosexual	4	1.1
Predominantly heterosexual, some homosexual	5	1.3
Predominantly heterosexual, slightly homosexual	1	0.3
Exclusively heterosexual*	1	0.3
	379	100.0

*This anomalous case involves a non-operated transsexual with a female identity.

The use of a computer to conduct the interview made it possible to gather data in sessions which included as few as four and as many as 18 individuals at one time. In view of the sensitive and intimate nature of the data, the technique avoids the interpersonal aspects of the interview process, reduces embarrassment, and although we cannot provide clear evidence it is our impression that it results in greater frankness. The technique also eliminates biases introduced by the interviewer and standardizes the questioning more effectively than does a personal interview. Fatigue on the part of interviewers on long interviews can be a problem, and that, too, is eliminated by the use of a computerized interview. Moreover, the novelty of being questioned by the computer was reported by subjects to make the process, which otherwise might have been intolerable, enjoyable. Interviews lasted on average 135 minutes; the length depended on the complexity of the participant's sexual career and the speed at which he was comfortable working. Though administered in group sessions, the interviews were individually paced, and participants could depart when they had finished. They were also allowed to take breaks for refreshments as often as they wished; most informants took at least one short break.

Variables

Dependent. The dependent variables in this study consisted of a set of 68 specific behaviors. While we had a total of 379 informants, after the first 198 had been processed the set of behaviors in the questionnaire was modified, so that in the end each informant answered questions about his participation in 40 different behaviors. We built in an overlap of 12 items, namely 12 of the more prevalent behaviors including those considered the riskiest for HIV transmission; this split design allowed us to investigate a larger number of sexual behaviors. Space limitations prevent us from reporting on the relationships between alcohol use and all of the sexual behaviors we investigated; therefore, in this analysis we report only on a subset of risky and possibly risky behaviors. Table IV contains a list of these behaviors and the prevalence of their practice in the GSRP cohort of men who had sex during the previous month.

Participants were asked: "When you have sex with someone, do you engage in [specific behavior]?" The possible replies were: a) "no, not now nor in the past;" b) "I used to, but not any more;" c) "I do it sometimes;" (d) "I do it regularly;" and e) "I do it always."

Another dependent variable was a composite sexual risk score. This score was calculated as follows:

Risk Score	Definition
0	No anal sex during the preceding month;
1	Anal sex (insertive or receptive) with a steady partner using a condom;
2	Anal sex (insertive or receptive) with a steady partner without a condom; anal sex (insertive or receptive) with other partners while using a condom;
3	Anal sex (insertive or receptive) without a condom with casual partners.

TABLE IV. Prevalence of sexual behaviors by relationship status.

| | Relationship status | | | | | | | |
| | Steady partner and monogamous | | Steady partner and nonmonogamous | | No steady partner | | Total cohort | |
Sexual behaviors	N	%	N	%	N	%	N	%
1. Anal sex: unprotected								
a. receptive	72/169	42.60	24/92	26.09	7/56	12.50	103/317	32.5
b. insertive	77/169	45.56	26/92	28.26	10/56	17.86	113/317	35.6
2. Anal sex: condom usage								
a. receptive	68/169	40.24	44/92	47.83	24/56	42.86	136/317	42.9
b. insertive	68/169	40.24	49/92	53.26	31/56	55.36	148/317	46.7
3. Fisting:								
a. receptive	5/169	2.96	0/92	0.00	0/56	0.00	5/317	1.6
b. insertive	8/169	4.73	6/92	6.52	1/56	1.79	15/317	4.7
4. Oral-anal contact:								
a. active	114/169	67.46	47/92	51.09	26/56	46.43	187/317	59.0
b. passive	125/169	73.97	70/92	76.09	43/56	76.79	238/317	75.1
(asked twice)	127/169	75.15	71/92	77.17	39/56	69.64	238/317	75.1
5. Fellatio: unprotected								
a. active	130/169	76.92	49/92	53.26	30/56	53.57	209/317	65.9
b. passive	138/169	81.66	67/92	72.83	40/56	71.43	245/317	77.3
6. Fellatio: semen ingestion								
a. ingestee	45/93	48.39	10/49	20.41	6/30	20.00	61/172	35.5
b. ingestor	42/76	55.26	13/43	30.23	7/26	26.92	62/145	42.8
7. Fellatio: use of condoms								
a. active	35/169	20.71	26/92	28.26	19/56	33.93	80/317	25.2
b. passive	35/169	20.71	26/92	28.26	16/56	28.57	77/317	24.3
8. Urolagnia								
a. receiver	5/93	5.38	3/49	6.12	3/30	10.00	11/172	6.4
b. donor	9/76	11.84	5/43	11.63	5/26	19.20	19/145	13.1
9. Deep kissing:	72/76	94.74	42/43	97.67	25/26	96.15	139/145	95.9

The numbers and percentages of men who fell into these different risk levels are shown in Table V.

Independent. Our alcohol-use variable was operationalized with four questions concerning respondents' alcohol consumption patterns. The questions, along with summary frequencies and percentages of possible answers to the questions, are presented in Table VI. We were interested in measuring the frequency of drinking, the amounts consumed on an average day, and the use of alcohol specifically in the context of sexual behavior. In addition we created an aggregate measure of alcohol use which we call the "drinking index." Scores on this index were calculated by assigning points to the responses to each of the four alcohol questions and adding them together. The alcohol variables are not independent of each other, to be sure, and the intercorrelations of these variables are shown in Table VII. While all of the correlations are highly significant, the degree of association found suggests that they are not mere reflections of each other.

Controlled. Analyses were done on the total cohort as well as on subgroups based on the individual's relationship status, as follows:

    a) men in a steady, monogamous relationship;
    b) men in a steady, nonmonogamous relationship;
    c) men with no steady partner;
    d) men who engage in casual sexual encounters (b+c).

Since the implications of risky sexual practices are different for men in these different categories, testing the hypothesis for each of these separate groups is important. In some previous studies relationship status has been ignored, while in others certain categories (e.g., men in a monogamous relationship) were eliminated from the analysis.

Statistical Techniques

Much of the research on the alcohol/risky-sex hypothesis appears to emphasize the avoidance of Type II error (i.e., acceptance of the null hypothesis when it in fact is false), often reporting results which "approach" significance. Inasmuch as our review of the literature suggests that the null hypothesis will need to be accepted rather than rejected, in our analysis we, too, decided to emphasize the avoidance of Type II error. This was accomplished by using the following strategy.

TABLE V. Sexual risk scores of men in the GSRP cohort.

Risk Score		n	%
0	No risk	142	37.5
1	Low risk	44	11.6
2	Moderate risk	164	43.3
3	High risk	29	7.6
	TOTAL	379	100.0%

TABLE VI. Responses to questions on alcohol consumption.

Questions	Responses	
	n	%
1. How often do you use alcohol?		
a. Not at all	25	7.9
b. Occasionally	161	50.8
c. Regularly	131	41.3
2. Which of the following situations describes you best? You normally drink:		
a. do not drink at all	25	7.9
b. <1 drink per day	175	55.2
c. 1–2 drinks per day	58	18.3
d. 3–4 drinks per day	39	12.6
e. 5–6 drinks per day	10	3.2
f. more than 6 drinks per day	10	3.2
3. The last time you drank alcohol before having sex, how many drinks did you have?		
a. did not drink before sex	109	34.4
b. 1–2 drinks	112	35.3
c. 3–4 drinks	55	17.4
d. 5–6 drinks	21	6.6
e. more than 6 drinks	20	6.3
4. Thinking about the times that you drink prior to or during sex, how many times were you drunk enough so that you were unable to drive a car?		
a. never	180	56.8
b. almost never	89	28.1
c. sometimes	31	9.8
d. almost half the time	13	4.1
e. almost always	4	1.3

N = 317 (subset of the total cohort: men who had sex during the previous month).

TABLE VII. Intercorrelations of alcohol-related variables.

	F10	F11	F12
F9	0.681	0.511	0.434
F10		0.537	0.425
F11			0.640

Note: All correlations in the table have a p < 0.0001; n = 379.
F9 = How often do you use alcohol?
F10 = How many drinks do you normally have per day?
F11 = The last time you drank alcohol before you had sex, how many drinks did you have?
F12 = Thinking about the times that you drank prior to or during sex, how many times were you drunk enough so that you were unable to drive a car?

Strictly speaking, most of our variables are measured at the ordinal level. It can be assumed, however, that these ordinal variables measure underlying continuous dimensions. Therefore, we will report both on measures of association that apply to ordinal and to interval variables. Our analysis started with chi square as a test of independence. This statistic measures the deviation of the actual cell frequencies from the cell frequencies that could be expected as a function of the marginal distributions. A significant chi square ($p < 0.05$) means that the bivariate variable distribution shows a pattern that differs from a pattern that would be obtained given independence. We took this measure as the main criterion to decide if a bivariate relationship was worth reporting in this study. For those bivariate relations with a significant chi square, we calculated tau c as an ordinal measure of association. We used this measure since the rows and columns of our different cross-tabulations differed. Using tau b would create difficulties in comparing our findings across tables since the upper limit of tau b is a function of the number of rows and columns. We do not have this handicap with tau c which can reach unity, or near unity, regardless of the number of rows and columns.

Given the likelihood that an assumption of linearity between alcohol variables and sexual behaviors is not a valid one (Wolman 1985), we also used eta.[1] Although statistical purists can object to the use of eta given that our dependent variable is not strictly an interval variable, we do include this measure because of its usefulness. Eta squared can be interpreted as the proportion of the variability of the dependent variable that can be accounted for by the independent variable. We contrast eta squared with Pearson's r squared, the latter indicating the magnitude of a linear relationship. Using the formula $(eta^2 - r^2)100/eta^2$, we calculated the proportion of the total association that is not linear. Summing up, in this study we report on those bivariate relationships that have a chi square $p < 0.05$ and the following measures, eta^2, Pearson's r^2, tau c, and the nonlinear proportion of the relationship. The thoroughness of our approach makes the presentation of results somewhat complex, but it is essential in order to provide a systematic and satisfactory test of the hypothesis; it also is an improvement over the statistical simplicity manifested in some previous reports in which the hypothesis was tested.

RESULTS

In our analysis we examined the relationships between individual sexual behaviors as well as overall measures of risky sex, such as a risk index based partially on the one used by Stall and his associates, and our drinking variables plus a drinking index; these analyses were carried out for the entire set of men who had had sex during the previous month and separately for each of the groups constituted on the basis of the type of relationship in which those in the group participated: monogamous steady partnership (monogamous), nonmonogamous steady partnership (nonmonogamous), and no steady partnership (singles) plus a group constituted by combining the nonmonogamous men and those without partners in order to look at a subset of all men who engage in casual sex (casuals). Before discussing these findings, however we shall present an overview of the sexual practices reported by the gay and bisexual men in our study and the prevalence of alcohol consumption by these men.

A. Prevalence of Risky and Possibly Risky Sexual Practices

Table IV provides detailed data on the frequency with which the men in this study engage in the sexual practices about which they were queried. Approximately one-third of these men continue to engage, at least on some occasions, in unprotected anal intercourse, both receptive and insertive, but the extent to which they do so is partially determined by their relationship status, with men in monogamous relationships being the most likely to do so (receptive = 42.6%, insertive = 45.6%) and single men the least likely (receptive = 12.5%, insertive = 17.9%). Approximately half of the men report engaging in receptive or insertive anal sex using condoms. Fisting is a relatively rare practice among these men, and the only ones in the sample who reported receptive fisting (n=5) were monogamous men with a steady partner. Rimming (oral-anal sex), in contrast, is quite prevalent in all three relationship groups, engaged in by 46%–77% of the men. Unprotected fellatio, both active and passive, is also widely practiced by men in all groups (54%–82%). Over one-third of the men report swallowing semen during fellatio or allowing their partner to do so, this practice being reported by approximately 50% of the monogamous men and 20% of the single men. Watersports (urolagnia), on the other hand, is engaged in by a small minority in all groups, 10% or fewer in all but the singles group in which 19% report being a donor in urolagnia, with fewer men overall reporting being urine receivers (6.4%) than donors (13.1%). Deep kissing is almost universally practiced (95.9%) by the men in the GSRP cohort.

B. Drinking Patterns

As can be seen in Table VI under 8% of these men abstain entirely from alcohol. Approximately 37% average one or more drinks per day, with 19% averaging three or more drinks daily. While 34% had not drunk immediately before their last sexual encounter, over 30% had drunk three or more drinks on that occasion. Inebriation to the point of not being in condition to drive an automobile was reported as occurring at least sometimes by approximately 15% of the subjects, while 57% reported never reaching this level of inebriation in conjunction with sex.

While the gay community in Belgium is not as well-organized and cohesive as in some other Western countries such as the United States and the Netherlands, nonetheless a gay subculture does exist, especially in the two major cities of Brussels and Antwerp. Much of the life of the community revolves around gay commercial establishments, the bars and the saunas, and it is common for men to meet sexual partners in such places where alcohol is served. In 1989 there were more than 150 gay bars and 14 gay saunas (where alcohol is also available) in the country, most of them concentrated in Brussels and the Flemish-speaking region of Belgium (Gmünder and Stamford 1990). Brussels and Antwerp supported 44 and 23 gay (or mostly gay) bars respectively. Wine, spirits, and non-alcoholic beverages are served, of course, but beer is the most popular drink, which should hardly surprise anyone given the superb quality and the rich diversity of beers produced in Belgium. See Table VIII for information on the prevalence of various locales used by these men for meeting sexual partners. Although two-thirds of these men deny meeting sexual partners in bathhouses, only 17% never make contacts in bars or discos.

Drinking is a convivial activity in Belgian gay bars, and while solo drinkers can be seen, it is more common to observe a high level of social interaction in such settings. Buying rounds for the group of friends with whom one is drinking is expected of everyone, and sending drinks to friends elsewhere in the bar or to a stranger as a way to "break the ice" is frequent. Though not usually boisterous in tone, the atmosphere in gay bars in Belgium, especially during the crowded hours of the night is often one of joviality. In addition to the large discos that exist, many bars have small dance floors. Although individual bars may close for a few hours each day, at any hour of the day or night some gay bars are open, at least in Brussels. The laws on bar closing times are more liberal in Belgium than in almost any other country, and many bars remain open until dawn, or until the number of customers has declined to one or two. Men may make the rounds of a set of favorite bars, often beginning in those where the prices of drinks are lower and ending up at the higher-priced discos late in the night. Backrooms or darkrooms, where on-premises sex takes place, continue to exist in some bars and discos.

Given the above findings, it is not surprising that sex and drinking co-occur to a considerable extent among gay and bisexual men in Flanders.

TABLE VIII. Type of public venues where individuals in the GSRP cohort go to socialize or to meet sexual partners.

Type of venue	n	%
Bars and discos		
Never	65	17.1
<1 time per month	122	32.3
1 to 4 times per month	132	34.9
>4 times per month	60	15.7
Gay organizations, meetings		
Never	165	43.6
<1 time per month	87	22.8
1 to 4 times per month	88	23.4
>4 times per month	39	10.2
Public cruising areas		
Never	227	60.1
<1 time per month	74	19.4
1 to 2 times per month	27	7.1
>2 times per month	51	13.4
Bathhouses		
Never	243	64.0
<1 time per month	107	28.3
>1 time per month	29	7.6

C. Drinking and Risky Sex: The Index Results

Sexual behaviors were aggregated to form a sexual risk index as described in the methods section. Correlations between the risk index and drinking variables are presented in Table IX. When we tested for relationships between the sexual risk index and our drinking variables, we obtained the following results. Self-reported frequency of drinking was related to sexual risk-taking only for the men with no steady partners, and in this instance, the correlation (tau c = -0.208, p < .05) was negative. Thus, single men who drank more frequently were less likely to engage in risky sex. It is worth noting that this was the strongest correlation of any between our drinking variables and the sexual risk index.

The average daily consumption of alcohol, too, was significantly correlated with the sexual risk index only for the single men, and again, the correlation was negative (tau c = -0.176, p < .05), indicating that the greater the alcohol consumption the lower the sexual risk score.

The number of drinks consumed prior to the last time the subject drank before or during a sexual encounter was unrelated to the sexual risk index for all groups in this cohort.

Significant correlations did emerge between the frequency of inebriation and sex for the monogamous men (tau c = 0.097, p < .05) and for the combined group of nonmonogamous and single men (tau c = 0.130, p <05) as well as for the total cohort of men who had had sex during the preceding month (tau c = 0.112, p < .05), though not for the single men nor for the nonmonogamous men considered separately. Inspecting Pearson's r^2 suggests that these correlations are low, accounting for less than 2% of the variance.

The risky sex index and the alcohol index were not significantly correlated for the sample as a whole, nor for any of the subgroups analyzed separately.

TABLE IX. Correlations between indicators of alcohol intake and the index for risky sex for the data on Flemish gay men.

Alcohol variable	Relationship group				
	A	B	C	D	E
F9	0.078	-0.008	-0.208*	-0.088	-0.004
F10	0.033	0.052	-0.176*	-0.040	-0.005
F11	-0.014	0.122	-0.043	0.056	0.035
F12	0.097*	0.109	0.152	0.130*	0.112*

*Kendall's tau c; p < 0.05
F9 = How often do you use alcohol?
F10 = How many drinks do you normally have per day?
F11 = The last time you drank alcohol before you had sex, how many drinks did you have?
F12 = Thinking about the times that you drink prior to or during sex, how many times were you drunk enough so that you were unable to drive a car?
Relationship Groups:
A. Monogamous men in a steady relationship (n = 169)
B. Nonmonogamous men in a steady relationship (n = 92)
C. Single men, no relationship (n = 56)
D. Men who engage in casual sex, B + C (n = 148)
E. Total cohort of men who had sex during past month (n = 317)

D. Drinking and Specific Sexual Behaviors

Table X presents the results of tests of hypotheses concerning the impact of drinking on specific sexual behaviors, ranging from high risk to possibly safe ones. We have included in the table only the results which were statistically significant at the .05 level of probability or lower. In this section we will review the results as they pertain to specific forms of sexual behavior.

1. *Anal Sex: Unprotected.*   Unprotected receptive anal intercourse has generally been found to carry the highest degree of risk for the transmission of HIV. Somewhat less risky but nonetheless highly dangerous is unprotected insertive anal intercourse. While the sexual risk index is heavily based on anal sex involvement, we also tested the hypothesis using the question of the extent to which the individual engages in unprotected anal sex, leaving aside relationship status and use of condoms which are built into the risky sex index. In our cohort, there were no significant relationships between unprotected anal intercourse (receptive or insertive) for any of our groups on any of the drinking indicators. In short, we find no evidence of an increase in unprotected anal sex by individuals associated with their drinking behavior.

2. *Anal Sex: Condom Usage.*   Condoms provide protection against the transmission of HIV, but given misuse and the potential for breakage, anal sex even with barrier protection is considered somewhat risky. The frequency of drinking was significantly correlated with insertive anal sex using a condom for single men in our sample, and receptive anal sex using a condom was positively associated with frequency of inebriation during sex for the nonmonogamous, the casual, the set of men who had had sex the previous month, and the total sample. But it should be noted that both the linear measure (r^2) and the nonlinear measure (eta^2) of the amount of the variance accounted for is minimal (ranging from below 1% to just over 8%).

3. *Fisting.*   While fisting need not involve the exchange of body fluids and therefore is not inherently a high-risk behavior, under certain conditions it can be a vector for the transmission of HIV and some studies have placed it in the highest risk category. In our data, there were no relationships between the drinking variables and involvement of fisting as the receptive partner. However, there were numerous statistically significant positive relationships between insertive fisting and drinking variables. The average number of drinks per day was associated with participation in insertive fisting for nonmonogamous men, for those who engage in casual sex, for the subsample of men who had had sex the previous month, and for the sample as a whole. For single men, insertive fisting was associated with frequency of drinking. The drinking index was correlated with insertive fisting for nonmonogamous men, for the casual sex subsample, and the subsample of all men who had had sex during the previous month. And finally, frequency of inebriation during sex was associated with insertive fisting for the total sample but not for the various subsamples considered separately. Some of these correlations are moderate in strength, but in all such instances the relationship is nonlinear. It appears, then, that with increased alcohol intake involvement in fisting increases to a point, and beyond that insertive fisting participation decreases.

4. *Oral-Anal Contact (Rimming).*   For the men in steady relationships (both monog-

TABLE X. Statistically significant associations between drinking variables
and sexual behavior variables by relationship group.

Sexual behaviors	N	Chi square	eta^2	r^2	Nonlinear %	tau c
					Statistics	
Alcohol question: How often do you use alcohol?						
1. Insertive anal sex, using a condom:						
Singles:	56	13.17*	.019	.003	83.9	ns
2. Insertive fisting:						
Monogamous:	169	13.91*	.015	.010	34.9	ns
Total sample:	379	12.76*	.008	.002	70.9	ns
3. Oral-anal (active):						
Singles:	56	15.04*	.110	.019	83.3	ns
Total sample:	379	12.68*	.010	.000	95.93	ns
4. Fellatio, partner swallows semen:						
Casuals	69	14.87*	.024	.002	89.9	ns
Last month	145	13.25*	.037	.015	60.2	.150*
Total sample	181	16.06*	.036	.019	48.2	.155***
5. Urolagnia, giving:						
Monogamous	76	15.98***	.175	.080	54.5	−.100*
Last month	145	14.14**	.057	.040	29.6	−.084*
Total sample	181	15.65*	.032	.026	18.9	−.065*
Alcohol question: How many drinks do you normally have per day?						
1. Insertive fisting:						
Nonmonogamous	92	37.45****	.201	.071	64.9	.073*
Casuals	148	32.24****	.118	.032	73.0	ns
Last month	317	34.49***	.035	.003	92.9	ns
Total sample	379	33.85***	.029	.001	96.2	ns
2. Oral–anal (active):						
Singles	56	28.53*	.140	.001	99.4	ns
3. Unprotected fellatio, active:						
Singles	56	25.22*	.284	.043	85.0	ns
4. Urolagnia, receiving:						
Nonmonogamous	49	28.12****	.544	.351	38.9	.220***
Casuals	79	17.94***	.227	.154	32.2	.175***
Last month	172	24.05*	.090	.022	74.9	ns
Total sample	198	24.69**	.084	.017	80.0	ns
5. Urolagnia, giving:						
Monogamous	76	26.15***	.264	.038	85.6	−.113*
6. Deep kissing:						
Singles	26	30.06*	.264	.018	93.0	ns
Alcohol question: The last time you drank alcohol before you had sex, how many drinks did you have?						
1. Fellatio, swallows partner's semen:						
Singles	30	21.35*	.090	.019	78.4	ns
2. Protected fellatio, active:						
Monogamous	169	26.37**	.067	.008	88.4	ns
Casuals	79	16.52*	.071	.003	95.5	ns
Last month	317	25.32*	.023	.006	75.0	ns
3. Urolagnia, receiving:						
Singles	30	12.41*	.414	.254	38.7	.249*
Nonmonogamous	49	17.68***	.361	.251	30.5	.210***
Casuals	79	28.87****	.365	.241	34.0	.221****
Last month	172	21.02**	.086	.012	86.4	ns
Total sample	198	19.51*	.073	.006	91.6	ns
4. Deep kissing:						
Singles	26	34.88****	.267	.000	100.0	ns
Last month	145	21.38*	.116	.000	99.7	.103*

(Continued)

TABLE X. (*Continued*).

Sexual behaviors	N	Chi square	eta²	r²	Nonlinear %	tau c
				Statistics		

Alcohol question: Thinking about the times that you drink prior to or during sex, how many times were you drunk enough so that you were unable to drive a car?

Sexual behaviors	N	Chi square	eta²	r²	Nonlinear %	tau c
1. Receptive anal sex, using a condom:						
Nonmonogamous	92	28.03**	.082	.021	75.0	.172*
Casuals	148	29.12***	.047	.020	58.1	.159***
Last month	317	27.05**	.023	.007	70.7	.090*
Total sample	379	31.73***	.021	.001	95.2	ns
2. Insertive fisting:						
Total sample	379	22.90*	.013	.003	79.5	ns
3. Protected fellatio, active:						
Singles	56	22.98***	.184	.079	57.2	ns
Monogamous	169	29.39***	.107	.024	77.9	ns
Casuals	148	20.41**	.076	.024	68.2	ns
Last month	317	41.86****	.054	.023	57.5	ns
4. Urolagnia, receiving:						
Nonmonogamous	49	9.49*	.194	.057	70.6	.148*
5. Deep kissing:						
Singles:	26	32.88****	.319	.008	97.6	ns
Drinking index:						
1. Insertive fisting:						
Nonmonogamous	92	51.64****	.284	.028	90.0	ns
Casuals	148	61.63****	.228	.016	93.2	ns
Last month	317	58.50*	.072	.001	98.2	ns
2. Fellatio, swallow partner's semen:						
Singles	30	48.31**	.647	.066	89.8	.199*
3. Unprotected fellatio, active:						
Singles	56	51.63*	.437	.070	84.0	.279**
4. Protected fellatio, active:						
Monogamous	169	76.01****	.122	.019	84.3	ns
Casuals	148	47.49*	.130	.012	90.7	ns
Last month	317	112.14****	.098	.016	83.5	ns
Total sample	379	75.62***	.066	.009	87.2	ns
5. Urolagnia, receiving:						
Nonmonogamous	49	37.40****	.763	.276	63.8	.217***
Casuals	79	40.91****	.518	.175	66.3	.207***
6. Urolagnia, giving:						
Monogamous	76	34.78*	.340	.028	91.8	ns
7. Deep kissing:						
Singles	26	45.09*	.424	.005	98.9	ns

*p < .05
**p < .01
***p < .005
****p < .001

amous and nonmonogamous) there were no associations between drinking and active or passive rimming, nor for the single men were there any associations with passive rimming. However, frequency of drinking and average daily intake of alcohol were significantly associated with active rimming for the single men, and frequency of drinking was associated with active rimming for the total sample. Though statistically significant, it should be noted that variance accounted for is 1% for the total sample, and for the single men it is 14%. The relationship, however, appears to be nonlinear, with almost all of the variance accounted for by the curvilinear aspect of the association.

5. *Fellatio: Unprotected.*   While documented cases of HIV transmission via fellatio are few and far between, despite the relatively high frequency of this form of sexual behavior among gay men, fellatio (active in particular) continues to be regarded as moderately risky, even in the absence of ejaculation if there is pre-ejaculate present. In our sample, insertive (passive) fellatio is unrelated to the drinking variables, but receptive (active) fellatio is significantly correlated with average number of drinks per day and the drinking index for the single men. For none of the other samples is there an association between drinking variables and active oral sex. Again, the two associations found between unprotected fellatio and drinking variables was not a linear one.

6. *Fellatio: Semen Ingestion.*   As noted earlier, fellatio is considered riskier when the fellator ingests semen if his partner ejaculates in his mouth. For none of our groups was semen ingestion by our subjects related to their drinking patterns. However, some of the drinking variables were related to whether or not our subjects' partners swallowed the subject's semen during fellatio. An increase in likelihood of semen ingestion by our subjects' partners was reported as follows: by single men who drank more the last time they had sex; by subjects who ranked high on the drinking index; by those who engage in casual sex and by those who had sex last month; and by the total sample if they drank frequently. Only in the case of the association between the drinking index and semen ingestion by the subjects' partners does the amount of variance accounted for exceed 10%, and in this instance, again, the relationship is nonlinear.

7. *Fellatio: Use of Condoms.*   Condoms cut down the risk when used in conjunction with fellatio. Protected active fellatio was significantly associated with the number of drinks consumed prior to or during the last encounter in which sex and alcohol were combined for the monogamous men, for those who engage in casual sex, and for those who had had sex during the previous month. Protected active fellatio was also associated with frequency of inebriation during sex for all groups except the total sample. And it was correlated with the drinking index for all groups except the single men. Variations exist in the amount of the variance accounted for by nonlinearity for these correlations.

8. *Urolagnia (Watersports/Golden Showers).*   Watersports are risky only if infected urine comes into contact with the mucosal tissue or breaks in the skin of the receiving partner. It is hardly surprising that watersports yielded not only more significant associations with drinking than did other sexual behaviors but also stronger associations in general. What is somewhat surprising is that for the monogamous men, the men who had sex last month, and the total sample, the correlations were negative, with half or more of the variance accounted for by linearity. However, these correlations were on the order of .10 or lower. Associations between receptive urolagnia and average number of drinks per day were moderately high and largely linear for nonmonogamous men and those who engage in casual sex; they were lower and less linear for the total sample and for those who had had sex the previous month. For monogamous men, participation in urolagnia as the urine donor appears to be related nonlinearly to average daily alcohol intake. Receptive urolagnia was significantly associated with the amount drunk the last

time the subject combined sex and alcohol for all samples, with notably higher associations for the single men, the nonmonogamous ones, and those who engage in casual sex. Likewise, receptive urolagnia is correlated significantly for the nonmonogamous men with frequency of inebriation during sex. The drinking index was associated with receptive urolagnia for nonmonogamous men and those who engage in casual sex and with donor urolagnia for the monogamous men.

9. *Deep Kissing.*   Deep (French) kissing is practiced by almost all the men in the GSRP sample. This behavior is generally considered safe, but it can carry some risk if there are cuts or sores in the mouth of one or both of the participants. Associations between three alcohol variables (amount drunk during the last encounter combining sex and alcohol; frequency of inebriation during sex; drinking index) and deep kissing were found for single men, with moderate levels of variance accounted for, albeit not in a linear fashion. The only other significant association on deep kissing was with the amount drunk during the last encounter combining sex and alcohol for the sample of all who had had sex during the previous month.

DISCUSSION

When we embarked on research on this topic in 1989, we based our expectations on the reports coming out of San Francisco, and expected that our test of the hypothesis of a relationship between drinking and risky sex would provide confirmation of its validity. Preliminary analyses of our data and an assessment of the literature published on the hypothesis since we began the work lead us to conclude that the hypothesis stood on very shaky ground. Given the importance of this issue for AIDS prevention programs, we were determined not to reject the hypothesis without being certain that it had been tested thoroughly and fairly. Consequently, we followed a strategy of data analysis intended to ferret out of our data whatever evidence we could find in support of the hypothesis. We can summarize our findings as follows.

When single men were considered separately there was no evidence that alcohol increased their involvement in anal sex. Indeed, to the contrary, those who drank more often and averaged more drinks per day participated less in unprotected anal sex. However, inebriation during sex was significantly associated with the sexual risk index for monogamous men, those who engage in casual sex, and the total sample of men who had had sex during the previous month. The correlations, though, were low and the amount of the variance accounted for was less than 2%. Moreover, when unprotected anal sex alone was analyzed (i.e., without confounding from considerations of relationship status and use or nonuse of condoms which were built into the risk index), there were no relationships between the drinking variables and unprotected anal sex. Having anal sex with condoms may be related to the degree of inebriation, but it should be underscored that the relationship is not linear and little of the variance is explained by the drinking variable.

It appears likely that involvement in fisting as the active partner is related to various dimensions of drinking, again nonlinearly. We would suggest that this is not a meaningful finding for prevention purposes inasmuch as fewer than 5% of the men in this sample engage in this practice, in most cases infrequently (and eight of the 15 men in the cohort who practiced insertive fisting were in monogamous relationships) and further because the practice itself is not likely to transmit HIV unless cuts or tears are present or semen is somehow introduced. Also, the practice is probably more dangerous for the receptive partner, and drinking was not related to receptive participation in this practice in any of our analyses.

Rimming is generally considered a high-risk behavior for HIV transmission, albeit at a much lower level than anal sex. While some drinking variables were correlated with rimming, the variables in question were the general ones, not those referring to drinking or inebriation in the context of sexual activity. In addition, the relationships that emerged were nonlinear and accounted for a small proportion of the variance in this behavior.

Unprotected active fellatio by single men is nonlinearly associated with the drinking index and with their average daily alcohol consumption, but not with drinking in the context of sex. Therefore, we believe that we can reject the hypothesis that drinking increases involvement in unprotected oral sex. This is confirmed by the lack of any association between drinking and swallowing the partner's semen, although drinking may be related to allowing the partner to swallow the subject's semen. This means that drinking is not related to an individual's own risk taking. Fellatio with the use of condoms is very low risk; therefore, the finding of some associations between this variable and drinking do not indicate an increase in risk taking with drinking.

On the basis of the multiple associations we found between drinking variables and urolagnia, we would not discount the possibility that drinking does increase this form of behavior. Being the donor in such activity carries no risk; being the receiver may entail minor risk. Only 6.4% of the men in the GSRP cohort engage in receptive watersports, and five of the 11 men who do so are in monogamous relationships. Thus, whatever the risk this practice involves, it is one that pertains to an exceptional few cases.

Deep kissing, in contrast, is a widespread practice, and it may be related, albeit again nonlinearly, to drinking prior to or during sex.

We conclude that the patterning of statistical results found in our data do not support the hypothesis of a relationship between alcohol use and risky sex. To the extent that any of our tests yielded confirmatory findings, it seems that the relationships were weak, usually curvilinear, and generally derived from data on relatively uncommon sexual behaviors, not from the highest risk practices. The net effect of alcohol consumption among these men was not an increase in sexual risk taking.

This study can be added to the list of studies discussed above in the literature review in which there was a failure to replicate the findings of the earliest research on the topic. We can speculate on the reasons behind these failures to replicate. The study designs varied, of course. When dealing with both alcohol and risky sex, we are faced with complex social phenomena, and in most studies operationalizing of these measures has been rather simplistic. In some cases, the alcohol question specified drinking in the context of sex, whereas in others it did not. Only rarely were multiple indicators of alcohol habits utilized. As noted in Table 1, the indicators of risky sex also varied, with some investigators even using data on multiple partners as the measure of riskiness. In the present study we have attempted to improve on former research designs by using diverse indicators of both the dependent and the independent variables. That we still did not find support for the hypothesis suggests that methodological differences may not account for the failures to replicate.

It is plausible to explain the failures by appealing to cultural differences in both alcohol and sex practices. This alternative would seems reasonable if the failures to replicate all occurred in one cultural context, while the confirmatory studies occurred in another. However, our Belgian results must be seen in the context of American studies which also failed to replicate. Indeed, neither the patterns of sexual behavior nor the drinking practices of the Flemish men are out of line with data reported from American studies. This is not to suggest that there are no differences in meanings attached to some of these behaviors, but we have no evidence of such inferred differences. The burden of proof for such differences and their impact on the proposed relationship would rest on those who would advance this interpretation.

Our findings underscore the necessity of taking into consideration in analyzing risky behaviors the relationship status of the participants in the research (Fitz-patrick et al. 1990). Unsafe sexual behavior between two men who test negative for HIV is not risk-free, of course, given the possibility of false negative test results, but such risky behavior in such partnerships is certainly lower on riskiness in an absolute sense. Some investigators have excluded men with committed monoga-mous relationships, but we believe that it is necessary to include them inasmuch as relationships do not always last forever, and many men who indicate that they are in monogamous relationships comply with rules of fidelity with differing degrees of success—while still considering themselves to be in a monogamous relation-ship. Gay relationships are not constructed on the same set of standard patterns as straight relationships, and it is not entirely clear how the participants in this study define a "steady partner." A steady partner could be someone with whom the participant lives and shares all aspects of life or it could be merely a person with whom he has sex on a fairly regular basis, a relationship sometimes referred to as one of "fuck buddies" in American gay culture.

To their credit, Stall and his associates (1986) noted that the relationship they found may not have been a causal one. And Stall (1988:84) has stated that "efforts to prevent the spread of further HIV infection within this [the gay] community which rely on preventing drug or alcohol use are probably inappropriate." Indeed, even if a relationship were to exist, numerous plausible non-causal interpretations could be made. For example, consider these possibilities. An individual who is inclined to engage in risky sex goes in search of a sexual partner; his search is quite likely to lead him to a setting where he is most likely to find a partner, a bar or bathhouse. He has a drink, picks up a "trick," and has sex. In this case the desire for risky sex may have driven his drinking rather than vice versa.

A plausible methodological explanation for a correlation between risky sex and alcohol in cultural contexts where both types of behavior are under attack is the likely co-occurrence of an unwillingness to admit to disdained behaviors. Cottler, Helzer, and Tipp (1990:220) state this possibility as follows: "It should be pointed out that an association between high risk substance abuse and high risk sexual activity may exist because the same persons who are willing to report high risk sexual activities are also willing to admit illicit drug use." The same is true of licit drugs such as alcohol when they are being discouraged as harmful.

Another possibility suggested by our data on the men in our sample who engage in casual sex despite being in a relationship is that a general personality trait involving stimulation-seeking is responsible for both the drinking and the high-risk sex. Having multiple sexual partners, drinking, and high-risk sex would all be, under this interpretation, manifestations of the need for excitement and high levels of stimulation. Evidence in favor of this interpretation exists. Fisher and Misovich (1990) found high sensation seeking to be associated with number of sexual partners, less fear of AIDS, and less AIDS anxiety. High sensation seekers show more interest in sex and they consume more alcohol (Zuckerman 1979). Their high-risk personalities make such individuals less likely to attend to prevention messages based on fear and "saying no" to risky behavior (Bolton and Good 1988).

Whether or not one finds a relationship may also depend on cultural interpretations of the influence of alcohol on behavior and on drinking patterns. Undoubtedly, the amounts consumed and the patterning of drinking may differ in different populations. It is possible that drinking is much more integrated into daily life in Belgium than it is in the United States, although fieldwork by the senior author in both cultures indicates that the differences in drinking and sexual behavior between urban gay populations in the U.S. and Belgium may be slight and that it would be unwise to exaggerate such differences. Nonetheless, it may be that there is a lower expectation in Belgium that alcohol will influence behavior, thereby reducing a possible expectancy effect.

One explanation that has been advanced to account for the reduction in the strength of the relationship or the absolute failure to find one in later studies can be ruled out, however, as the reason for our failure to replicate. It could be argued that educational campaigns stressing the alcohol/risky sex connection may be responsible for the disappearance of the correlation found presumably before gay men knew about the hypothesized connection of risky sex to alcohol consumption and if involvement in risky sex and alcohol consumption have both declined, it may be more difficult for investigators to detect the continued presence of a relationship. In Belgium, though, not only has risk-reduction education not been as intense as in metropolitan areas of the U.S., but little attention has been paid to the alcohol factor in the educational campaigns that have been carried out.[2]

We might ask, Why is it important to clarify this issue? On the surface it might seem that it would do no harm to stress a causal link between alcohol and risky sex even if that linkage is weak or non-existent. We believe it is extremely important because of its implications for prevention programs. Alcoholism is certainly widely perceived to be a problem in many gay communities (Nardi 1982; Cabaj 1989; Dickmann 1990; Hellman et al. 1989; McKirnan and Peterson 1989a; Paul, Bloomfield, and Stall n.d.; Stall and Wiley 1988), and if stressing this connection did not reduce HIV transmission, at least it might yield other benefits to the health of gay men.[3] It is often noted that alcohol-related problems even in the age of AIDS kill more gay men than does AIDS. But in fact there may be serious dangers inherent in placing any emphasis on this presumed association, no matter how much it appeals to common sense and no matter how neatly it fits our folk models about how alcohol makes one do things one would not otherwise do (the "demon rum made me do it" syndrome).[4]

First, if the association is not causal, then this variable could easily be perceived as just another hypothesized co-factor which comes out of a moralistic approach to medical problems (Herek and Glunt 1991), and this could lead to a rejection of the entire package of risk-reduction messages. Second, stressing alcohol may distract educators from what should be the focus of AIDS prevention programs, the promotion of healthy and pleasurable erotic lives (see Taylor, this issue). Just saying no to everything is not likely to work (Shernoff and Bloom 1991). This distraction may be as counterproductive as the message to "stop being promiscuous" has been (see Bolton 1992a, this issue). The number of partners with whom one engages in sex is irrelevant to HIV transmission if the lessons of safer sex have been internalized and for people who practice safe sex consistently. This issue is not merely one of priorities; rather, it is a question of how complicated an educational program one wants to have and which strategy is most effective (see Petrow 1990 and Mays, Albee, and Schneider 1989). Should one focus attention on the limited set of seriously risky behaviors, or should one dilute that focus by dwelling on a broad range of related but definitely peripheral factors. Our view is that it is better to focus on risk behaviors, especially unprotected anal intercourse, and to emphasize the positive aspects of safe behaviors (Catania et al. 1989).[5]

Scientists and the media have bombarded people in industrial nations, especially the United States, with information about the harmful effects of all kinds of behaviors. Alcohol, in particular, has been singled out for attention. Not only is it dangerous to drink and drive, but alcohol, it is stressed, causes fetal damage, contributes to degenerative diseases, and so forth. Notices about the dangers of alcohol are posted wherever alcohol is sold in the U.S. A saturation point may be reached and people may then ignore all risk warnings. Thus, it would seem that HIV prevention should avoid all but the most essential "prohibitions" and concentrate on empowering individuals to enjoy safe sexual activities.

This is not to argue that anti-alcohol education might not be important. Since alcohol appears to be an immunodepressant, it is possible that its long term effects have an impact on susceptibility to HIV infection for individuals who do not practice safe sex. And it may certainly be detrimental for individuals who are seropositive, although some studies have found no relationship between progression of HIV disease and alcohol or recreational drug usage (van Griensven et al. 1990; Schechter et al. 1989; Haverkos 1990; Pillai and Watson 1990; Lifson et al. 1990). But providing information on these potential dangers is different from attempting to explain risk taking by placing the blame on alcohol, an explanation which may be all too congenial to individuals who engage in risky behavior, allowing them to exculpate themselves and rationalize their behavior. In fact, this psychological process may be responsible for the findings that support the hypothesis inasmuch as they occur in populations exposed early to both AIDS and AIDS-prevention campaigns.

Furthermore, by emphasizing alcohol as a risk factor, one runs the risk of exacerbating the problem by reinforcing the folk theory of a linkage between sex and alcohol; this, we suggest is risky business and needs to be thought through carefully. If this is the case, emphasizing alcohol may be positively dangerous, increasing rather than reducing the likelihood of risky sex by giving people an excuse for engaging in such behavior that they otherwise would not have. Though this may seem counterintuitive, if alcohol is discussed at all in HIV-prevention campaigns, the message should probably be that alcohol **does not** cause risky sex.

In other words, the need is to undermine the cultural myth that perpetuates risky behavior. This approach has been adopted by some Australian AIDS educators (see Figure 1).

This suggestion is made on the basis of the following considerations. Alcohol is a depressant which has complex associations with patterns of sexual behavior which are not due to an enhanced sexual response following drink. Quite the reverse is true. As Wilson and Lawson (1978:358) note: "Dose-related studies have shown

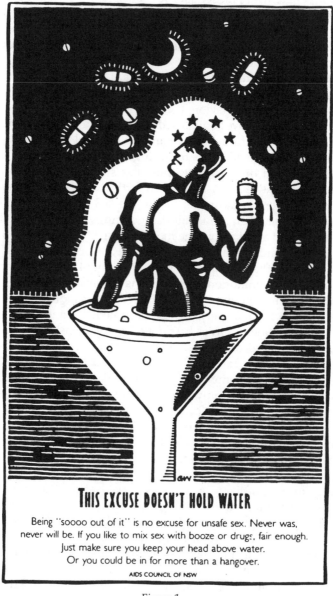

THIS EXCUSE DOESN'T HOLD WATER

Being "soooo out of it" is no excuse for unsafe sex. Never was,
never will be. If you like to mix sex with booze or drugs, fair enough.
Just make sure you keep your head above water.
Or you could be in for more than a hangover.

AIDS COUNCIL OF NSW

Figure 1.

that there is a significant negative linear relation between sexual arousal and blood alcohol level" in both male and female drinkers. Further, sexual response tends to decline among those who have been heavy drinkers over a long period. Both male and female sexual dysfunction results from chronic alcohol abuse (Briddell and Wilson 1976). Reviewing the literature on this subject, two sexologists conclude:

It appears that the erotic effects of moderate amounts of alcohol are due largely to our psychological interpretation of our physical state and to disinhibition. . . . Both men and women believe that alcohol acts to reduce sexual inhibitions. . . . If we view alcohol as a sexual or social lubricant, we are more likely to engage in sexual behavior when under its influence. Disinhibition of sexual response comes about only because drinking allows us to attribute our sexual behavior to the effects of alcohol rather than to ourselves—"alcohol made me do it" is the standard excuse. Thus it is the denial of personal responsibility that may prompt us to engage in behaviors that we would enter into more slowly, if at all, under normal conditions. [Allgeier and Allgeier 1991:511]

AIDS prevention should attempt to destroy our folk theories instead of turning them into self-fulfilling prophecies.

The disinhibitory effects of alcohol may account for the studies which did find a relationship between drinking and risky sex. Consider that confirmation comes primarily from studies on heterosexual adolescents, among whom both anxieties over sexuality and the need to provide excuses for their behavior are found. The studies are less consistent for adult heterosexuals, and mostly disconfirmatory for homosexuals. Gay men past the coming-out phase are probably among the least inhibited segments of the population, and therefore are not likely to need excuses for their sexual activity. The AIDS crisis, however, may have raised the inhibition level of gay men due to the risks inherent in sexual behavior in these times. In fact, this may account for the Stall et al. (1986) results inasmuch as this study was done early in the epidemic when fear of sexuality may have been at a peak in San Francisco's gay community, an epicenter of the pandemic. As safe-sex knowledge has been reinforced since then, fear of having sex has undoubtedly subsided and the inhibitions which may have contributed to their results may have dissipated in large measure. Evidence for this assertion can be found in the explosion of safer-sex venues in San Francisco in recent years (see Taylor and Lourea 1992, this issue).

An additional danger lurks on the horizon. We are all too familiar with the hysteria surrounding bathhouses which were blamed for spreading AIDS; a re-run of this scenario but with bars instead of baths as the scapegoats is not difficult to imagine, at least in less enlightened places where calls have already been heard for the closing of bars. Though defeated, legislation to close gay bars was introduced in at least one state (Indiana). Given the results of our study and others which have failed to confirm a relationship between alcohol and risky sex, such an attack on gay institutions would be as unwarranted as were the attacks on bathhouses, and as ineffective in combatting the spread of HIV. It is important to remember that the beginning of the modern gay liberation movement occurred in 1969 when gay men in New York City responded to police harassment at the Stonewall Inn by rioting and fighting back. Yet even today police attacks on gay bars are not uncommon in the United States, including metropolitan areas with large gay populations such as Los Angeles. HIV-prevention campaigns which target drinking will have to take

356/[218]   R. Bolton et al.

into account the historical context and cultural symbolism of drinking and bars for the gay community.

Finally, we must ask why so much attention has been focussed on alcohol as a co-factor, and, indeed, why it was so readily accepted as a significant cause of risky sex in the absence of more than a smattering of supportive evidence. We suggest that there are numerous reasons. First, such an approach fits neatly into the ethos of the 1980s in the United States, which condemned all forms of mind-altering experiences, and argued that the solution to many problems from teenage pregnancy to drug addiction was to simply say no. Second, alcohol was a major target of scientists interested in risk. Third, support for risk research on AIDS could be obtained from already existing granting agencies concerned with drug abuse, e.g., the Alcohol, Drug Abuse, and Mental Health Administration of the Department of Health and Human Services. Fourth, addictionology had become an aggressively expanding field, encompassing now even the controversial phenomenon of "sexual addiction" (another manifestation of the anti-pleasure ethos of the decade). The influence of the field of addictionology on HIV prevention research is hard to exaggerate. The latest dubious concept from that field to be drawn into the AIDS prevention arena is "relapse" (e.g., St. Lawrence, Brasfield, and Kelly 1990; Stall et al. 1990a). Fifth, it was easier to draw on existing theories (e.g., the much-vaunted Health Belief Model) developed for the study of domains other than sexuality than to create new ones or to obtain funding for research based on the more relevant field of sexology (Frayser 1990; Wellings et al. 1990).

Lorion (1990) has pointed to some valuable lessons that need to be learned by HIV researchers if they are to improve risk-reduction efforts. We can note only two of his insightful observations. He suggests "avoiding the glow of street lamps," referring to the joke about the man who was looking for his keys under the street lamp because that's where the light was. Unfortunately, AIDS researchers have not ventured into the darker areas where the keys to risk reduction are likely to be found. Specifically, they have done almost no research on the dynamics of sexual encounters (Bolton 1992b). In this area, research is more difficult to carry out (it cannot be done using phone survey methodologies, for example, the ultimate form of "phone sex"), and funding is difficult to obtain (Gagnon 1988).

Lorion also advises investigators to "question the obvious." Alcohol as a risk factor is much too obvious, not because of scientific knowledge but because of cultural predispositions and beliefs about alcohol. In AIDS research, the obvious has often turned out to be wrong, e.g., "drug addicts won't change their behavior," "poppers cause AIDS." The connection between alcohol and risky sex has been elusive because, once again, the obvious is probably wrong.

ACKNOWLEDGMENTS

The research reported in this paper was sponsored by the AIDS Reference Center of Ghent State University, Ghent, Belgium. The Commission for Educational Exchange between the United States of America, Belgium, and Luxembourg and the Research Committee of Pomona College provided additional support. The authors would like to thank Ron Stall for his detailed comments on an earlier draft of this analysis and for providing the New South Wales illustration and to Gail Orozco for her assistance in preparing the manuscript. Earlier versions of this paper were presented at the annual meetings of the Society for Cross-Cultural Research, Claremont, February 1989 and the Southwestern anthropological Association, Long Beach, April 1990.

NOTES

1. From the tables it is clear that an important component of the relationships (based on the chi squares that are significant) is not linear. To obtain more insight into the nature of these relationships, we performed one-way analyses of variance in which we tested for polynomial trends. In these analyses the categories of the variable measuring the amount of alcohol subjects drink before having sex was used as the grouping variable and the frequencies of sexual practices as dependent variables. Rank ordering the means of the dependent variable per category of the grouping variable, we see that for some sexual practices frequencies rise when drinking becomes heavier but at the highest drinking intensities frequencies decline again. For these variables the quadratic terms are significant. However, these findings cannot be interpreted in a straightforward manner. Tests for homogeneity of variances (Cochran's C) indicate that variances across categories are not equal. It becomes impossible to determine whether significant differences between groups result from differences of means or differences of variances. These findings lead us to the following conclusion. Most samples of gay men within the context of AIDS research are not truly representative and probably do not reflect known population characteristics. In addition, variables such as alcohol consumption, drug use, and sexual behavior do not have normal distributions. Taking into account these considerations, researchers should be extremely vigilant in interpreting the results of statistical techniques that are based on simplified models of the nature of relationships such as the linear model.
2. Nagy, Hunt, and Adcock (1990) report the results of a study done on adolescents in which it was found that AIDS knowledge was lower among those who drank alcohol than among abstainers. This finding would support the claim that drinkers do not seek out or do not attend to information about risk behaviors. Future studies on the alcohol/risky sex hypothesis should control for AIDS knowledge. If the connection between alcohol and risky sex has been "disappearing," this could be the result of drinkers finally becoming informed about AIDS risks due to repeated exposure to information as the epidemic progresses.
3. Though widely perceived as a problem in many gay communities and by alcohol researchers, the rate of alcoholism in this population, sometimes estimated to be as high as 30%, may have been exaggerated, in part because of the expectation that gay men would respond to the stresses they encountered in a homophobic society by escaping through alcohol, and in part because of methodological deficiencies in the early studies which were often based on samples drawn from bar patrons. More recent investigations using more diversified samples of gay men indicate that 10% of gay men are problem drinkers (Martin 1990a) and that heterosexual and homosexual men do not differ significantly in their drinking patterns (Stall and Wiley 1988).
4. We should note that the problem of chronic, serious alcohol abusers is a separate issue and one which should not be ignored. In the case of such individuals, for example those in treatment, it may indeed be appropriate to deal with the question of how their sexual behavior is affected by the use of alcohol (Ottomanelli et al. 1990; Silvestre et al. 1989; Westermeyer et al. 1989; Windle 1989).
5. HIV-prevention campaigns may need to incorporate messages about the effects of recreational drugs other than alcohol, however, since the evidence that such drugs may indeed be associated with high risk behavior is stronger than the evidence for alcohol, although this effect may also be disappearing (Martin 1990b) and future work may find that this is another nonproblem. Targeting users of recreational drugs means focussing on a smaller segment of the gay population, not only in Belgium but also in the United States and probably everywhere.

REFERENCES CITED

Allgeier, E. R., and A. R. Allgeier
  1991   Sexual Interactions. Third Edition. Lexington, MA: D.C. Heath and Company.
Bagnall, G., M. Plant, and W. Warwick
  1990   Alcohol, Drugs and AIDS-Related Risks: Results from a Prospective Study. AIDS Care
         2(4):309–317.
Bell, A. P., and M. S. Weinberg
  1978   Homosexualities: A Study of Diversity Among Men and Women. New York: Simon and
         Schuster.
Bolton, R.
  1992a AIDS and Promiscuity: Muddles in the Models of HIV Prevention. Medical Anthropology
         14(2,3,4):145–223.
  1992b Mapping Terra Incognita: Sex Research for AIDS Prevention, An Urgent Agenda for the
         Nineties. IN The Time of AIDS: Social Analysis, Theory, and Method. G. Herdt and S.
         Lindenbaum, eds. Newbury Park, CA: Sage.
Bolton, R., and J. Good
  1988   Playing Safely: A Cross-Cultural Analysis of AIDS Posters. Paper presented at the Annual
         Meeting of the American Anthropological Association, Phoenix, November.
Brendstrup, E., and K. Schmidt
  1990   Homosexual and Bisexual Men's Coping with the AIDS Epidemic: Qualitative Interviews with
         10 Non-HIV-Tested Homosexual and Bisexual Men. Social Science and Medicine 30(6):713–720.
Briddell, D. W., and G. T. Wilson
  1976   Effects of Alcohol and Expectancy Set on Male Sexual Arousal. Journal of Abnormal Psychol-
         ogy 85(2):225–234.
Cabaj, R. P.
  1989   AIDS and Chemical Dependency: Special Issues and Treatment Barriers for Gay and Bisexual
         Men. Journal of Psychoactive Drugs 21(4):387–393.
Catania, J. A., T. J. Coates, S. M. Kegeles, M. Ekstrand, J. R. Guydish, and L. L. Bye
  1989   Implications of the AIDS Risk-Reduction Model for the Gay Community: The Importance of
         Perceived Sexual Enjoyment and Help-Seeking Behaviors. IN Primary Prevention of AIDS:
         Psychological Approaches. V. M. Mays, G. W. Albee, and S. F. Schneider, eds. Pp. 242–261.
         Newbury Park, CA: Sage.
Coates, T. J., R. D. Stall, J. A. Catania, and S. M. Kegeles
  1988   Behavioral Factors in the Spread of HIV Infection. AIDS 1988, 2(suppl 1):239–246.
Cottler, L. B., J. E. Helzer, and J. E. Tipp
  1990   Lifetime Patterns of Substance Use among General Population Subjects Engaging in High Risk
         Sexual Behaviors: Implications for HIV Risk. American Journal of Drug and Alcohol Abuse
         16(3–4):207–222.
Darrow, W. W., H. W. Jaffe, and J. W. Curran
  1988   Behaviors Associated with HIV-1 Infection and the Development of AIDS. IN AIDS 1988:
         AAAS Symposia Papers. R. Kulstad, ed. Pp. 225–235. Washington, DC: American Association
         for the Advancement of Science.
Detels, R., P. English, B. R. Visscher, L. Jacobson, L. A. Kingsley, J. S. Chmiel, J. P. Dudley, L. J. Eldred,
and H. M. Ginzburg
  1989   Seroconversion, Sexual Activity, and Condom Use Among 2915 HIV Seronegative Men Fol-
         lowed for up to 2 Years. Journal of Acquired Immune Deficiency Syndromes 2:77–83.
Dickmann, K.
  1990   A House with 12 Steps. Edge, No. 172, pp. 31–38.
Doll, L.
  1989   Alcohol Use as a Cofactor for Disease and High-Risk Behavior. Paper presented at the Alcohol
         and AIDS Network Conference, Tucson, Arizona, April 27–29.
Ebbesen, P., M. Melbye, and R. J. Biggar
  1984   Sex Habits, Recent Disease, and Drug Use in Two Groups of Danish Male Homosexuals.
         Archives of Sexual Behavior 13(4)291–300.

Ekstrand, M. L., and T. J. Coates
  1990   Maintenance of Safer Sexual Behaviors and Predictors of Risky Sex: The San Francisco Men's Health Study. American Journal of Public Health 80(8):973–977.
Fisher, J. D., and S. J. Misovich
  1990   Social Influence and AIDS-Preventive Behavior. *IN* Social Influence Processes and Prevention. J. Edwards, R. S. Tindale, L. Heath, and Posavac, eds. Pp. 39–70. New York: Plenum.
Fitzpatrick, R., J. McLean, J. Dawson, M. Boulton, and G. Hart
  1990   Factors Influencing Condom Use in a Sample of Homosexually Active Men. Genitourinary Medicine 66:346–350.
Frayser, S. G.
  1990   The Cultural Context of Sex Research and AIDS Prevention. Paper presented at the Annual Meeting of the American Anthropological Association, New Orleans, November.
Gagnon, J.
  1988   Sex Research and Sexual Conduct in the Era of AIDS. Journal of Acquired Immune Deficiency Syndromes 1:593–601.
Gmünder, B., and J. D. Stamford, eds.
  1990   Spartacus '90/91 Guide for Gay Men. 19th Edition. Berlin: Bruno Gmünder Verlag.
Gómez, R. D., M. V. Arango, G. Velázquez, and B. Orozco
  1990   Factores de Riesgo de Infección en Usuarios de un Programa de Control del VIH, Antioquia, Colombia. Bol. Of. Sanit. Panam. 108(3):181–197.
Haverkos, H. W.
  1990   Nitrite Inhalant Abuse and AIDS-Related Kaposi's Sarcoma. Journal of Acquired Immune Deficiency Syndromes 3(Suppl. 1):47–50.
Hays, R. B., S. M. Kegeles, and T. J. Coates
  1990   High HIV Risk-Taking Among Young Gay Men. AIDS 4(9):901–907.
Hellman, R. E., M. Stanton, J. Lee, A. Tytun, and R. Vachon
  1989   Treatment of Homosexual Alcoholics in Government-Funded Agencies: Provider Training and Attitudes. Hospital and Community Psychiatry 40(11):1163–1168.
Herek, G. M., and E. K. Glunt
  1991   AIDS-Related Attitudes in the United States: A Preliminary Conceptualization. The Journal of Sex Research 28(1):99–123.
Hingson, R. W., L. Strunin, B. M. Berlin, and T. Heeren
  1990   Beliefs about AIDS, Use of Alcohol and Drugs, and Unprotected Sex among Massachusetts Adolescents. American Journal of Public Health 80(3):295–299.
Jackman, J.
  1978   Missing the Ports O Call. *IN* Lavender Culture. K. Jay and A. Young, eds. Pp. 150–154. New York: Harcourt Brace Jovanovich.
Judell, B.
  1978   Sexual Anarchy. *IN* Lavender Culture. K. Jay and A. Young, eds. Pp. 135–139. New York: Harcourt Brace Jovanovich.
Kelly, J. A., and J. S. St. Lawrence
  1990   The Impact of Community-Based Groups to Help Persons Reduce HIV Infection Risk Behaviours. AIDS Care 2(1):25–36.
Kelly, J. A., J. S. St. Lawrence, H. V. Hood, and T. L. Brasfield
  1989   Behavioral Intervention to Reduce AIDS Risk Activities. Journal of Consulting and Clinical Psychology 57(1):60–67.
Kelly, J. A., J. S. St. Lawrence, T. L. Brasfield, A. Lemke, T. Amidei, R. E. Roffman, H. V. Hood, J. E. Smith, H. Kilgore, and C. McNeill, Jr.
  1990   Psychological Factors That Predict AIDS High-Risk Versus AIDS Precautionary Behavior. Journal of Consulting and Clinical Psychology 58(1):117–120.
Kelsey, J.
  1978   The Cleveland Bar Scene in the Forties. *IN* Lavendar Culture. K. Jay and A. Young, eds. Pp. 146–149. New York: Harcourt Brace Jovanovich.
Kraft, P., J. Rise, and B. Traeen
  1990   The HIV Epidemic and Changes in the Use of Contraception among Norwegian Adolescents. AIDS 4(7):673–678.

Kus, R. J.
1987   Sex, AIDS, and Gay American Men. Holistic Nursing Practice 1(4):42–51.
Leigh, B. C.
1990a   Alcohol Use and Sexual Behavior in Discrete Events: II Comparison of Three Samples. Paper presented at the Alcohol Epidemiology Symposium, Kettil Bruun Society, Budapest.
1990b   The Relationship of Substance Use During Sex to High-Risk Sexual Behavior. The Journal of Sex Research 27(2):199–213.
Lifson, A. R., W. W. Darrow, N. A. Hessol, P. M. O'Malley, J. L. Barnhart, H. W. Jaffe, and G. W. Rutherford
1990   Kaposi's Sarcoma in a Cohort of Homosexual and Bisexual Men. American Journal of Epidemiology 131(2):221–231.
Linn, L. S., J. S. Spiegel, W. C. Mathews, B. Leake, R. Lien, and S. Brooks
1989   Recent Sexual Behaviors Among Homosexual Men Seeking Primary Medical Care. Archives of Internal Medicine 149:2685–2690.
Lorion, R. P.
1990   Evaluating HIV Risk-Reduction Efforts: Ten Lessons from Psychotherapy and Prevention Outcome Strategies. Journal of Community Psychology 18:325–336.
MacAndrew, C., and R. B. Edgerton
1969   Drunken Comportment: A Social Explanation. New York: Aldine de Gruyter.
Marshall, M., ed.
1979   Beliefs, Behaviors, and Alcoholic Beverages. Ann Arbor, MI: The University of Michigan Press.
Martin, J. L.
1986   AIDS Risk Reduction Recommendations and Sexual Behavior Patterns among Gay Men: A Multifactorial Categorical Approach to Assessing Change. Health Education Quarterly 13(4):347–358.
1990a   Drinking Patterns and Drinking Problems in a Community Sample of Gay Men. IN Alcohol, Immunomodulation and AIDS. D. Seminara, R. R. Watson, and A. Pawlowski, eds. Pp. 27–34. New York: Alan R. Liss Corp.
1990b   Drug Use and Unprotected Anal Intercourse Among Gay Men. Health Psychology 9(4):450–465.
Martin, J. L., and D. S. Hasin
1991   Drinking, Alcoholism, and Sexual Behavior in a Cohort of Gay Men. IN AIDS and Alcohol/Drug Abuse: Psychosocial Research. D. G. Fisher, ed. Pp. 49–67. New York: The Harrington Park Press.
Mays, V. M., G. W. Albee, and S. F. Schneider, eds.
1989   Primary Prevention of AIDS: Psychological Approaches. Newbury Park, CA: Sage.
McCoy, H. V., C. McKay, L. Hermanns, and S. Lai
1990   Sexual Behavior and the Risk of HIV Infection. American Behavioral Scientist 33(4):432–450.
McCusker, J., A. M. Stoddard, J. G. Zapka, M. Zorn, and K. H. Mayer
1989   Predictors of AIDS-Preventive Behavior among Homosexually Active Men: A Longitudinal Study. AIDS 3(7):443–448.
McCusker, J., J. Westenhouse, A. M. Stoddard, J. G. Zapka, M. W. Zorn, and K. H. Mayer
1990   Use of Drugs and Alcohol by Homosexually Active Men in Relation to Sexual Practices. Journal of Acquired Immune Deficiency Syndromes 3(7):729–736.
McCusker, J., J. G. Zapka, A. M. Stoddard and K. H. Mayer
1989   Responses to the AIDS Epidemic Among Homosexually Active Men: Factors Associated with Preventive Behavior. Patient Education and Counseling 13:15–30.
McKirnan, D. J., and P. L. Peterson
1989a   AIDS-Risk Behavior among Homosexual Males: The Role of Attitudes and Substance Abuse. Psychology and Health 3:161–171.
1989b   Alcohol and Drug Use among Homosexual Men and Women: Epidemiology and Population Characteristics. Addictive Behaviors 14:545–553.
1989c   Psychosocial and Cultural Factors in Alcohol and Drug Abuse: An Analysis of a Homosexual Community. Addictive Behaviors 14:555–563.
1989d   Tension Reduction Expectancies Underlie the Effect of Alcohol Use on AIDS Risk Behavior Among Homosexual Males. V International Conference on AIDS, Montreal, June.

Miller, H. G., C. F. Turner, and L. E. Moses, eds.
  1990   AIDS: The Second Decade. Washington, DC: National Academy Press.
Molgaard, C. A., C. Nakamura, M. Hovell, and J. P. Elder
  1988   Assessing Alcoholism as a Risk Factor for Acquired Immunodeficiency Syndrome (AIDS).
         Social Science and Medicine 27(11):1147–1152.
Morgan Thomas, R., M. A. Plant, and M. L. Plant
  1990   Alcohol, AIDS Risks and Sex Industry Clients: Results from a Scottish Study. Drug and
         Alcohol Dependence 26:265–269.
Nagy, S., B. Hunt, and A. Adcock
  1990   A Comparison of AIDS and STD Knowledge Between Sexually Active Alcohol Consumers and
         Abstainers. Journal of School Health 60(6):276–279.
Nardi, P.
  1982   Alcoholism and Homosexuality: A Theoretical Perspective. Journal of Homosexuality 7(4):9–
         25.
National Institute on Alcohol Abuse and Alcoholism
  1991   Research on Relationships Between Alcohol Use and Sexual Behaviors Associated with HIV
         Transmission. Program Announcement, PA–91–75
Newman, F.
  1978   Why I'm Not Dancing. *IN* Lavender Culture. K. Jay and A. Young, eds. Pp. 140–145. New York:
         Harcourt Brace Jovanovich.
Ocamb, K.
  1989   AIDS and Alcohol: The Deadly Connection. Frontiers (October 6):21.
O'Reilly, K.
  1988   Risk Behaviors and Their Determinants. *IN* AIDS 1988: AAAS Symposia Papers. R. Kulstad,
         ed. Pp. 245–250. Washington, DC: American Association for the Advancement of Science.
Ostrow, D. G., M. J. VanRaden, R. Fox, L. A. Kingsley, J. Dudley, R. A. Kaslow, and the Multicenter
AIDS Cohort Study (MACS)
  1990   Recreational Drug Use and Sexual Behavior Change in a Cohort of Homosexual Men. AIDS
         4(8):759–765.
Ottomanelli, G., T. H. Kramer, B. Bihari, J. Fine, S. Heller, and J. A. Mosely
  1990   AIDS-Related Risk Behaviors Among Substance Abusers. The International Journal of the
         Addictions 25(3):291–299.
Paul, J. P., K. A. Bloomfield, and R. Stall
  n.d.   Gay and Alcoholic: Epidemiological and Clinical Issues. Unpublished ms.
Paul, J. P., R. D. Stall, and F. Davis
  1989   Sexual Risk for HIV Transmission in a Gay Male Substance-Abusing Population. Poster
         presentation at the V International Conference on AIDS, Montreal.
Penkower, L., M. A. Dew, L. Kingsley, J. T. Becker, P. Satz, F. W. Schaerf, and K. Sheridan
  1991   Behavioral, Health and Psychosocial Factors and Risk for HIV Infection among Sexually Active
         Homosexual Men: The Multicenter AIDS Cohort Study. American Journal of Public Health
         31(2):194–196.
Petrow, S., ed., with P. Franks and T. R. Wolfred
  1990   Ending the HIV Epidemic: Community Strategies in Disease Prevention and Health Promo-
         tion. Santa Cruz, CA: Network Publications.
Pillai, R., and R. R. Watson
  1990   Response to 'Alcohol, Sex and AIDS.' Alcohol & Alcoholism 25(6)711–713.
Pittman, D. J., and C. R. Snyder, eds.
  1962   Society, Culture, and Drinking Patterns. Carbondale, IL: Southern Illinois University Press.
Plant, M. A.
  1990a Alcohol, Sex and AIDS. Alcohol & Alcoholism 25:293–301.
  1990b Sex Work, Alcohol, Drugs, and AIDS. *IN* AIDS, Drugs, and Prostitution. M. Plant, ed. Pp. 1–
         17. London: Tavistock/Routledge.
Plant, M. L., M. A. Plant, and R. Morgan Thomas
  1990   Alcohol, AIDS Risks and Commercial Sex: Some Preliminary Results from a Scottish Study.
         Drug and Alcohol Dependence 25:51–55.

Pleak, R. R., and H. F. L. Meyer-Bahlburg
  1990   Sexual Behavior and AIDS Knowledge of Young Male Prostitutes in Manhattan. The Journal of Sex Research 27(4):557–587.
Read, K. E.
  1980   Other Voices: The Style of a Homosexual Tavern. Novato, CA: Chandler & Sharp Publishers.
Rolf, J., J. Nanda, J. Baldwin, A. Chandra, and L. Thompson
  1990–91   Substance Misuse and HIV/AIDS Risks Among Delinquents: A Prevention Challenge. The International Journal of the Addictions 25(4A):533–559.
Schechter, M. T., K. J. P. Craib, T. N. Le, B. Willoughby, B. Douglas, P. Sestak, J. S. G. Montaner, M. S. Weaver, K. D. Elmslie, and M. V. O'Shaughnessy
  1989   Progression to AIDS and Predictors of AIDS in Seroprevalent and Seroincident Cohorts of Homosexual Men. AIDS 3:347–353.
Shernoff, M., and D. J. Bloom
  1991   Designing Effective AIDS Prevention Workshops for Gay and Bisexual Men. AIDS Education and Prevention 3(1):31–46.
Siegel, K., L. J. Bauman, G. H. Christ, and S. Krown
  1988   Patterns of Change in Sexual Behavior Among Gay Men in New York City. Archives of Sexual Behavior 17(6):481–497.
Siegel, K., F. P. Mesagno, J.-Y. Chen, and G. Christ
  1989   Factors Distinguishing Homosexual Males Practicing Risky and Safer Sex. Social Science and Medicine 28(6):561–569.
Silvestre, A. J., D. W. Lyter, R. O. Valdiserri, J. Huggins, and C. R. Rinaldo, Jr.
  1989   Factors Related to Seroconversion among Homo- and Bisexual Men after Attending a Risk-Reduction Educational Session. AIDS 1989(3):647–650.
St. Lawrence, J. S., T. L. Brasfield, and J. A. Kelly
  1990   Factors which Predict Relapse to Unsafe Sex by Gay Men. Poster presented at the VIth International Conference on AIDS, San Francisco. Abstract F.C.725.
Stall, R.
  1988   The Prevention of HIV Infection Associated with Drug and Alcohol Use During Sexual Activity. In AIDS and Substance Abuse. L. Siegel, ed. Pp. 73–88. New York: Harrington Park Press.
Stall, R. D., T. H. Coates, and C. Hoff
  1988   Behavioral Risk Reduction for HIV Infection Among Gay and Bisexual Men: A Review of Results from the United States. American Psychologist 43(11):878–885.
Stall, R., M. Ekstrand, L. Pollack, L. McKusick, and T. J. Coates
  1990a   Relapse from Safer Sex: The Next Challenge for AIDS Prevention Efforts. Journal of Acquired Immune Deficiency Syndrome 3(12):1181–1187.
Stall, R., S. Heurtin-Roberts, L. McKusick, C. Hoff, and S. W. Lang
  1990b   Sexual Risk for HIV Transmission among Singles-Bar Patrons in San Francisco. Medical Anthropology Quarterly 4(1):115–128.
Stall, R., L. McKusick, J. Wiley, T. J. Coates, and D. G. Ostrow
  1986   Alcohol and Drug Use During Sexual Activity and Compliance with Safe Sex Guidelines for AIDS: The AIDS Behavioral Research Project. Health Education Quarterly 13(4):359–371.
Stall, R., and J. Wiley
  1988   A Comparison of Alcohol and Drug Use Patterns of Homosexual and Heterosexual Men: The San Francisco Men's Health Study. Drug and Alcohol Dependence 22:63–73.
Taub, D.
  1982   Public Sociability of College-Aged Male Homosexuals: The Gay Bar and Cruise Block. Sociological Spectrum 2:291–305.
Taylor, C. L., and D. Lourea
  1992   HIV Prevention: A Dramaturgical Analysis and Practical Guide to Creating Safer Sex Interventions. Medical Anthropology 14(2,3,4):243–284
Temple, M., and B. Leigh
  1990   Alcohol and Sexual Behavior in Discrete Events: I Characteristics of Sexual Encounters Involving and Not Involving Alcohol. Paper presented at the Alcohol Epidemiology Symposium, Kettil Bruun Society, Budapest.

Turner, C. F., H. G. Miller, and L. E. Moses
  1989   AIDS, Sexual Behavior and Intravenous Drug Use. Washington, DC: National Academy Press.
Valdiserri, R. O.
  1989   Preventing AIDS: The Design of Effective Programs. New Brunswick, NJ: Rutgers University Press.
Valdiserri, R. O., D. Lyter, L. C. Leviton, C. M. Callahan, L. A. Kingsley, and C. R. Rinaldo
  1988   Variables Influencing Condom Use in a Cohort of Gay and Bisexual Men. American Journal of Public Health 78(7):801–805.
Van der Graaf, M., and R. Diepersloot
  1989   Sexual Transmission of HIV: Routes, Efficiency, Cofactors and Prevention. A Survey of the Literature. Infection 17(4):210–215.
Van Griensven, G. J. P., E. M. M. de Vroome, F. de Wolf, J. Goudsmit, M. Roos, and R. A. Coutinho
  1990   Risk Factors for Progression of Human Immunodeficiency Virus (HIV) Infection among Seroconverted and Seropositive Homosexual Men. American Journal of Epidemiology 132(2):203–210.
Vincke, J., R. Mak, and R. Bolton
  1990   Gay Service Research Project (een multidisciplinair onderzoek): Eerste Rapport. Ghent, Belgium: Rijksuniversiteit Gent.
Vincke, J., R. Mak, R. Bolton, and P. Jurica
  1991   Factors Affecting AIDS-Related Sexual Behavior Change among Flemish Gay Men. Unpublished manuscript.
Weinberg, M. S., and C. J. Williams
  1974   Male Homosexuals: Their Problems and Adaptations. New York: Penguin Books.
Wellings, K., J. Field, J. Wadsworth, A. M. Johnson, R. M. Anderson, and S. A. Bradshaw
  1990   Sexual Lifestyles Under Scrutiny. Nature 348(2):276–278.
Westermeyer, J., M. Seppala, S. Gasow, and G. Carlson
  1989   AIDS-Related Illness and AIDS Risk in Male Homo/Bisexual Substance Abusers: Case Reports and Clinical Issues. American Journal of Drug and Alcohol Abuse 15(4):443–461.
Wilson, G. T., and D. M. Lawson
  1978   Expectancies, Alcohol, and Sexual Arousal in Women. Journal of Abnormal Psychology 87(3):358–367.
Windle, M.
  1989   High-Risk Behaviors for AIDS among Heterosexual Alcoholics: A Pilot Study. Journal of Studies on Alcoholism 50(6):503–507.
Winkelstein, Jr., W., D. M. Lyman, N. Padian, R. Grant, M. Samuel, J. A. Wiley, R. E. Anderson, W. Lang, J. Riggs, and J. A. Levy
  1987   Sexual Practices and Risk of Infection by the Human Immunodeficiency Virus: The San Francisco Men's Health Study. Journal of the American Medical Association 257(3):321–325.
Witomski, T. R.
  1986   Gay Bars, Gay Identities. IN Gay Life: Leisure, Love, and Living for the Contemporary Gay Male. E. E. Rofes, ed. Pp. 201–209. Garden City, NY: Doubleday & Company.
Wolman, T.
  1985   Drug Addiction. IN Pathophysiology in Psychosocial Disease. M. Farber, ed. Pp. 277–285. New York: Macmillan.
Zielinski, M. A., and C. Beeker
  1989   Drugs, Alcohol and Risky Sex among Gay and Bisexual Men in a Low-Incidence Area for AIDS. Paper presented at the Annual Meeting of the American Public Health Association, Boston, MA, November.
Zuckerman, M.
  1979   Sensation Seeking: Beyond the Optimal Level of Arousal. Hillsdale, NJ: Erlbaum.